By Echo Heron
Published by Ivy Books:

Nonfiction
INTENSIVE CARE: The Story of a Nurse
CONDITION CRITICAL: The Story of a Nurse Continues
TENDING LIVES: Nurses on the Medical Front

Fiction
MERCY

The Adele Monsarrat, R.N., medical thrillers
PULSE
PANIC
PARADOX

CONDITION CRITICAL

The Story of a Nurse Continues

Echo Heron

IVY BOOKS • NEW YORK

An Ivy Book
Published by The Ballantine Publishing Group
Copyright © 1994 by Echo Heron

www.ballantinebooks.com

Library of Congress Catalog Card Number: 93-49058

ISBN 0-8041-1335-1

First Hardcover Edition: July 1994
First Mass Market Edition: July 1995

OPM 15 14 13 12 11

For Mary Catherine Bianchi, my true sister, in honor of forty years of devoted friendship and unconditional love.

Acknowledgments

For those who hung in there with love and support, I wish to thank:

Simon Day Heron, Janey O'Hara Justice, Catherine Murray Barnes, Colette Coutant Trembly, The Rexford Herons and the Scotia Salatos, Andra Loy Carson, Marty DeLaney, Laura Gray, Linda Stone, Kaye Manly-Hayes, Nancy J. Evans, Rinelle Shay, Margie Dingfelder, Nancy Schuepbach, Lee M. Eldridge, Robin Morgan, Michael J. McClure, Mary Dale and James Scheller, James 'Doc' Nelson, Julie Griewe, Mary Sean Young, Elinor Mazzucchelli, Marlene Glaser. And to Christine Mason, for all her tender, loving care, ER expertise, and those unbelievable biscuits!

For their technical advice, support, and the sharing of themselves in the process, many thanks to: yet again, Thomas M. Meadoff, M.D. physician extraordinaire, Dolores Miniaci, R.N., Susan Moore, R.N., Donna Diers, R.N., Patricia Benner, R.N., Glen R. Justice, M.D., Jean Touroff, Dominick Abel, my agent, and to Leona Nevler, my editor.

And, special thanks to Mill Valley Library's reference staff for their willing and wonderful help—even on the weirdest of questions.

Author's Note

I have written this book to describe for the reader my experiences, thoughts, and feelings about my life as a critical care nurse. Like many writers, I have borrowed from true incidents and have based many of the scenes contained in this book on real life events that either I have observed firsthand, or that firsthand observers have described to me. With the exception of a few individuals (for example: Janey Justice, my son Simon, David, and me), I have used fictitious names and characteristics for all the patients, family members, doctors, and other health-care providers, hospitals, schools, and institutions portrayed here. In some cases I have also combined characteristics from several individuals and have altered the chronology of events. Thus, this book is not intended to record events as historical fact, nor is it meant to focus criticism on any particular group, individual, or institution. Any resemblances the reader may imagine they discern are unintended and entirely coincidental.

PROLOGUE

SHE SINGS SOFTLY to the teenager with the crushed skull while documenting the inevitable fraying of his hold on life. She tends to his broken young body, whispering questions she knows will go unanswered forever. "Can you hear us?" "Did you feel any pain?" "What was your last thought?"

It is only a matter of hours before death renders her powerless as his life flows through her hands and into her heart. Later, with his soul still fresh in her keeping, despair comes to fill her sleepless night, tormenting her with the sounds of his mother's pleadings—"Oh God, why my son? Please, not my son." Then comes the vision of a weeping sister too young to understand why her favorite brother no longer laughs or calls her his little bratty.

Whether or not this nurse has yet found that delicate balance of compassion and hopelessness, detachment and intimacy, she will choose, of her own free will, to return again tomorrow. Her need to nurture is not something she can turn away from, no matter how much it hurts. As a healer, she sees only that she may be given the chance to steal a child away from death, or perhaps it will be her touch alone that will soothe the fears and aches of some ancient soul.

And when she wipes the sweat of suffering from your face, she is not concerned with whether you are a Jew or a Catholic, a Protestant or an atheist, but only that you are freed from your pain. When she holds you in her arms delivering you to the peace of death, her thoughts are not of whether you lived in a cardboard box or in a castle, but that you have comfort and

1

dignity. When she ministers to your broken body, she does not care about the color of your skin, but only that you are made whole. When you are afraid, she speaks with gentle understanding, unmindful of whether you are a prostitute or a priest, for she herself knows well the singular loneliness of fear.

That intimate stranger at your bedside is not only your nurse, she is your sister, your mother, your confessor, and your healer. It is not the medicine or the treatment that cures your ills; it is her caring that heals.

Nurses see things, the afterimages of which will haunt them for the rest of their lives. But they are not hardened monsters. On the contrary, they each carry a courageous and sympathetic heart inside them always, so that when you look into a nurse's face, you are looking into the face of human compassion; a human being who still sends a silent prayer each time a siren sounds.

And you, the layperson, you who live on the "normal" side of life, in the end you always ask: "How can nurses bear to do what they do? Why do they keep choosing to face the sorrow and the horror day after day? How can they continue to care when it hurts so much?"

In answer, there is one universal truth about the true giver: Nurses are able to do what they do because they are rich in the gifts of healing, compassion, and love.

ONE

"Nurses ... we speak with our eyes, teach with our hands, comfort with our presence."

EUNICE K. M. ERNST, R.N.

RUNNING BACK to Mr. Keiller's room under a mountainous pile of clean linen, I noticed bubbles oozing out from the sides of my nursing shoes—the result of having doused them with an excessive amount of germicidal soap and not gotten it all out in the rinse. I made the mistake of stopping long enough to brush away the suds, thus making myself accessible instead of a moving blur. Mrs. Norman's son headed straight for me, like an arrow going for a sitting duck.

Mrs. Norman had been my patient on and off since she was admitted to Redwoods Memorial's coronary care unit two weeks earlier with a large myocardial infarction, otherwise referred to as an MI or, simply stated for the layperson, a heart attack.

Mr. Norman wore the slightly mortified, pursed-lip look of someone who was about to ask if he had bad breath or if something not quite socially acceptable was caught between his teeth. Instinctively, I knew he'd chosen me to ask not only because the laundry was straining my arms, but because the lingering cloud of orange foam around my shoes put me at a slight disadvantage.

For a moment I thought about ducking into the patient's room immediately to my left and closing the door, but I knew Mr. Norman would wait until I came out. He was, like his mother with the call bell, a consistently persistent person. Besides, I couldn't afford the time to play cat and mouse; Redwoods Memorial's CCU was in its usual state of pandemonium and, as usual, we were understaffed.

3

The four-bed acute and fourteen-bed intermediate units were almost full—a result of the emergency room having done its job too well. Nine of the present seventeen patients had been admitted since eleven A.M., and it was only four-thirty in the afternoon. What really put the finishing touches on the chaos were the five patients in intermediate CCU who were more than sick enough to be on the acute side.

True, there were the three intermediate patients who were stable enough to be turfed out to other units, but the process of contacting all the doctors involved on each case, then convincing each of them that their patient was ready to move on, was as time-consuming as getting chewing gum out of a wool shag carpet.

Plus, we were having to reckon with the minor din coming from Mrs. Watson's room. Dr. Cramer's raised voice floated out into the hall carrying exclamations such as "Blast!" or "Moron!" and inquiring as to where the hell was a qualified CCU nurse when you needed one, damn it!

If this weren't enough, the patients on intermediate seemed to be having a call bell contest among themselves. Since the three P.M. shift change, the nurses figured each patient was using his call bell an average of five times per hour. That worked out to be one and a half call bells going off every minute. That's a lot of bells for three nurses to answer.

Of course, then there was Mrs. Guasco's heart, which had stopped twice since noon. The code blue team was waiting for the third alarm, but all that had happened was Mr. Keiller's second attack of diarrhea—partly in the bed, partly on the floor to the bathroom, and partly on my shoes. It was a code brown of monumental proportions.

Mrs. Norman's son was close. I could hear his wheezy, asthmatic breaths coming at a rate of about thirty per minute. The need for avoidance overwhelmed me and I stepped into room 18. Mr. Tyler, the resident patient, was sitting on the toilet, concentrating on the small bubble that was headed down his IV line toward the entry site in his arm.

I waved and smiled.

He waved back and strained.

With no one except a nurse, I thought, would this sort of private event be shared so freely. Nurses, to be sure, have intimate encounters of the third kind.

At my back, the anxious presence of Mr. Norman tapped.

"Excuse me, miss, but I was wondering if I might ask you something?" he asked.

Ah. The old redundancy trick; a man after my own heart.

In the name of propriety, I pulled room 18's door closed with my foaming foot and peered over the top of my laundry. Mr. Norman was a nondescript guy. Overall, he had the aura of a beaten dog about him—a man who blended in to the point of evaporation. He would have been perfect as an undercover agent for the CIA. At this particular moment in time, however, he wore his khaki leisure suit large, and his anxiety like a neon sign.

"Shoot," I said, trying to appear receptive over the top of the laundry. My arms were beginning to tremble under the weight of the sheets.

Mr. Norman was wringing his fingers as though he had an invisible Chinese finger trap attached to a couple of them. "I didn't know who else to ask." He looked toward his mother's room.

"Here I am, the original Answer Woman," I said. I began to perspire. I had a feeling Mr. Norman could string it out for a long time.

"I've got to talk to somebody about this, and well ... I mean, who better to ask than a nurse, right?"

"Well, that depends. If it's a question about pork bellies and the stock market ..." Levity, I thought, might get him to ease up on the Chinese finger trap before he pulled his fingers out of their sockets.

Mr. Norman didn't even simper. As a matter of fact, he looked so grave, I had a fleeting fear that he was going to tell me he'd injected his mother with a lethal dose of potassium chloride or that she had fallen out of bed.

"I mean, nurses must hear and see a lot of ... well, I bet you young ladies see just about everything, right?"

"And then some." I shifted the laundry onto my hip and gave a toothy, encouraging grin; one I hoped would prompt him to get on with it. Past Mr. Norman's left ear, I spied Dr. Cramer glaring around the hallway, stalking a nurse.

With a jerky, extremely quick movement, Mr. Norman brought my attention back by moving his face very close to mine. Nose to nose, in a decidedly gloomy tone, he whispered, "Flatulence."

"Uhn huh. I see." I nodded. "Flatus. I have a bachelor's degree in flatulence." I chuckled.

Mr. Norman held on to his worry face for dear life.

"Well, what I mean is . . ." He hesitated, faltered, then hitched up his mouth in an expression of extreme concern. "My mother. She has it. Bad."

"Bad," I repeated. In nursing school they always told us if you couldn't think of anything to say, repeat the patient's last word or statement.

"Oh, thank God you understand!" He stopped with the fingers and brightened up. "Mother and I were wondering if there's some sort of surgical procedure we might pursue that—"

The snort of laughter was headed up and out just as I pulled it back and forced it to return to the place between the throat and the nose where those particular snorts lived. "You know, Mr. Norman, I don't think surgical intervention for flatulence would really be feasible for your mother. She *is* eighty-seven, and, well, after a certain age, everybody's sphincter control kind of loosens up, and—"

"What about plastic surgery?" he asked, pressing on undaunted. "I heard on the Geraldo show about this procedure where they take a charcoal filter . . ."

I sighed. Daytime talks shows were at it again. So many people had the strangest healthcare notions born of either Phil or Oprah or the seriously lacking Geraldo. Geraldo *would* get excited over some bogus surgical procedure involving the implantation of a rectal muffler.

"Mr. Norman, even if there *is* some surgery for the correction of flatulence, I seriously doubt that your mother would be a good surgical candidate. She's elderly, she's got some major pulmonary problems, and she's recovering from her third heart attack in as many years."

Mr. Norman let his shoulders slump into the major depression position. "It's so embarrassing when Mom and the rest of the gang do the town, you know."

"Do the town?" I asked, eyebrows rising off the forehead scale of surprise. We were talking about an eighty-seven-year-old cardiac invalid. Being the member of a gang "doing the town" didn't exactly fit the profile. Bingo on Wednesday nights at St. Adolphe's, perhaps, but for Mr. Norman's mother, even that was pushing limits.

Plus, Mrs. Norman was a woman seriously afflicted with what I called the Fluff My Pillow syndrome, or the lift-me-carry-me-feed-me-and-wipe-me personality type.

"Oh yes, Mother is quite the social butterfly." He smiled weakly. "A gassy butterfly, but still a butterfly."

"Mr. Norman," I said firmly. The guilt about leaving Mr. Keiller sitting buck naked at his sink was making me antsy. Besides that, Dr. Cramer, all six feet four of him dressed in scrubs, was down by the nurses' station leaning his forehead against the wall with his arms crossed. He wasn't kicking the wall very hard, but enough to scuff the new paint. "Have your mother try some antiflatulence drugs—most over-the-counter antacids will do. If that doesn't work, try controlling it with diet. Cut out the cabbage, carbonated beverages, beans, and onions . . . you know, the usual gas-producing foods."

"So you don't think a charcoal rectal-filter implant would be right for Mother?" Mr. Norman asked, not quite listening. "Maybe if we built her up with some vitamins before surgery?"

"No, Mr. Norman."

"No, huh?" His words came out as a downtrodden croak—a child looking into an empty Christmas stocking.

"No."

I waited until Mr. Norman did the dejection shuffle back into his mother's room, then ran on tiptoes past Dr. Cramer, who was still kicking the wall and mumbling. Like a giant lizard tongue, a long, hairy arm shot out with the speed of lightning and caught me around the neck. I'd forgotten he was a pitcher for one of the local baseball teams.

He drew me close enough so I could see that the inside of his thick glasses were heavily steamed.

"*Where* are all the CCU nurses?" he asked.

Dr. Joseph Cramer, sometimes known as "the Mumbler," was a partner in what the CCU nurses referred to as the Cardiology Cartel, one of the area's four cardiology groups. At that moment, he was also known as "the doc in the box," meaning he was the cardiologist assigned to be in the hospital all day. He was the troubleshooter, the doctor on call, the man to whom all cardiac questions were addressed.

"Well, Joe, I can only guess that the few of us who have been left on the unit are busy dealing with doubled work loads."

"What do you mean, the ones who're left?" His dark lashes made chicken scratches in the steamed surfaces of his glasses as he blinked. "Where are the rest of them?"

"Floating, as usual." Two hundred pounds of pure tooth

pressure ground into the rubberized surfaces of my tooth guard—the contraption that kept my teeth from being gnashed into nubs during those extra-stressful grinding moments. Floating was a subject I could get bitter about with very little encouragement. It was one of the many down sides of nursing, although there was a stray (and strange?) nurse hither and yon who actually enjoyed it. The policy differed a bit from hospital to hospital, but basically it meant that the management had the right to take nurses out of their home units and reassign them to work in patient care areas foreign to their specialty of practice. Though she or he was not trained in the specialty of that unit, the nurse was expected to pick up a full patient assignment and be perfectly competent.

More often than not, this practice created problems. For instance, it is a certainty there will be bedlam for both staff and patient when a nurse from the newborn nursery is floated out to work in the geriatric psych ward. Or, for a medical/surgical nurse—one who is used to working with the less critical, more chronically ill patient—being assigned to acute CCU, then given a patient in critical condition on a respirator, arterial and Swan Ganz lines, and four IVs with a different cardiac drug running into each one, would be like suddenly finding oneself on Evel Knievel's motorcycle in midair over the Grand Canyon.

The same went for the critical care nurse who worked the acute units such as intensive care, coronary care, or emergency department. When floated out to the general medical/surgical floors, the nurse would often be assigned as many as ten patients, then required to do procedures and treatments she hadn't performed since nursing school. Inevitably, the critical care nurse would lag behind schedule, thus throwing everyone else into a tizzy.

And to top it all off, nurses who floated out to other units frequently got dumped on. The floating nurse could almost always count on being assigned the most difficult or time-consuming patients whom everyone else had grown tired of dealing with.

While this practice of floating sometimes proved perilous to the patient, it was considered a wise business strategy because it saved the hospital corporation money by eliminating the need to "rent," at higher cost, extra nurses from an agency or hire more benefited staff nurses.

"Floating?" Joe asked. Had he learned the same last-word maneuver in med school?

"Yes, floating. Sent out of the unit. You know how it goes, Joe—you might find some of our nurses bumbling around in the orthopedics ward, tripping over traction pulleys and trying to find the zipper on somebody's full-body cast, and then again you might spot one in pediatrics wandering around asking how you tell the front from the back of a diaper. Hell, you might even discover one of them doing filing in the administrator's office. It's been known to happen."

"But we need them here," he grumbled between clenched teeth. "I just had to insert an arterial line practically by myself, and it wasn't pleasant for anyone—I made sure of that."

I smiled. Part of what made Joe Cramer an eccentric was his triple-sec sense of humor. Those who recognized it as a sense of humor at all loved him; those who took it personally, stepped around him when he approached.

"I want a nurse!" He enunciated each word very slowly, filling it with annoyance. "I want a CCU nurse and I want one now."

"Hey Joe, I've told you a million times—talk to management. Until you can get them to staff us adequately, which I estimate will be a cold day in hell, you'll have to make do with what you've got—just like the rest of us."

From the pants pocket of his scrubs, Joe Cramer pulled a pocket-sized black book and quickly jotted something in his linear scrawl.

Dr. Cramer's black book was famous among Redwoods personnel. No one knew what he wrote in the thing, but he was never without it. It was rumored that he would sometimes stop right in the middle of a procedure to write a line or two, then reglove and continue on.

I looked down at my shoes while he scribbled. The border of suds was now a good two inches thick around each foot. That reminded me of Mr. Keiller's diarrhea and the fact that I had placed a call to his cardiologist over an hour ago.

It was par for the course that Dr. Meyers, the most difficult physician to deal with in the Cartel, would not respond to a nurse's call, since he regarded us as bothersome and useless . . . like gnats. I might have let it go for another hour or so, but Mr. Keiller had begun to have some premature ventricular contractions, a cardiac arrhythmia that could be as ominous as Times Square after midnight.

When the black book was finally slipped back into the physician's pocket, I spoke. "By the way, do you know Mr. Keiller, the angina patient of Dr. Meyers?"

"Who?" (The On-Call Physician's Standard Response Number One.)

Of course, I didn't *really* expect that Dr. Meyers would have given report on his patients to the doc in the box. It was always so much easier to have the nurse stop what she was doing and take precious time to give the full report instead.

"He's fifty-eight, history of angina, hypertension, and one MI about a year ago. He has a new onset of PVCs that Meyers has been treating for two days with quinidine. It hasn't affected the PVCs much, but it's sure made a difference to the man's bowels. The diarrhea started today and it ain't pretty. I need you to order another antiarrhythmic. How about some Procan?"

"I don't want to mess with anyone else's orders. This isn't my patient." (The On-Call Physician's Standard Response Number Two.)

"Yes, I know, Joe, but you *are* the doc on call. Meyers isn't calling me back, and Mr. Keiller's next dose of quinidine is due now."

"Wait until I'm off call." (The On-Call Physician's Standard Response Number Three.) "Give the quinidine for now until you talk to Meyers."

"Wait a minute. You mean to tell me . . ." I paused, fitted a muzzle over the sharp fangs of my voice, and continued, ". . . you'd let this poor guy suffer with diarrhea for another twelve hours rather than change one of Meyers's orders? Isn't that taking the holy brotherhood a little too far? I'm disappointed in you, Joe."

I shoved the pile of linens at him. "Tell you what. Why don't you go in there and give him the quinidine and then come by about ten tonight, when he's stooling all over the room, and *you* can dance with the mop."

Wearing an expression of disgust, Joe tried to give me back the linens. I stepped away and put my hands on my hips. The muzzle slipped from my voice.

"This is such typical BS, Joe. We end up being the bad guys because you boys don't want to offend each other. Now I have to give Mr. Keiller the quinidine *knowing* he's going to have diarrhea but I can't do a thing about it. Sure, I suppose I could tell Mr. Keiller the truth and take the risk he'll refuse the quinidine, but then his PVCs would increase and . . . voilà! A code blue versus a code brown. And then, of course—"

"You know, Heron, for someone who blows bubbles with her feet, you're a real pain in the neck."

I tapped my bubbling foot impatiently. Down the hall, an IV pump alarm bleeped, and there were three patient call bells ringing at the same time. One of them was Mr. Keiller's.

Joe gave a theatrical and painful sigh. "All right. Give Procan seven hundred and fifty milligrams every six hours, but discontinue the drug after six A.M. tomorrow. Meyers can take it from there."

Joe's expression said he expected me to get down on my knees in praise.

I rolled my eyes. "Oh gee, thank you, doctor, O mighty ruler, master, sir, but while you're here there's just one more thing . . ."

Dr. Cramer handed me back the pile of linens and headed toward Mrs. Watson's room. "No more requests, Heron. I have to go play God now."

I thought about Mrs. Norman and her son having to deal with the gases that be, and addressed the back of his neck. "Certainly the great and powerful Cramer can grant an antacid order for Mrs. Norman?"

"Who?"

"Arrrggh!"

"Okay, okay, order whatever you want."

Smiling, I stamped the suds from my shoes and ran toward Mr. Keiller, who was standing naked in his doorway making frantic motions for me to hurry.

Considering it was only seven P.M., I was ahead in the time-versus-nurse game. Mr. Keiller had been washed down and put in a fresh gown for a fourth time, except now he was resting in bed with a small bedpan under him at all times. Mr. Shirinian, my post-operative gallbladder/congestive heart failure patient, had been stabilized. Mrs. Norman had been ambulated (jet-propelled was more like it) and fed dinner along with her eleven pills. Mrs. Guasco had coded and didn't make it to go for a fourth try. My two stable pulmonary edema ladies in beds 14 and 15 were fed and given their diuretics, which, of course, ensured that their call bells would be ringing up a storm, first one, then the other, with requests to get on and then off the bedpan. Mrs. Englewood had been treated with morphine for chest pain and bolused with lidocaine for a short run of ventricular tachycardia.

Through the window behind the nursing station, the fading June sun gave a warm golden glow to everything below. On the exercise path across the road, people jogged and roller-skated their way through rings of orange and gold haze.

These were Normal People. Normal People had nothing to do with the frailties and infirmities of the human body. Normal People weren't required to put in a ten-hour day but get paid for eight, or to work every other weekend plus holidays. In short, Normal People would never, ever feel comfortable discussing blood, feces, and mucus over dinner.

Not that I couldn't be out there with them. Nobody was forcing me to work the evening shift. I had been working the swing shift for ten years and, in fact, guarded the position carefully. For me, the alternatives—day or night shifts—were worse than death.

The graveyard shift people, those who worked from seven or eleven P.M. to seven A.M., perpetually looked so tired and pale, I always had a desire to pop an iron pill into their mouths or yawn for them. On the other hand, the day nurses, the ones who came in at seven A.M. and left at either three or seven P.M., looked downright worked to the bone. What with bed baths and dealing with all the docs at once, serving two meals, doing cardiac teaching, and dealing with the walking wounded known as the family, not to mention actually taking care of the patients themselves, was it any wonder?

The swing shift people had the best of all worlds. Although a person's social life could be ruined, nobody's biorhythm got upset, and the main traumas of the day shift—constant exposure to the doctors' moods and attitudes—were over for the most part before the shift began.

My stomach growled loudly, causing Sandy, the nurse in charge, to turn. "Why don't you go eat while you have the chance? There's a hot heart in ER that may need to go to the acute side and you're the one up for the next admit."

I didn't argue. Nurses who worked critical care learned early on to eat when the chance came or deal with the hunger and hypoglycemia later on. Those of us who had tried eating while on duty found it a messy and sometimes hazardous business trying to sneak bites of sandwiches (kept out of sight in the desk drawers or under a monitor) while on the run between patients.

The CCU refrigerator, a limitless source of strange biology experiments and other faulty-storage surprises, was packed to its Freon tubes with a variety of brown paper bags and half-filled jars. In a hidden corner on the bottom, behind the fifteen-year-old bottle of green something that no one ever, ever touched, I found my airtight plastic container of salad.

Eyes and ears closed to the sounds of call bells and alarms, I went to the room used for the insertion of temporary pacemaker wires and let the heavy door shut behind me. The sudden peace and silence that inevitably shocked my ears enveloped me. Hopefully, no one would need temporary pacing for the next thirty minutes, so I could eat and worry in peace.

I was pouring the usual no-calorie, no-flavor dressing over my healthier-than-God salad, when the jar of peanut butter and box of crackers stashed in my locker magically called out my name. As if summoned by sirenic wizards, I automatically stood and headed toward the locker room.

Screw the healthy stuff, I thought. I'd have carbos, starches, and fat for dinner.

Except as I reached for the door, my mother's ghost stood at the gate of my mind, hands on hips. She stopped me cold. A truly stubborn force, therapy and libraries of self-help books had yet to erase all her negative tapes from my mind.

"You're not a young woman anymore, Echo," she said with that authoritative, slightly British tone I knew so well.

Reluctantly, I had to agree with her; my hairdresser was beginning to drop hints about dye jobs.

"After thirty-five it's all downhill. Calories don't just evaporate into thin air anymore," she went on, shaking her finger.

I noticed the fat on her upper arm and knew her to be an authority.

"Listen, Mum, I need the protein."

"Pfft. Peanut butter is nothing but fat."

"I'm over five feet six inches tall and weigh a hundred and eight pounds. People tell me I'm too skinny."

"They're lying. Just three years ago you weighed a hundred and six. And don't forget the chest pain you have when you're stressed—clogged arteries from all the peanut butter. Besides, you don't look so good anymore. Soon you'll be losing estrogen. Broken bones and heart disease will follow. You'll wrinkle early like your father's family. Why, a massive stroke is just around the—"

I laughed at the absurdity of her arguments and snapped her off. Three minutes later, five peanut-buttered crackers in hand, I was back at my salad.

When I was at the searching-for-crumbs-and-piercing-stray-pieces-of-lettuce stage of my meal, I decided I'd stalled long enough—it was time to do some serious worrying.

From the deepest regions of my uniform pocket, I pulled a wad of well-worn pages titled "June–July/1987 Publicity Tour—Heron," and studied them for the fifteenth time that day. My stomach tightened at the word "publicity," sending an ache of protest throughout my gut.

Almost two years since the day I was put into dumbfounded shock over the news that my book proposal had been accepted, *Intensive Care: The Story of a Nurse* was a 370-page reality, sitting on bookstore shelves.

Wonderful, except for this one clause in the contract that stated something about the author being more or less obligated to promote the book on what was known as a "book tour." This meant, my agent calmly explained, going on TV and radio and talking to thousands—no, millions of people at a time.

But . . . But . . . didn't the publicity department realize that I'd had a problem with stage fright since I was a kid?

Don't worry, they said, you'll get over it.

Yeah, except I had never been able to speak to more than two people at a time—even in the privacy of my own living room—without freezing up.

Don't worry, they said, you'll get over it.

But didn't they know that writers are the most reclusive and inarticulate people on the face of the earth?

Don't worry, they said, you'll get over it.

Didn't they know I'd most certainly faint or do something equally embarrassing the second I knew I was on camera?

Don't worry, they said, you'll get over it.

But I'm just a small-town girl—a nurse, for Christ's sake. I don't know anything about television; don't even watch the damned thing. And besides, didn't they know that I was frequently guilty of blurting out whatever came to the space where my mind used to be?

Don't worry, they said, just get over it and hurry up.

Except I wouldn't get over it, and the prospect of talking glibly—let alone at all—on the *Today* show filled me with indescribable terror. I had horrible visions of throwing up all over Bryant Gumbel's perfectly pressed suit and then falling into Jane Pauley's lap in a dead faint.

I'd never forgotten the young starlet I'd seen on the Jackie Gleason show when I was a child, who froze onstage and had to be carried off before a live audience. Certainly I would match her and go one better, especially since I'd gone and written this autobiographical book that had a full-sized close-up of my face on the back cover.

To get a feel for the torture, I'd been watching the talk shows for a month. Everyone appeared to be totally at ease. It seemed that *anyone*, even housewives from Idaho or Minnesota, could get up in front of a million viewers and let it all hang out—with jokes and quick, clever rhetoric.

Did they get special drugs before the show? I wondered. Or were all talk show participants, in fact, professional actors?

I looked at the date of my first interview: a local noon news show scheduled to take place in three days. It was, thank Buddha, only four minutes long, but the words after the date read, "LIVE INTERVIEW." My ulcer spasmed and kicked.

I allowed myself to look at the next item on the list and saw that scheduled two days later was a very popular local radio talk show. Radio wasn't so bad; at least people wouldn't be able to point me out on the street as easily.

Swallowing my misery whole, I scanned the second, then the third page of the schedule and broke into a cold sweat. CNN. The *Today* show. *Hour Magazine*. Suddenly the salad, all five crackers, and the old-fashioned, extra-crunchy style were knocking at the back of my throat to be let out, away from an ulcer gone berserk.

I can't go through with it, I thought. That's all there is to it. I'll refuse. Simple enough.

Resolved, I walked to the bathroom, gagged a few times, washed my face and hands, and returned to work. In this year of harmonic convergence, I and my ulcer would be perfectly at peace regardless of outside stresses trying to throw in a few wrong notes.

Oh yeah.

Sandy was watching for me in the wide-view mirror hanging over the nurses' station. The second I stepped into the hallway, she motioned to me to hurry it up; there was bad news that I needed to hear right away. In light of my worries over the publicity tour, any bad news she had for me was going to be a piece of cake.

Before I even got close to the nursing station, I could hear the commotion coming from the acute side. Peeking around the double doors, I saw several of the CCU nurses talking at once and running in and out of bed 2 as if it were Grand Central. Dr. Cramer saw me, frowned, and hurried into the room concealed from view by blue curtains. It was always a sign of bad trouble or impending death when the curtains were drawn all the way around a room.

Sandy spoke rapidly, her voice a decibel above normal. "I've put you in charge of bed two, who is a thirty-one-year-old woman in active labor. Dr. Cramer suspects a cardiac tamponade. She's in shock, without a palpable blood pressure. Fifteen minutes ago, she had a V fib arrest and had to be shocked three times. The baby is in distress with a heart rate of seventy." Sandy stared at me with what I thought was almost a malicious glint in her eyes, as if to say, "So whaddaya gonna do about it, huh?"

"But ... why isn't she in labor and delivery? I mean, how soon is the baby coming? Is there an OB-GYN man in there? What about a cesarean? What about ICU?" I realized immediately that in my panic, I was desperate to turf this crisis to another department.

Having a labor patient in CCU was as rare an occurrence as finding an eohippus grazing in your backyard. Every brain cell I owned that had anything pertaining to labor and delivery stored in it had deserted its post or been misplaced. All I could come up with were vague techniques such as checking for the cord around the infant's neck, easing out the shoulders one at a time, and performing a maneuver called "massaging the fundus"—none of which were of any use to the patient in bed 2.

Somewhere in the back of my mind I heard, clear as day, Prissy in *Gone with the Wind* screaming in that cat-yowl voice, "I don't know nothin' 'bout birthin' babies, Miz Scarlett," and started to laugh a hysterical, mentally unhealthy type of laugh. It broke the panic spell.

Gathering my wits, I dashed over to the acute side, not at all surprised that the code bell over bed 2 went off the second I ran through the double doors.

I grabbed the crash cart, rolled the two-hundred-pound cabinet over my foot, said the *F* word, and pushed it crazily toward the room. The sweat made my hands slip on the push bar, and I tripped over my own injured foot. I flung back the curtain to find four nurses and Dr. Cramer huddled around the bed, yelling and waving their arms—except no one appeared to actually be *doing* anything for the patient.

My eyes went automatically to the bedside monitor, which showed a very fine ventricular fibrillation, then to the patient. Through the wall of nurses, I saw a wisp of blond hair and an absurdly huge belly that was hard to miss even under the heavy brown bedspread. The pregnant abdomen looked very much like a mound of earth where something—a giant sequoia perhaps—had been planted and was ready to sprout forth. From the bottom of the blanket, two small feet stuck out—clad in clean white tennis shoes. That no one had even bothered to remove the patient's shoes infuriated me, but my adrenaline was priming me for more serious action.

Joe pointed at me and shouted, "You! Do CPR."

The question of why the bloody hell no one had initiated CPR before I got there crossed my mind, and as I jumped onto the bed and threw back the bedspread, I was already composing an incident report: *"The patient was in full cardiac arrest with an assortment of no less than five medically trained morons surrounding her doing nothing except flapping their arms and lips, apparently for no other purpose than to create wind."*

I was on the second paragraph when the patient's "belly," an immense silver helium balloon in the shape of a star, floated toward the ceiling. Flabbergasted, I looked down at the patient and saw Resusi-Annie, our CPR practice dummy. One of her floppy arms hugged a bottle of champagne to her removable plastic chest.

I looked back at the balloon. On it was a message written in Sandy's unmistakable perfect hand: "Congratulations from CCU. Hope you sell a million copies!"

I looked into the faces of my fellow nurses Pia, Sandy, Risen, and Nealy and thought of how they had become my surrogate, West Coast family; my sisters and brothers, mothers and fathers. I had gone to school with most of them, and knew their fears and joys. At one time or other over the years, we had cried on one another's shoulders, bitched among ourselves, been held and comforted and pulled out of tight spots by one another.

Pia, the youngest and closest to my heart, hugged me. "Isn't it exciting?" she whispered. "You're an official authoress, going on national TV with all those people listening to what you have to say."

I looked at her to make sure she wasn't being cruel, saw her sincerity and forced a smile. Inside, my stomach flipped over and bounced into my throat.

At 10:27 P.M. the phone rang. "That's my new admit," I said without looking up from Mr. Keiller's chart.

It was not a Jeane Dixon moment, only that we had not had an admission for almost six hours. This was too good a deal; it stood to reason our dues would be an end-of-shift admit.

Sandy answered, listened for a second, glanced at me, and raised her eyebrows. I signed off the chart and automatically headed for room 11/12, which had recently been vacated due to Sandy's and Risen's excellent turfing efforts.

After making sure the room was set up for admission, I went back to get an abbreviated rundown on the new admit from Sandy.

"The patient is on his way up from ER," Sandy said, her eyes still fixed on her charting. She was in a hurry to finish before night shift report was due. "He's a twenty-five-year-old endocarditis patient of Dr. Cramer's. He has a two-year history of IV drug abuse and goes by the name of Charlie. Temp is 101.6. ER started an IV. They're running in his first dose of penicillin as we speak. He's in sinus tach at a hundred, BP is one-ten over sixty, and—"

The double doors opened and a float nurse came into the unit pushing a wheelchair. At first glance, the person propped up in the chair looked like a scared twelve-year-old boy. His haunted, tired expression left no doubt in my mind that Dr. Cramer had already told him that endocarditis, a bacterial infection of the inner lining of the heart, was fatal unless treated quickly with antibiotics.

While the nurse wheeled him to his bed, I looked over Joe's orders and then went back to room 11/12. I found Charlie half sitting, half slumped on the side of the bed. He was still wearing his jeans and socks.

"Why didn't you get into bed?"

"Didn't want to get your clean sheets all messed up," he whispered without opening his eyes. "Haven't had a bath with soap for"—he sighed—"two months. Been too sick. No money."

"Can you sit up so I can help you off with your clothes?"

I gently pulled at the perspiration-soaked patient gown that covered his upper body.

Charlie attempted to move, but was too weak to pull himself up. "So thirsty. If I could have some water, maybe I . . ."

I poured a glass of ice water and put the straw to his lips. He pulled at the straw. The effort was just enough to bring up a mouthful of water. He caught his breath, then pulled again, this time with more strength. When the glass was drained, he opened his eyes. "Thank you. Haven't been able to get much to eat or drink."

"Do you think you could sit up now?"

Charlie nodded. Little by little, with my arm slipped under him, we managed to get him into an upright position. In my arms he felt like a small, sleepy child. The flimsy blue gown fell off his shoulders. Underneath, his emaciated body was streaked with dirt. His arms and the backs of his hands were dotted with purple-and-red needle tracks—not as bad as some I had seen, but in a few years he would be as scarred as the worst of them.

Only the area around his IV had been wiped clean, leaving the white patch of skin contrasting sharply with the gray.

He turned his eyes toward the bathroom, where the shower door stood open. The sparkling white tiles of the stall were an invitation to cleanliness.

"Christ," he croaked, "I'd do anything for a shower."

His expression was that of one making a last wish.

It took about a second to weigh out the pros and cons: He was on bed rest orders, and he was too debilitated to possibly stand in the shower for more than a few seconds. Yet . . . if I gave him a bed bath, it wouldn't be half as satisfying or relaxing to him, plus I wouldn't be able to wash his hair, and he wanted a shower so badly . . .

Two months?

Well, if I got it together quickly . . .

Leaning him back on the bed, I ran to the station and picked up some one-pint cartons of orange juice, asked Nealy to call the supervisor and tell her to bring up a dinner for my patient, dodged Sandy's questions as to why Charlie wasn't on monitor yet, got more towels and bath soap, loaded them into one of our small wheelchairs, and ran back to the room.

After boosting his energy level with a couple of glasses of orange juice, Charlie was able to stand long enough for me to slip off his pants and transfer him into the wheelchair. With a towel draped over his lap for the sake of modesty, I filled my pockets with packages of shampoo and soap, washcloths, and two razors, then wheeled him into the shower, IV and all.

At first I tried to help out with the scrubbing by reaching around the shower door, but that was pretty awkward, besides the fact that I was getting soaked. I finally figured what the hell, took off my shoes and socks, threw on a shower cap, and stepped into the shower with him.

I washed him down, starting at the top of his head, working the soap over the skeletal shoulders. He was so skinny, it was pathetic. I saw that he was nothing but bones and, once the dirt was off, pale as paper.

He was terribly weak, so that I had to lift his arms and legs to clean in the hidden places. In an abstract way, he reminded me of a sick deer, or some large starving animal, and it made me more tender and stronger at the same time. This could be my son, I thought, and perhaps if my son were ever to be in need this way, someone would provide a similar measure of comfort for him.

At first Charlie literally groaned with pleasure at the warm water and the smell of soap and shampoo; then he started to giggle. Had someone entered the room, seen my shoes and socks, and heard the sounds coming from the shower, there would have been raised eyebrows and wild rumors, I'm sure.

Finally he began to bawl.

As he cried, I looked at the needle tracks and the bones, and I listened to the scared sobs about how he didn't want to die, and that he was so sorry . . .

"You aren't going to die, Charlie." I washed out the infected spaces between his toes as gently as I could. "You'll feel pretty good in a few days. What I'm worried about is that you'll forget how bad you felt today." I stared into eyes that were filled with pain. "I'm afraid you won't remember not wanting to die."

"No," he said quietly, "I'll never forget this. I'm not going back to that life ever again. I won't. I promise to God, I won't."

I toweled him dry, put him into a clean gown, retaped his IV, got him into bed, hooked him up to the monitor, then toweled myself off as best I could. I'd have to borrow a dry scrub dress from labor and delivery.

As I was finishing Charlie's physical assessment, Risen came in bearing a tray loaded down with food. Except as the tray passed, I could see and smell that the food was definitely not from the Redwoods kitchen; this food looked and smelled edible.

I recognized a steaming helping of Nealy's homemade pasta primavera; next to that was a small bowl of the chicken noodle soup that Sandy had been saving all shift. The huge piece of angel food cake with peach glaze was unmistakably from Pia's dinner.

Risen set down the tray and from his shirt pocket pulled out a banana. As tired as I could see he was, he patiently began to spoon soup into Charlie's mouth.

Between bites of pasta and soup, Charlie started to cry again.

"Why are you people doing this?" he asked. "Why are you so good to me?"

"Because," answered Risen, "we have faith in the living."

By the time I changed into dry scrubs and returned to the nurses' station, Sandy had retired to the nurses' lounge to report off to night shift. Nealy was watching monitors, waiting for report to end.

"Hey, thanks for the food. What happened to the supervisor? I thought she was supposed to bring up a dinner."

Nealy shook her head. "The supervisor wouldn't get a dinner for the patient because she said he's a street person and doesn't have any insurance." The nurse pursed her mouth. "I guess all that meant to her was that the guy doesn't deserve to eat, so we decided to put something together out of what we each had left over from our dinners. I mean, the man is sick and starving." Nealy shrugged. "Since when did the price of a slice of bread and a lousy bowl of soup outweigh compassion?"

"Never happen in this unit," yawned Risen, setting down Charlie's dinner tray and falling into the chair next to me. The tray was so devoid of food, it looked like the plates had been washed. "Not with this particular group."

I yawned, then Nealy, the power of suggestion ever strong.

"Yeah," said Nealy, laughing, "we're all such suckers."

"Not suckers," I said. "Human. We're all just very human."

I sat up and turned on the light. It was three-thirty A.M., and my mind felt like a shorted-out blender. Over my bed, the purple ribbon tail of my silver balloon waved cheerily, reminding me I should be optimistic and confident. Exhausted, I flipped it the finger.

Mooshie, also known in softer, sillier moments as Mommy's Kuka Man, Brown Buddha, and Mushu Pork with Pancakes, yawned and stretched his lithe cat body to an amazing length.

I yawned, stretched in a stiffer fashion, and faced him. His round gold eyes leveled mine in that earnest, straightforward way overfed cats sometimes have. He briefly rested his germ-laden feline paw on my mouth as if to say, "Don't start with that Mommy's-little-soldier routine—I'm not in the mood," and jumped off the bed to go in search of less active mattresses. I did not take this rejection personally. As the adult kitten of a dysfunctional litter, Mooshie, like many cats, was an avoidance addict to the max.

Picking up the pen writers were always supposed to keep handy at their bedsides, I opened a fancy leatherbound book to the first blank page.

It has been said that most brilliant plots and ideas for books come to writers during sleep. That worried me because I had been suffering from insomnia for some time. Did this mean I would have to start worrying now about writer's block, too?

At the top of the page I wrote, "Things I Worry About Lately That Keep Me Awake Nights."

1. *The book tour. (Can't go into detail right now or I'll throw up.)*

2. *What will the hospital administration's reaction to the book be, especially the parts that show them for the moneygrubbing asses they are? Will I be burned in effigy, or perhaps lynched in person? Will they sue me?*

3. *What will the doctors' reactions be to finding out that many of them have been portrayed in a realistic, less than flattering light; i.e., still stubbornly believing that the M.D. stands for Medical Deity?*

4. *What will other nurses think? Could I lose my license?*

5. *Will my father have a heart attack when he reads the parts about my personal life?*

6. *Could I be happy living in China where no one knows (or can pronounce) my name?*

7. *Is loneliness fatal?*

* * *

Calmly, I went over the list with an objective, middle-of-the-road eye—just as my therapist instructed. I went over it again, and then once again.

I'm not a religious person, so when I found myself on my knees beseeching God's help, I convinced myself that no one I knew personally would read the book anyway, so there was nothing to worry about.

Feeling somewhat relieved, I went to the kitchen to make myself a cup of hot tea, softened with plenty of milk and honey.

"Have a bad dream?"

At the deep voice, I started, dribbling honey over Mooshie, who was busy marking my ankles with the scent glands purportedly located in the vicinity of his ears. In the dim light of the kitchen doorway stood my sixteen-year-old son, Simon, sleepily scratching his bony chest, which sported a trio of hairs he'd named Boris, Valiant, and Lucky Larry.

It never ceased to amaze me how silently Simon could move around for such a tall person. I studied the six-foot man in pure wonder, as if he were my own private miracle. Had he *really* once been a toothless rug rat whom I carried around under one arm and whose diapers I changed?

Being the divorced single mother of an adolescent was an experience I found educational and certainly very stimulating, rather like wading through the Everglades in the dead of night without a flashlight. Not only had Simon taught me patience, but he'd also forced me to take food-shopping frugality seriously; he ate such huge quantities of food, and so often, that I periodically felt the need to take out a loan just to cover dinner.

My communication skills had expanded also. Simon introduced me to a unique vocabulary not yet found in any dictionary ("Hey Ma! Watch me bloto fruckspin this dweeber!"). He also gave many in-home demonstrations on mental telepathy by phone. For hours at a time he monopolized the line, neither party saying a word but just breathing into the mouthpiece.

He was my constantly unfolding mystery, like a biology lab project gone awry. As a child of the seventies, Simon turned out completely differently than I expected. I knew by the time he was ten, Si wasn't going to be the Ivy League type of son who played tennis with his buddies on Saturday mornings. He would never be a member of the student council, nor would he be the perpetrator of sit-ins because he believed in politically tenuous and radical causes.

No, the son I had borne was an artistic, verbally absent, and crotchety eighty-seven-year-old hiding in a sixteen-year-old's body. At times, he could be Mother Teresa in disguise; other times, he was Freddy Krueger in the horrible flesh.

Artistic was fine, even when the nerve-jangling Jimi Hendrix guitar practice went far into the night.

Old before his time was all right too. His innate wisdom never failed to make me feel as though I were at a disadvantage—like being on a seesaw with someone heavier than myself.

Even crotchety was understood, considering his age group and its American-teen hormonal traumas. It was the verbally absent that got to me, the never knowing what was going on inside that adolescent steel trap of a mind.

Simon's father, Patrick, who often helped shoulder parenting responsibilities, once made the observation that Simon and I related to each other in a variety of ways—brother and sister, best friends, Siskel and Ebert, Oscar and Felix.

As two distinctly different personalities, I thought it admirable that Simon and I shared such a complete understanding and acceptance of one another. It was thus on his sixteenth birthday when I gave up the control over him that I never had.

Now I stopped staring at my son (Tip to Parents of Teens: Staring at adolescents drives them up a wall) and wiped the honey off Mooshie's head with a sponge.

"Yes, Simon, I am not only having but I am also *living* a bad dream. It's called a book tour."

"Huh?"

"I'm worried about the tour," I said, and sat down at the rickety kitchen table with my hot milk tea. "I hate being a public person. I'm afraid I'm going to throw up or faint on TV."

There was silence while Simon considered me with what was either infinite compassion or the conviction that his mother actually was from a different planet. "Why would you want to throw up and faint on TV?"

"I don't *want* to, Si, I'm just worried I might because I'm terrified I'll make a fool of myself in front of millions of people. That's all."

"Well, when the cameras go on and the spotlights are beating down on you and all those millions of TV viewers are judging you by what you say, make believe you're at home alone talking to yourself like you usually do."

I narrowed my eyes. "Is cruelty an affliction of your particular age group, or are you harboring deep-seated rage against your mother? Go to bed. I want to suffer alone."

Simon shrugged, opened a quart of milk, drank it in three swallows, and headed for his room. A few seconds later, he stood again in the kitchen doorway.

"Ma?"

"Yeah?"

"Do me a favor—if any of the interviewers ask, tell them you don't have any children."

I finally fell into a troubled sleep about five-thirty A.M. The dream was in color and took place on the Great Wall of China. The hospital's administrator was chasing me with a summons, and behind him were a group of angry doctors wielding ungreased proctoscopy tubes and shouting my name. As I ran past the viewing audience, I noticed the cameras marked "*Today* show" getting the whole episode live.

Horrified by the spectacle, Simon, my father, and co-workers looked on, vowing to interviewers that they'd never seen me before in their lives.

TWO

> "Nursing puts us in touch with being human ... Without even asking, nurses are invited into the inner spaces of other people's existence ... for where there is suffering, loneliness, the tolerable pain of cure, or the solitary pain of permanent change, there is a need for the kind of human services we call nursing."
>
> DONNA DIERS, R.N.

I AWOKE WEDNESDAY MORNING on the other side of black. The reddened indentations on my palms, left by my fingernails, were a sign that I had worried during my sleep. This fact was further evidenced by the too familiar ache that was now kicking my stomach around like an old soccer ball. Bleary-eyed, I located the bottle of ulcer medication on the bedside table and swallowed one of the bitter tablets dry.

Through the cobwebs of a mind fouled by inadequate sleep came the daily question of which role I would play when I finally pulled out of my horizontal posture and made a stab at the vertical one.

I slid my feet into the overstuffed slippers with the miniature nursing caps on the toes and padded toward the bathroom. On the way, I stepped on Mooshie, who was posing as a fur rug. In true feline melodrama, he yowled like a noon whistle, sprang up, rolled over, and flew halfway up the wall, his tail exploding into a bottle brush with an erection.

Startled from drowsiness, I echoed his yowl, tripped over his retreating body, and sprawled, hip first, onto the floor. I stared up at the hallway ceiling. At least I had gotten my daily accident out of the way.

Just as I had chronic bad hair days, I had body injury days—every day. For the past two years I had become a major threat to my own physical safety. I fractured, I punctured, I burned, I lacerated, I bruised. My trips to the emergency room were so numerous, I was sure the staff suspected me of self-abuse of the traumatic sort.

Some days I woke up wondering what mishap would befall my body that day: Today I might burn the hair off one side of my head. Tomorrow it could be the tearing of some essential tendon, or I might get off easy with a simple concussion.

It seemed I'd heard something about clumsiness and a faulty memory being signs of perimenopause, but I couldn't remember exactly what had been said. In order to keep track of tidbits like that, I had recently taken to writing everything down in what I called my memopause book.

I reached into my purse, near which I had conveniently fallen, and pulled out my appointment book. The square for Wednesday indicated I was scheduled to fulfill my on-call, part-time obligations as an emergency room nurse. Feeling better instantly, I gathered myself off the floor. ER was an experience not to be missed.

Working emergency room had a lot of up sides to it. It was interesting and exciting; one had to be ready to lend oneself to whatever came through the doors—from scrapes to rapes, hemorrhoids to gunshot wounds. Plus, there was only a minimal amount of charting required, a duty I hated even more than cleaning slimy, food-caked dentures.

Unlike CCU nurses, whose specialty centered around dysfunctions of the heart and lungs, the ER nurse tended to all parts of the body; every illness, trauma, and psych problem that walked into our arena had to be taken care of, and taken care of quickly. It was, as Gus—one of the ER staff nurses—often said, the git-along-you-ol'-doggies system—"Git 'em in and git 'em out quick as greased pigs can slide down a chute."

Not that the job was totally thornless. ER nurses stayed on their feet and running all shift. If you had back problems, which most nurses do, an eight-hour shift could be a painful hell; twelve could be crippling. Besides that, there was always a hint of danger in the air. Who knew *what* was going to walk in off the street?

In every city or town, the emergency room is thought of as the clinic of last resort by every indigent and mentally unstable person for miles around. To too many of these people, an emergency room means instant cure for all the ills of mankind. And when that help isn't delivered, people can get pretty testy. I have personally known two nurses who were murdered in parking lots as they came off shift—one stabbed in the back, the other shot in the head, both crimes committed by disgruntled patients.

Working the ER was like going to the movies or a museum of social history. It was, for sure, the gallery in which to view human frailties in the raw.

In the trauma room, sometimes referred to as the "doom room," the man on the gurney appeared calm, even somewhat removed from what was going on around him. Sarah, ER's evening charge nurse, moved quickly to catch something that had fallen off the gurney, and slipped in a puddle of his blood. Instinctively, the patient grabbed for her, setting his IV bag swinging on its pole. The scene of the wounded reaching out to help the healer, framed itself in the moment.

I'd stopped by the trauma room mainly out of curiosity, but also to offer my help and let Sarah know that Gus and I were reporting for duty.

As I stepped close to the gurney, Sarah turned on me with the speed of light. "Careful of the bowel!"

The urgency in her voice froze me in midstep. Following her gaze, I blinked in disbelief and leaned in for closer inspection.

From the gaping wound that stretched from the crest of one of the man's hipbones straight across his abdomen to the other, protruded several delicate loops of pink bowel. One loop dangled onto the mattress. My childhood memory bank instantly coughed up a recollection of standing outside an ancient butcher shop window where loop after loop of dark red and pinkish-gray sausage hung from wires, attracting flies.

I looked to Sarah for some explanation, but she was already moving about the room in a brisk, businesslike manner. It was so Sarah—unruffled, stepping over pools of blood with the kind of composure that came from working in the emergency room since the beginning of time.

She dropped several packages of sterile gauze into a basin of saline solution, then expertly opened a pair of surgical gloves, fitting them over her hands without contaminating the outside—a feat not always easily accomplished. "Our friend here tried to commit hara-kiri with a turkey-carving knife," she said. "He didn't quite make it, I'm glad to say."

The patient closed his eyes and sighed. "Can't do anything right."

"Oh, come on, Bill." Sarah diligently rinsed off the man's bowel and wrapped the exposed sections in the wet gauze. "There's too much out there to live for." She paused, and in place of a more physical touch, inserted into her voice that certain gentleness that belonged only to nurses; it was the soft, rounded sound of compassion. "There are still things like sunsets, love, and warm summer days to look forward to, you know."

The man turned his face to the wall, his broad shoulders shaking. He tried to hide his face, but the IVs had been placed at the crooks of his arms, making it impossible for him to bend his elbows.

I moved to the head of the gurney and lightly stroked his hand. "It's going to get better from here," I said, my intuitive feelers reading the essence of the man. I've never been sure what to call this ability to walk around inside other people's skin, but I did know that being in the trenches for any length of time caused some nurses to develop a sixth sense of knowing what was in store for the people they took care of. It was rather like being able to predict when the phone would ring, or what song was going to play next on the radio. I knew that this man's pain would not pull him down again; he would learn from what he had seen in the darkest part of himself and go on.

When his shoulders relaxed, he asked for a Kleenex, promising Sarah he wouldn't blow too hard and push out any more intestine.

His vital signs were remarkably normal, considering. Sarah told me the man had miraculously (he'd used a recently sharpened ten-inch carving knife) missed all his major blood vessels and organs. As far as anyone could tell, his bowel hadn't even been nicked.

I touched his shoulder. "You can always tell people you got into a knife fight with a midget."

"Either that," said Sarah, "or that you were thinking of becoming a surgeon and wanted to practice."

From the pile of clothes on the counter, I saw that he had been wearing new khakis and a T-shirt imprinted with the picture of a dolphin and a whale swimming side by side. The logo read, "Save Our Friends in the Sea." I looked into the man's careworn face and felt his pain and the exhaustion of his spirit. Catching his eyes with mine, I thought, *How could you do this? Life is too short, too precious. Scream, beat your chest, cry, run naked through the streets, anything but this.*

The man shivered.

Automatically, I went to the linen warmer and pulled out two hot flannel blankets. I wrapped one around his upper body, avoiding the wound. I was winding the other around his legs when Dr. Mahoney, our ER doc du jour, stuck her head through the door. "How's our butcher trainee doing in here?"

I laughed at her irreverence, checking to see if the patient had taken offense. He was smiling, which was the way most people responded to Susan Mahoney. The woman was one of those rare humans who could get away with having an outrageous and distinctively peculiar personality, no sweat.

"His vital signs are more stable than mine," I said.

"In your case that's probably not saying much, Reverb." Although I had shown Dr. Mahoney my driver's license, passport, and library card, she refused to believe Echo was my true given name. As a result, she'd nicknamed me Reverberation, explaining that it was as close as she would go to Echo. As for my sister Storm, Dr. Mahoney wouldn't allow me to mention her name at all, insisting I refer to her only as Miss Lillian. "However," she went on, "I want to be the first to inform you that there are several casualties out here who are in need of your services."

"What's the CH level?" Sarah asked, delicately placing a loop of gauze-covered bowel on the sterile towel situated on the man's abdomen.

Susan's head disappeared, then reappeared a minute later. "Level two and a half and climbing," she announced, and was gone.

Dr. Mahoney and Dr. Menowitz, our other senior ER doc, had developed the Redwoods Memorial Emergency Department Chaos Level Chart late one weekend night when things were slow. Any other combination of doctors would have been sleeping on the bunks in the ER docs' lounge, but Dr. Mahoney refused to sleep in the same room with Dr. Menowitz: she insisted that he made such strange and horrible noises when he slept, it conjured up hideous images in her mind of turning on the light and finding him devouring the lower half of his face.

Thus, instead of sleeping, the two devoted their free time to the creation of ideas and inventions that centered around the needs of an emergency room. One night they assembled a machine made from a broom handle, tape, weights, and a five-gallon bucket, which proved quite effective for popping dislocated shoulders back into their sockets. Another time they produced an inexpensive, comfortable, nonslip, no-fuss joint immobilizer. Their best effort, however, was the Chaos Chart.

If one went by the Redwoods Memorial Emergency Department Chaos Level Chart, Chaos Level One represented low stress no-brainers like minor burns and cuts, a (yawn) bloody nose or two, ingrown toenails, gastrointestinal upsets with minor electrolyte imbalances, flu and sore throat boredom, contact dermatitis, fecal impactions, migraines, and mildly colicky babies who belonged to overreactive parents.

Level Two included rapes and other sex-related traumas, conscious overdoses, beatings, burn patients needing to be transferred to the burn unit, chest pains with arrhythmias, kidney stones, minor amputations, mildly violent psych cases, multiple large broken bones, conscious motorcycle and auto accident victims, respiratory distress patients, and screaming children of any age.

Level Three encompassed unconscious overdoses, stabbing and shooting traumas, CPR in progress, diabetic comas, amputations of major limbs, bad head or spinal injuries, burn patients with acute respiratory problems, respiratory patients who were blue or gray in color, flatline patients, blood pressures lower than 60, and heart rates lower than 30.

Level Four included more than any two of Level Three happening at the same time.

I took quick inventory of the main room and saw that all six beds were filled. At the far end, the door to the ten-by-seven pelvic room, popularly known as the "orifice room," was closed, meaning it too was occupied. Both beds in the surgical suite were in use, and I already knew what was in the trauma room. It was a full house.

Ileta, our clerk, stared suspiciously at the closed curtain of bed 4, located directly in the middle of the emergency department, not five feet from her desk.

"Something funny going on in there," the middle-aged woman whispered, never taking her eyes off the curtain.

Ileta had been chief evening clerk since the recent and sudden departure of Irene, Redwoods's ER clerk of twenty years.

Poor Irene had been the innocent victim in a series of three unfortunate ER events. First, there was the afternoon when one of our more rancorous repeaters, Wheelin' Wilma, chased her down with her wheelchair and bit her on the arm for refusing to let her use the ER phone to call her sister in Toledo for a chat.

We had just calmed Irene down, assuring her she didn't need a rabies vaccination, when the very next evening, a lady who came in for a sore throat walked over to her desk, gave her a low-down and deadly look, and said, "I warned you that I'd find you someday, Mildred. You've got to stop seeing Ed."

We managed to get the switchblade knife away from the woman, but not before Irene had pulled a muscle in her back jumping over the counter.

A week later, Irene came off medical leave. Within a day or two, she was her old, easygoing self again—right up until the psych patient we were holding for the crisis unit jumped on her desk and relieved himself all over her brand-new patient ledger book.

The way it was told to me, Irene gathered up her things then and there. "A bite, a sprained back, okay," she said, drying off, then throwing her phone headset and bits of erasers into her bag. "Those sorts of things I can handle, but urine on my new ledger book? I'm sorry, that's my limit!"

She straightened her shoulders, yanked a loose wisp of gray hair out of her eyes, and marched down the black runner out the automatic door. No amount of pleading, vacation time, money, or promises of bulletproof walls around her desk could lure her back to the department.

Ileta knew all about the trials and tribulations of her predecessor and was always cautious of patients who came within four feet of her desk. Sometimes she was even jumpy around the ER personnel, especially Dr. Menowitz, Redwoods's own ER doctor from hell, the brooding and occasionally caustic physician who, in fact, had the heart of a misguided poet.

"Get this lady on the road outta here," Ileta said, pointing a short brown finger at the pile of charts in a plastic milk crate marked "Nurse" situated next to the overflowing crate marked "Doctor." "She's making my hair stand up on the back of my neck."

I glanced at the back of Ileta's neck and saw that the hairs there were indeed sticking up—along with the rest of her moderately short Afro.

Mrs. Wade's chart was on top of the "Nurse" pile. This meant she had been brought back from the waiting room and put on a gurney, but her vital signs and the initial assessment of her problem had not yet been completed by a nurse. Under the "Reason for Visit" space, the sixty-five-year-old Mrs. Wade was quoted as saying she had not had a BM since eight that morning.

Under the "Present Medications" column, she'd written: "Ex-lax, Dulcolax, Swiss Kriss"—she had starred this one and written, "The best!"—"Fleets, Doxidan, DOSS, Metamucil, and Elixir of PowerPrune."

Oh God, I thought, bowel mania has hit Fog City. First Mrs. Norman, then a bowel loop flasher, and now a bona fide bowel baby.

Bowel babies are notorious among nurses. Every nurse and doctor has dealt with at least a hundred of them, long before he or she is even out of training. Although you could find bowel babies of all ages (I'd actually met a ten-year-old bowel baby when I did my pediatric rotation), the largest concentration seemed to be among people born in the first third of the century—say, around 1910 to 1930.

Now, I don't know what was going on at that time, except that Woodrow W. was president and the first double no-hit nine-inning baseball game in the major leagues was played between the Chicago Cubs and the Cincinnati Reds in 1917, but there had to have been some strange information given out to new mothers on the subject of toilet training, because those tots, who were now our older patients, were absolutely obsessed with their bowels and the moving of them.

I had, during my ten years as a nurse, sat and listened to hundreds of bowel babies go on and on *ad nauseam* about the frequency, size, color, and shape of their bowel movements. And God help us if a day was missed. That was, in the mind of the bowel baby, a monumental disaster, equaling the devastation of finding out one had been infected with AIDS. Their whole life was simply ruined, and pass the Ex-lax, please.

Well, *somebody* had to listen to Mrs. Wade, and since I was the only on-call, part-time ER nurse, I figured Sarah and Gus had probably had their share of listening to accolades of what the human body could produce in the way of waste.

I threw back the curtain, which was my first mistake. I should have announced myself, then asked if I could open the curtain *before* I barged in. That way, I would have given Mrs.

Wade a chance to compose herself and I would have been spared the sight of her, sans clothing, crouched and balanced on the balls of her feet, on top of the gurney. She was straining like a sumo wrestler, so that the veins in her perspiring forehead stuck out large and blue. Her right hand was cupped under her quite broad hindquarters, ready to catch should something fall.

I wasn't sure of what to say. "Whoops" wasn't quite strong enough, but "Christ on a bicycle! What the Sam Hill do you think you're doing?" didn't seem right either.

"Oh. Hi. Mrs. Wade?"

She startled, then in a rather dainty manner—one that didn't seem possible considering her size—got off the gurney, fashioned for herself a togalike garment out of the cover sheet, and sat down. It all seemed entirely proper.

I asked the obvious. "Are you having a problem, Mrs. Wade?"

"Oh yes, and I can't tell you how this upsets everything." Mrs. Wade had a high, gushy kind of voice, like the E string of a violin plucked underwater. "I usually make three times a day like clockwork, but today I missed my noontime. I *never* miss my noontime."

I didn't need to ask noontime what.

"It's almost four P.M. and I'm feeling unwell already." Her eyes got teary. "This is terrible, terrible." She grasped my hand with the same hand she'd had under her, and I kicked myself for not wearing gloves. Nowadays nurses, especially ER nurses, wore exam gloves routinely. I did, however, notice that her hands were cold and clammy. Upon closer inspection, I also saw that her skin was a dusky gray color.

"Mrs. Wade, I need to take your blood pressure and pulse, and then I'll make sure the doctor sees you as soon as possible."

She let me do what I needed, while she wiped away the perspiration that dripped from her face and neck. I was not surprised to find her blood pressure 200 over 100 and her pulse 110 and irregular.

I stepped back and looked at her. Overweight, short of breath, clammy. The plot was thickening. "Hey Mrs. Wade, are you having any pain anywhere right now?"

Her hand went exactly to the center of her chest. "Aches like the dickens. It's gas. I've had it since noon when I couldn't make."

I forced myself to walk, not run, to the cardiac monitor and wheel it back to bed 4. The instant she saw the monitor, Mrs. Wade went quietly crazy. I acted as nonchalant as I could, hurrying in slow motion, keeping my voice as level as a funeral director's. "Let me see, I need you to lie down here so I can hook you up to the monitor. Then we can see what your heart is doing . . ." Mrs. Wade grabbed my hand again. It was even clammier than before.

"Gawd help me," she said, clasping our hands to her clammy chest. "Ma was right—I didn't make and now I'm going to die."

Careful not to give in to outright laughter, I smiled reassuringly. "Not at all, Mrs. Wade. I just need to make sure everything is perfect before the doc comes over, okay?"

Mrs. Wade relaxed a bit. "Oh, well, in that case . . ."

"Would you like some oxygen?"

She tensed again and I added, in a confidential way, "It sometimes helps with, you know, moving things along."

She was elated with my bold-faced lie. "Oh really? I didn't know oxygen could be used for *that*."

"Latest medical data," I hastened on, only slightly ashamed of myself. *"New England Journal of Medicine."*

Mrs. Wade was so excited when I slipped the O_2 prongs into her nose, I felt like I was strapping her in for a ride at Disneyland. The monitor bleeped unevenly even, every third beat a premature ventricular contraction. Combined with high blood pressure and chest pain, arrhythmias like this weren't to be ignored. Calmly, I told Ileta to call lab and get a stat EKG and CCU bloods.

After I further perjured myself by telling Mrs. Wade there was an intravenous drug that would help her heart relax, thus making her bowels relax, I slipped an IV into her arm, hung a bottle of dextrose and water, then slowly injected a bolus of lidocaine. Her PVCs cleared almost at once. I followed this with sublingual nitroglycerine for her "gas" pain and took her blood pressure again.

I found Dr. Mahoney in the surgery room suturing a long scalp laceration on a young man in his late teens.

"Like I said, Mark, the next time you want to attempt a Frankenstein's monster look-alike injury, aim lower for the forehead."

The patient smiled uncertainly and looked to me for verification that the woman sewing up his head was perhaps not quite balanced. I shrugged and nodded.

"Dr. Mahoney, we've got a sixty-five-year-old diaphoretic chest pain of four-hour duration in bed four. BP was two hundred over a hundred, pulse of a hundred and ten, and trigeminal PVCs. Fine rales at the bases." I lowered my voice. "She's a very anxious bowel baby."

Susan tied off the final stitch. She'd done a sewing job worthy of a top-notch plastic surgeon. In two months the young man wouldn't even be able to find the scar to brag about. "Not Myrtle W., is it?"

I nodded.

Dr. Mahoney sighed. "Old Myrt and I go way back. She's a hard-core laxative addict with bad coronary artery disease. She denies both conditions. Get an EKG and CCU bloods. Start an IV of dextrose and water and give seventy-five milligrams of lidocaine and sublingual nitro."

"Already done," I said apprehensively. With Dr. Mahoney I never knew how far I could go. Granted, the nurses in CCU had standing orders that covered us in certain emergency situations, and because of that, I was used to acting on my own. But in other departments, for a nurse to take it upon herself to do things without either written or, in the case of ER, verbal, explicit orders from a physician was always risky.

There were physicians whose egos could not deal with a nurse acting without his or her direct guidance, but some were more relaxed about the issue, especially if the nurse in question had proved herself competent. The doctors at the other end of the spectrum actually welcomed and encouraged a nurse to do what she thought best, knowing that it would make their lives easier in the long run.

Susan shot me a brief, unreadable glance. "My, my. Haven't we been busy practicing medicine."

I smiled uncertainly, not knowing if she was angry or pleased. "She's cleared out her PVCs and her BP is down to one-fifty over ninety. On the ten scale, her pain has gone from a six to a one."

Susan nodded and pinched her patient's cheek. "Do you need a tetanus shot, kid?"

Wide-eyed, the teenager jumped off the gurney and headed for the door. "Naw. Say no to drugs and all that shit, you know? Besides, it doesn't hurt that bad. I mean, I hate shots. I really hate—"

I grabbed him by the shirt and pulled him back into the room. "Tetanus is a shot you need to prevent you from getting lockjaw, which is fatal. We'll find out if you've had one in the last ten years. If so, you go free. If not, it's over quick—like a bee sting."

The patient was clearly skeptical of the words "bee sting" as he again headed toward the door.

"Listen kid," Susan said. "The shot is good for ten years. If we give you one today, that means you can keep jumping out of the backs of trucks until you're well into your twenties. You'll have a full ten years to keep trying for that Frankenstein look."

Sarah's bowel-hanging suicide attempt was taken off to surgery. Mrs. Wade, of a different kind of bowel fame, was rolled up to CCU, chatting all the way about the beneficial properties of Swiss Kriss. She had refused to be admitted to the heart unit until Dr. Ostermann, the most even-tempered and likable member of the Cardiology Cartel, promised her she could have any and all the laxatives she wanted. I could only hope that she and Mrs. Norman would not be roommates.

The rest of the afternoon was peppered with the usual nice-weather-end-of-school casualties, like baseball and track traumas. Then there was Gus's blushing young couple who came in with matching severe cases of contact dermatitis on their private parts from frolicking in a ravine rampant with poison oak. The deep-scrapes-full-of-road-dirt bicycle injuries came in numbers, although all of them together were not as time-consuming as the hysterical twenty-three-month-old with a chin laceration whom Sarah had to wrestle into a full-body restraint known as the papoose board.

Gus and I were finishing up with the last bicycle victim when Rescue 56 paramedics came in with a housepainter who had fallen from a third-story scaffold. On the stretcher, her head and neck were completely immobilized by a variety of braces, wide tape, and sandbags. These precautions prevented further trauma to the spinal cord, possibly making the difference between movement and complete paralysis, and, at times, even life and death.

With utmost care, the paramedics and I transferred the slender woman from the stretcher to the gurney. She weighed about as much as a sack of wet feathers.

"This is Kathy McCormack, age twenty-seven," said Russ,

Rescue 56's senior paramedic. "She took a major nosedive of about twenty-five feet a half hour ago." He hung the patient's IV bag on the hook over the trauma bed.

"Better than the water slides at Marine World," the woman mumbled. The wide strips of tape scrunched in the sides of her mouth.

"The first-floor awning was bent in half, so we're pretty certain she hit that before she hit the ground. No one actually saw her fall, but her co-workers estimated she was unconscious for about five minutes after they found her. She says she remembers rolling herself onto her back at some point, although she doesn't remember falling.

"She was oriented when we first got there," Russ went on, "but seems to come in and out of consciousness. Her BP was ninety over sixty, heart rate was ninety without ectopy. Her breathing in the field was pretty labored at first, then, after we got her in the rig, she evened out. There's a three-inch laceration on the back of her head and a fractured left collarbone."

Kathy groaned and wet her lips. "I've got a horrible headache." Her speech was slightly slurred. "If you'd let me sit up for a few minutes, I think I'll be okay. I'm so thirsty. Can I get some Dr. Pepper?"

I smiled at the specific request. "You can't have anything to drink or eat for a day or two, but we'll make sure you get some Dr Pepper when you can."

Slipping my fingers into the cup of her right hand, I squeezed. There was absolutely no response.

"My arms feel funny," she said, and in her voice was a faint note of repressed hysteria.

Russ leaned close to my ear. "She doesn't move anything below the neck to command," he said, more softly than a whisper.

"Did I fall on a nerve or something?" she asked, her eyes wide. "Can I please sit up for a minute?"

"We can't move you at all until Dr. Schupbach gets here. Try to hang in there for a little while longer. Everything is going to—"

I stopped, realizing I was going to fall back on using the phrase nurses used a million times a day. This time, I couldn't say it was going to be all right, because this time, I didn't think it would.

She looked at—no, she looked through me, and a lump formed in my throat. Unable to talk, I massaged her hand, speaking to her with my eyes. I told her what she already knew.

I waited for my throat to ease. In my mind, she was experiencing the worst thing that could ever happen to anyone. Ever since I took care of my first paraplegic in nursing school, I'd had nightmares about losing my ability to walk, run, or move freely that were of sweat-and-scream proportion. Never in my career had I been able to care for a quad or a paraplegic patient without going home praying to Buddha, the Virgin Mary, and Muhammad to save me and mine from that fate. From the time Simon was old enough to understand, I'd given him all my emergency-room-nurse speeches about how motorcyclists made up the largest number of paras and quads (never neglecting to mention that scaffolding workers, divers, roofers, and drunks diving into pools ran a close second). I told him he could do *anything*—come home after curfew, turn his amplifier to max, bring girls into his room and close the door, drop out of school—all as long as he promised that he would not buy a motorcycle while I was alive.

I turned back, smiling. "We don't know what's going on yet, but the docs will let you know as soon as they do."

"Do me a favor?" she asked.

"Anything." I meant it; my guilt over not being able to turn back the hands of time or make magic medicine and have her jump up and dance a jig made me believe I would do anything.

"Come down closer."

I put my ear next to her lips.

"Tell me . . ." Her voice broke, she sucked in air. "I got kids. I've got too much to do. Tell me I'm not going to be in a wheelchair. Please."

The ache returned to my throat with such force, I had to retreat behind my internal overload wall. If I allowed myself to be pulled in emotionally, I would be useless to her.

Instead of answering right away, I held Kathy's hand and tuned out the sound of her crying, making lists in my mind of what I needed to do for my patient. But my mind, refusing to stay on the practical end of the business at hand, wandered off to the philosophy section. Had it always been this woman's fate to have her life change course entirely in one split second?

After witnessing thousands of the senseless tragedies life handed out to people, I borrowed an old saying as a coping mechanism: Everything happened for a reason. And that included children dying, murder, and young mothers becoming quadriplegic.

But how could there possibly be a reason for the tragedy this woman would now have to face?

"Listen." I took a corner of the bedsheet and wiped the tears from her eyes. "With accidents like yours, we never know for sure what's going to happen. What we *do* know is that mind over body can be a powerful force. Think in terms of movement. Believe you can make things happen."

I sensed the strength and the fighting spirit of the woman and felt better. After all, who really knew what bounds the human spirit could break?

Kathy returned to us from the scanner more lethargic than before. She seemed only dimly aware when Dr. Schupbach shaved a strip of her long strawberry hair, ear to ear. In what seemed like a medieval torture ritual, he took a pair of sharp-pointed tongs and screwed the ends into the sides of her skull. When properly hooked up to traction, these tongs would completely immobilize her head and neck. The physician used no anesthesia, and although Kathy felt nothing except pressure, the rest of our scalps ached just from witnessing the procedure.

I noticed that Dr. Schupbach handled the sheared tresses with care, wrapping them in a sterile towel. Later, when Sarah presented the morbid package to Kathy's husband, I would understand this was a practice of courtesy—in the event Kathy did not survive, the mortuary would need the hair to fill in the shaved area.

After Kathy was safely transferred to ICU, Dr. Schupbach came back to take another look at Rescue 56's field report.

"So?" I asked.

"Hard to say," he said. "Her injury is at C five-six level. On the scanner, the cord looks normal, but she's partially fractured the bodies of five and six vertebrae. It's not subluxed and there's no encroachment on the spinal canal."

"Okay, so in English, what does that mean in terms of future mobility?"

"It means we aren't going to know how much function she'll get back until the swelling goes down. It's going to depend on how much actual nerve damage there is. With things like this, you never know until you know for sure."

"Tell me something, doc. Have you ever seen somebody with a bad spinal cord injury defy all the odds and come out walking on their own?"

Dr. Schupbach thought for a moment, standing stock-still. His glasses were Coke-bottle thick and the glare from the fluorescent lights was blotting out his eyes entirely. The overall effect was something distinctly reminiscent of Daddy Warbucks.

"Actually," he said slowly, "I have seen something like that once. It was a freak case down in Bakersfield."

Leaving his last statement hanging in the air, we both laughed. Bakersfield was a strange kind of place where a lot of freak things could, and probably did, happen.

"There was this young kid, twenty-two or so, who hit the back of a parked big rig going about fifty miles an hour on a motorcycle. Helmet or not, the impact should have decapitated him altogether, but instead, it snapped the kid's neck like a twig. He was a mess. We didn't think he had a snowball's chance in hell at surviving, let alone ever moving a muscle in his body.

"But eight months later, he walked out of the hospital without so much as a cane. None of us believed what we were seeing.

"To this day I still don't know how that happened. I mean, we would look at the X rays and then back at the kid, and it shouldn't have been possible." Dr. Schupbach turned back to the paramedic's report. "It was as close to a living miracle as I've ever seen, which is why no one should ever predict outcomes . . . even when they seem to be staring you in the face."

By six o'clock we usually knew what the blue plate special of the evening would be. Mostly it was turning out to be a laceration-and-angina kind of night. Sarah, Gus, and I assisted with no fewer than ten suturings of lacerations, caused by everything from a fishhook to a Skil saw, plus we admitted four chest pains to the CCU over the course of two hours.

At seven P.M., Sarah was relieved by Don, another ER regular, and Dr. Mahoney was relieved by Dr. Menowitz, the undisputed terror of Redwoods Emergency Department. A graying version of Harpo Marx with a prominent, hooked nose, Dr. Menowitz made his appearance carrying a plate heaped with at least two cans of cold pork and beans. That distinctive arrangement of victuals was covered with a frosting of brown cafeteria ketchup. He set the plate down on the six-by-ten-inch space meant as the doctor's work area, and wolfed down the mess as though he hadn't eaten anything solid for years.

Everybody who worked in ER was used to this spectacle and generally looked away, either to be polite or to keep from being sick. I once timed his mastication speed at 140 chews per minute. It had to be a record of some kind.

"Pork?" I said, raising my eyebrows in Molly Goldberg–like disapproval. "A Morton Menowitz eating pork with his beans and ketchup? *Oy vey.* You'll give your mother a heart attack."

"You want I should eat schmaltz maybe?" He shrugged, not slowing his chewing speed one beat. Unwilling to risk his reputation as Dr. Irascible, Dr. Menowitz looked around to make sure no one was watching, then leaned over to give me a peck on the cheek. "Congratulations. How's it feel to be in the public's myopic eye?"

I tensed and went paranoid instantly. "What do you mean in the public eye? I'm not in the public eye. Why do you say that I'm in the public eye? Did you hear or read something? Was something mentioned?"

Dr. Menowitz stopped chewing and regarded me in wonder. "Whoa! Relax, pony. I didn't *mean* anything by the question— it's just that I saw a display of your book in the bookstore a couple of days ago and I read a review of it in the paper."

The reality of the situation hit like a lead medicine ball to the solar plexus. It was verified—my face and name were on a book in which I had heedlessly spilled my guts about my life, my job, and all my private thoughts and fears. As I breathed, there were people out there somewhere who were actually going to read, or perhaps had already read, the thing.

My temples grew hot with panic, and for a minute I thought I was going into shock. What the hell could I have been thinking of when I wrote the damned thing? Why had I been so sure of selling only one copy?

I put my head in my hands and groaned.

"What's wrong?"

"I'm embarrassed."

Dr. Menowitz resumed chewing at his accelerated speed and yet managed to speak at the same time. "Why are you embarrassed? I read it in one sitting. Of course, I especially liked the parts about me, even though you did make me look like Snively Whiplash. Actually . . ." He trailed off as if to reevaluate what he was going to say.

I held my breath, while my ulcer geared up. Was he going to say, "Actually, I was thinking of suing you"? Or "Actually, it was the worst book I've ever read"? Morton Menowitz was not only a voracious reader, he was a vicious reader as well.

"Actually, I really liked it and I'm jealous as hell that you're published and I'm not."

I exhaled, heart pounding in my throat. Of course, he was only being kind, but thank Buddha anyway.

"By the way, who was Dr. Drigely? Several of us were trying to figure out—"

I went back down the panic-paranoid roller coaster and sucked in another breath. "*Several* of us? What do you mean several?"

"Dr. Kin, Dr. Gillespie, and Dr. Kelsic. We decided it was—"

"You mean *they* read it too?" My voice had gone thin and high. All I could think of was my dream the night before about being chased with proctoscopy tubes by a gang of angry physicians.

"Oh yeah, there's two copies going around the doctors' lounge with—"

Gus's huge mass of dark hair appeared around the corner of the thin partition, followed by her head. "Oh, and get this." She pulled a face. "Our dear assistant director of nurses wasn't watching where she was going yesterday on her way out of the building and ran right into me. A copy of your book fell out from under her coat. I thought for sure she was going to have a stroke on the spot.

"I stayed as cool as a refrigerated turnip. 'Say,' I said, 'isn't that *Intensive Care*?' and she starts doing dither exercises with her hands, flapping them around like hunted wild geese and stuttering to beat the band. 'I—I—I—f-f-found it on m-m-m-m-my d-d-d-desk. I'm not go—go—going to read it, of course, b-b-but I will see that it's disp—disposed of properly.' "

We all laughed, but inside I was having ulcer panic that wasn't to be believed. Zantac. Where the hell was my Zantac? The doctors were reading it, *and* the administration? Oh dear God, I thought, I'll never be able to work as a nurse again in this town or the next.

It must have been around nine when the shit hit the fan, so to speak. Through the pneumatic doors staggered six food poisonings explosively leaking from both ends (Mrs. Wade would have been positively green with envy), all of whom had eaten at the same restaurant earlier in the evening. There were two more bad lacerations, a man with canker sores, an Alzheimer's patient who escaped from a nursing home and was found sitting naked in the Mill Valley library, an eighteen-year-old who thought the warts on his penis were insect bites, two more anginas, a twenty-two-year-old woman in her eighth month of pregnancy with genital herpes, a migraine followed by a minor auto accident, and a ten-month-old with a raging fever.

Don and I were running back and forth from the waste sinks with alternately full and empty bedpans and emeses basins, while Gus went from bed to bed starting IVs. Running one step ahead of us, Dr. Morton Menowitz oversaw it all, directing us as if we were the army of brooms in "The Sorcerer's Apprentice."

Minutes after arrival, the ten-month-old had a convulsion, which sent the parents into hysteria. The mother clung to me, weeping, while the father seemed to be in shock to the point of not being able to move. I unwrapped the three wool blankets and two flannel sleepers, explaining that it wasn't uncommon for young children with high fevers to have convulsions. I gave the parents a bucket of cool water and told them to sponge the child down. This was another first-year-nursing-school lesson—give the walking wounded a simple task to lessen anxiety, like asking the prospective new father to boil water for the impending birth.

I took the next chart off the top of the slowly diminishing pile of those patients yet to be seen, and noticed that the chart under it bore the same last name.

Whisper and Rainbow Hanes. Fifteen and seventeen years of age, respectively. Address: General Delivery, San Rafael. Under "Reason for Visit" they had both written in childish scrawls, "Lost Time."

I rolled my eyes. Couldn't there be one night in ER without a crackpot case? Now I had two: a couple of stoned-out children of children from the flower child era.

I walked toward the waiting room, envisioning the story I was sure I was going to hear about how they were abducted by some aliens and taken for a spaceship ride to the star cluster of Pleiades where they met up with Shirley MacLaine and Whitley Strieber who got them stoned and made them drink milk from alien cows which gave them this strange rash and obliterated their memories . . . blah blah blah.

To that story they would add that they'd been gone for three days and hadn't had anything to eat and could I please give them a bowl of soup, some Kwell, and bus fare and they'd be on their way?

On the other side of the pneumatic doors, the industrial-strength fluorescent lights lit up the full waiting room like a stage. Two elderly women and one ancient man sat in the orange plastic chairs, all studying their hands the way old people sometimes do while they practice their infinite-patience skills.

On the tiled floor, a young woman in hiking garb lay moaning while a young man held a bag of ice to her thigh, which was swollen and purple with what looked like a bad black widow bite. A group of five Iranians, all dressed alike in black pajama outfits, paced around a wheelchair that held a visibly ailing old woman who was almost certainly the grandmother.

A handsome young black man with a bloody shirt and a superficial knife wound to his cheek, sat in the corner with two sullen friends, one of whom had an arm in a makeshift sling soaked through with blood. All three wore the same red and black patch over their hearts reading, "Bullets 'n' Blades."

Off to the side of the switchboard booth, way out of synch with his fellow sufferers, was a man in a tuxedo, leaning against the wall doing a pretty good imitation of Meade Lux Lewis whistling "The Whistling Blues."

No one fit the description of a couple of teenage girls with alien-produced rashes. On my way to check out the ladies' room, I walked past the dark lobby, which had been closed since eight-thirty P.M., and entered the dimly lit corridor. Out of the corner of my eye, I saw movement low to the ground. Instinctively, I crouched and put my back to the wall.

From the shadows of the lobby floor, two bundles of filthy rags unfolded and walked gracefully toward me. Into the dim light emerged two sets of tired green eyes and identical heads of stringy copper-colored hair. For a reason I could not fathom at that moment, their faces were familiar.

The girls were both malnourished and covered with filth, but what struck me dumb was the fact that the thin faces, even streaked with dirt, were absolutely gorgeous.

The taller of the two young women stepped forward and spoke with the authority of one used to being in charge. "Are you looking for us?"

"Rainbow and Whisper?"

She nodded solemnly, as though I had said it was time for her walk to the gas chamber. The younger girl whimpered and pushed close to the older one, knocking her off balance. The tall girl pushed her away, not in a cruel way but more out of a need to show they were not afraid.

"I'm Rainbow, but they call me Rainy, and this is my sister Whisp. We want to be seen together?" There was an uplift of her voice so that the statement came out more like a question.

I was about to deny them with the excuse that it wasn't standard procedure, when I realized why they were familiar. It was the shadows of pain and fear behind their eyes: the identifying phantoms familiar to the victims of misuse. These two had been raised on plenty of misery.

"Okay," I said, changing my mind, "I'll make sure you can be together, but you need to tell me what you mean by 'lost time.' "

The younger girl grabbed her sister's arm. In her eyes I saw suspicion of the world at large shining through as a hard green glint of distrust. "Don't, Rainy," she begged. "Don't tell. They're gonna call the cops. Let's just go, okay? Please?"

Rainy took her sister by the shoulders and at first I thought she meant to shake her, but instead she pushed the hair out of her face, a few loose strands at a time. "Shhh. Remember what I told you?"

They locked eyes for a moment, and with a sigh, the smaller girl leaned against her sister in resignation.

At length, Rainy faced me squarely. "We've been raped by some guys," she said in a tired voice. "I think we were drugged. I'm sure it started two nights ago, but Whisp thinks it was just last night."

There was a moment's pause. Rainy shuffled her feet, looking almost like she might scream or cry out in frustration. "They beat up on me too," she said, pulling up her shirt to expose her young breasts. One was scraped and bruised, and the other looked as though the nipple had been partially torn away. Red-and-purple welts covered the rest of her chest and abdomen.

Gently, I pulled her shirt back down and silently counted to ten. "Okay," I said without further comment, "follow me."

Both of them walked to the pelvic room slumped at the shoulders and hanging their heads, hiding behind the reddish curtains of their hair.

After the girls were settled, I slipped back out into the main room and instructed Ileta to call rape crisis for a volunteer to come down. From the supply carts, I gathered two of the unmarked cardboard boxes that were our rape kits and two pelvic exam packs. When I returned the girls were sitting on the exam table, each with an arm around the other's shoulder.

I handed them each a warm blanket, a clean gown, and a brown paper bag marked "Evidence," and asked them to carefully remove all their clothes, including socks and shoes, and put them in the bags.

To preserve modesty, I turned my back and busied myself with breaking the official police seal on one of the boxes. On the top of the box I wrote the exact time and date and signed my name. The odd assortment of contents I removed and placed on the counter: a two-by-two gauze pad, a fine-tooth comb, a wooden pick, several glass slides, swabs of various sizes, envelopes, several laboratory tubes, and an official rape report form.

While I labeled each item with Rainbow's official patient ID number, I asked them about their parents.

"Our father died of an overdose of heroin when we were little, and our mother . . ." Rainy left off and Whisper continued without a pause ". . . used to live in Las Vegas with her boyfriend until a couple of months ago, but we don't know where she is now."

Rainbow resumed. "I'm an emancipated minor. I work . . . well, I used to work at Taco Bell. I've been taking care of my sister since our mother left. We mostly live wherever we can, but sometimes we get to stay with friends. When I get extra money, we rent a room at the Last Stop for a week, but I don't like leaving Whisp there by herself."

The Last Stop Motel lived up to its name. It was one of those run-down California places of the forties, all dingy and cracked pink stucco with a rusted-out barbecue pit in the concrete back patio that no one ever used. The Last Stop was so depressing that the locals even avoided driving by the place.

More than a few of the stabbings, shootings, and overdoses that rolled through the pneumatic doors originated there. Situated right on the main drag, it was the place streetwalkers favored for conducting their business.

"We're done," they said in unison. They had one blanket wrapped around their legs, the other around their shoulders. I was surprised they hadn't tried to share a gown.

I stared into the two pretty faces. It was, to put it in sixties speak, a mind-blowing sight to see a couple of tired old souls staring out of the faces of beautiful children—children who were already more than half beaten down and all used up.

They both gagged while chewing on the dry gauze pads and spit them into individual envelopes marked "Saliva Sample," though something struck them funny about scraping under their ragged fingernails and depositing the minute bits of dirt into the envelopes marked "Nail Scrapings." We avoided each other's eyes when I ran the fine-tooth combs through their pubic hair and carefully placed them inside the envelopes marked "Hair Samples." The blood sample tubes, laboratory slides, and culture plates were left for Dr. Menowitz to use when he did their physical and pelvic exams.

I was halfway down the first page of the identical rape reports, checking, or not checking, the boxes.

"So, was either of you forced to perform fellatio?"

They looked at each other, then back at me, their faces blank.

I squirmed. Walking two kids through the dark alley of clinical sexual vocabulary wasn't a pleasant prospect.

I jiggled my pen, giving them plenty of time to save me from having to explain the question.

"Fellatio?" Rainy asked. The repeating-the-last-word scheme seemed to be universal.

I began feeling warm behind the ears, willing myself to stop the blush spreading down under my chin. "Ah, do you remember if any of the men put his penis in your mouth?"

"You mean, did they make us give them blow jobs?" asked Whisper matter-of-factly.

"Yes," I said. The blush was to my neck and traveling downward. "That is what I mean."

They both nodded. I checked the fellatio boxes, went to the next item on the list, and mentally cringed. "Did any of the men perform cunnilingus on you?"

I got the blank stare again. A light blush spread over my chest.

I cleared my throat. "Ah, you know, did any of the men put his mouth on your genitals?"

"You mean, did they eat—"

"Yes," I said quickly.

Again they both nodded and I checked off the boxes.

"Did you both experience vaginal penetration?"

Dual affirmatives.

"Was there anal penetration?"

Whisper and Rainbow conferred in low voices. Rainy nodded yes, Whisper, no.

"Condoms?"

No. None.

"Were foreign objects introduced into . . ." I hesitated. I knew Whisper would have questions about this one, and sighed. "Okay, what they're asking here is, did the men put anything other than their—"

Rainy either noticed the red blush of my neck or sensed my discomfort, because she cut me off before I could finish the question.

"I don't think they did," she answered, then made a gesture with her hand as if she were a crossing guard holding back a line of cars. "Can I just tell you the whole story? Maybe you can answer the questions better if you hear what happened. Would that be okay?"

I nodded, relieved that my task had been made easier.

Rainy took a breath and closed her eyes for a moment, the way I'd seen people do before they make their first bungee jump.

"Monday night we were hanging out at the Quik Stop on Front Street. It was around eight o'clock, because *MacGyver* was on the TV in the store.

"So these three guys drive up in this really hot car and they start talking to us and ask if we want to go for a ride. They said they were going to take us to a nice restaurant for dinner and then rent some movies. They said they lived in a big house up on Mount Tam, and if we wanted, we could go up there and watch movies with them and they'd take us home whenever we wanted."

"They lied to us," Whisper interrupted, her eyes dilated with rage. "I hate them. If I ever see them again, I'll kill them." Her smooth, childish hands gripped the side of the gurney. The tips of her fingers were pink where she had bitten her nails almost down to the quick.

I nodded for Rainy to continue. Satisfied that I was paying attention, she took another breath and resumed.

"So we rode around for a while, and they had some vodka and Coke mixed up in a thermos that they gave us. I drank about half a cup of the stuff before I started feeling fucked up. Not drunk, but dizzy and sleepy.

"I was in front and I told the guy who was driving to stop the car and let us out, but he wouldn't do it. Whisper was in the backseat, and I saw that she was totally out. The two other guys had all her clothes off and they were doing all this dirty stuff to her, like sticking their fingers in her and sucking on her. I tried to make them stop, but I couldn't talk or move or anything.

"I know they put drugs in the drinks, 'cause we didn't drink enough to make us drunk, and the stuff tasted real weird—like it was spoiled. I must've passed out after that, 'cause I woke up on a mattress in a room like a log cabin. I don't remember how we got there."

Rainbow hesitated, and I could tell from the slight wrinkling of her chin that she was on the edge of crying. Whisper and I stayed quiet, waiting with her. When she began again, it was in a fainter voice.

"The first thing I saw was all these really bright lights and a video camera and there were white sheets hung up on the walls. I got scared because I thought we'd been in an accident and I was in a hospital being operated on. When I woke up more, I realized that the assholes were filming themselves raping us. I was real cold and they were crushing me so I couldn't hardly breathe. Two of them were going at me at the same time, and the other one was trying to make me give him a blow job. They were hurting me real bad, so I couldn't move so good.

"I made believe I passed out again, but I was watching them through my eyelashes. I wanted to remember what they looked like so I could give descriptions.

"Then one of them stops with me and goes into another room. In a few minutes he comes back carrying Whispy. She was all white with her eyes rolled back in her head and I really thought she was dead. I thought they'd killed her." The girl's voice broke. "That's when I went crazy. I started screaming real loud and trying to get over to Whisp. One of them took a belt and began to strap me, but I wouldn't shut up, so they gave me a shot in my arm and I passed out again.

"I don't remember anything else until we woke up this morning out in Lagunitas. We were lying by the road covered up with a bunch of grass and dirt."

"Just like animals," murmured Whisper.

The despair in the child's voice made me ache; a new low on my Man's Inhumanity to Man Scale had been hit. When I finished filling in the forms, I asked if they could think of anything else to add.

Both girls thought for a few seconds. Then Whisper shyly raised her hand. The innocent gesture made me smile.

"Would their license plate number help?"

I stared, incredulous. "You got their license plate number?"

"Sure," she said, brightening. "I memorize license plates all the time. It's like a game; me and Rainy sometimes have contests to see who can remember the most plates the longest. I memorized it before we even got in the car."

I noted the plate number on the forms, thinking of how happy the sheriff's department was going to be, when Whisper slid off the gurney wringing her hands. "What's going to happen to us now?" she asked, uncharacteristically direct.

"Well, Dr. Menowitz is going to come in and examine you both. He'll ask more questions, take some samples from your vagina, and have the lab draw your blood. We'll probably give you some antibiotics to make sure you don't get any infections. Then we'll fix up any other injuries you have.

"After we're done with that, a woman from the rape crisis center is going to come in and talk to you, bring you some clothes, and probably take you to her home. A police officer will want to ask you some more questions to help them find the men who did this to you. After that . . ."

Whisper shook her head. "No, not that," she said. "I mean, what's going to happen to *us*? How're we gonna be decent now? It's like we're ruined, you know? People are gonna think we're bad, like the whore girls at the Last Stop."

The sounds of the child's hopelessness and bewilderment cut through my outrage. On instinct, I took one delicate chin in each hand and studied the two sets of green eyes.

"Listen to me. You are not ruined, and this doesn't make you whores. Something bad happened to you, but that doesn't make you bad. You didn't make this happen, it just happened, like when people have accidents.

"For a while you'll feel crummy, then you'll be angry and maybe even have nightmares about what happened, but you will make it out the other side.

"It took courage to come in here and tell what happened to you. You have integrity and you care about each other. That's more than a lot of people have."

They sat motionless, silent as leafless trees. Their eyes told me nothing. "Do you understand what I'm trying to tell you?" I asked. "You are both going to be okay because you're survivors. You did the right thing. You deserve medals for being so brave."

I stopped out of frustration. There was so much damage to

be repaired. Who was going to care enough to get them through? "I guess the most important thing for you to know and believe is that you both deserve to be loved and have good things in your lives."

My words bobbed in the air, then drifted away.

Simultaneously, the two of them began to weep.

Thursday
3:30 A.M.

Can't sleep again, only this time it's not the tour. When I close my eyes, I see those two girls. They will never get to grow up, they will only grow old. I want to know what is going to happen to them. I convince myself they'll be okay, that they'll bounce back with the resilience of youth. Except I keep hearing them cry, and it feels like knives going through my chest. And then when I think that this happens every day in cities and towns all over the world, my insides shrivel up. What the hell happens to these people?

I close my eyes and I see the lady housepainter's eyes when they tell her she'll never walk again. I wonder how her husband will react, and if her friends will stay by her.

I close my eyes and I hear more clearly all their voices, pleading, broken, hurt.

I close my eyes and I try to see myself from their eyes and I wonder if they can see how much they affect me. All anyone ever has to do is look.

I close my eyes and look down the well of my heart.

Will it ever go dry?

THREE

"Doctors are authorized by the states to prac-
tice medicine, which is to diagnose, treat, pre-
scribe, and operate ... on disease, not people.
Everything else is nursing."

DONNA DIERS, R.N.

THE INFAMOUS POET WAS LED IN on a gurney surrounded by an
ER nurse and three San Quentin prison guards. Three guards
meant he was a bad dude—a death row prisoner.

When the SQ prisoners came in with only one guard, it
meant they were lightweights—nonviolent criminals, having
perhaps stolen some insurance money from little old ladies or
maybe embezzled a few bucks from the company. Two guards
signified something more serious, like armed robbery. Three
guards meant homicide and worse. The only time I'd ever seen
four guards was the time the warden came in as a patient.

The man in the bed accidentally grazed my hand as I readjusted the monitor wires crisscrossing his chest. The brief
contact with those icy fingers sent shivers through to my
bones. I didn't want to touch him again, but at present I was
the person responsible for keeping him alive.

I ground my teeth into my tooth guard until my jaw ached,
took his vital signs, and increased the rate of dopamine dripping through his intravenous line. If the medication did its job,
it would inch his blood pressure up to an acceptable range.

Behind me, the three guards watched every move I made—
standard operating procedure whenever a nurse was in the
room with the prisoner. There were times when I wondered if
this precaution was actually for the nurse's protection and not
the prisoner's. Or it might have been that the guards were sim-

ply curious, or maybe they thought we were going to slip the prisoner a weapon or a map of the best escape routes.

Not likely, I thought. Not today, and especially not with this particular prisoner.

Max was forty-five—young to be a cardiac repeater with two MIs under his belt. But then again, the lines in his face revealed that he had lived hard, and from the stories I'd been told by the prison nurses, life on San Quentin's death row wasn't easy.

In truth, Max was a cardiac lost cause. The doctors had tried everything, but none of the medications prescribed had been able to control his chronic hypertension or the persistent arrhythmias and chest pain. His present visit was a result of a syncopal episode, or a brief loss of consciousness. It was almost certain that he had passed out due to prolonged runs of any one of the variety of deadly cardiac arrhythmias he was known to have.

I considered myself lucky that Max had never been assigned to me before. He was different from the other SQ prisoners. Where the others were, for the most part, a jivey and lively group, this man was perpetually sullen. Speaking only to let his needs be known, he rarely looked directly at anyone, but when he did, it definitely made you stop and think about who you were dealing with.

That the eyes are the windows of the soul is certainly true for those who suffer. When I look into the eyes of, say, a dying patient, I most often see either the desperate pleading of someone living half in and half out of that disturbing other world, or a mysterious tranquillity.

Max's eyes had neither of those traits. Reflected in his was the same impenetrable quality as that of every murderer I'd ever attended, except Max's were a bit colder than the usual garden-variety killer's. That these cold eyes were the last thing the people he murdered had seen seemed enormously cruel.

His hair was the other thing that bothered me almost as much as the eyes. Separated into oily clumps, the shoulder-length mane looked as if the last time it had seen shampoo and water was years back. With Max, this might have very well been the case, his theory on personal cleanliness being that all the great intellectuals never bathed. It was one of his many secret quirks that dated back to his early teen years.

I checked his blood pressure again, disturbed to find it still hanging low despite the increased dopamine. Taking a quick overall inventory, I let my nurse's sixth sense do all the sensing it needed. Okay, so he didn't look good, but he didn't look that bad either. Then again, there was something not quite right here.

Halfway through my taking his blood pressure a third time, his bloodless fingers tore the cuff off and threw it across the room. One of the guards immediately stepped closer to the bed, so I could just see him in my peripheral vision.

"Don't squeeze my arm like that," Max said evenly, fixing me with a stare. He used his eyes like weapons. "What is the problem, Miss . . . ?" He looked for my name tag, apparently having forgotten the hospital's policy that required all nurses to cover the last names on their tags or not wear one at all when caring for a San Quentin prisoner.

"You can call me nurse," I said flatly, feeling trapped by those eyes. "Your blood pressure is low and you're having some irregular heartbeats. I'm running a couple of medicines through your IV, one to make your blood pressure come up and one to calm your heart down."

The man made a choked sound that I thought might have been laughter. "Don't waste your energy," he said, and gazing off toward the clock, he recited (hand on heart, no less), "The black heart tires of carrying its weight, and it is with sweet death I shall soon keep my date."

This bit of theatrics seemed to conflict so much with his bitter manner that I was left waiting expectantly for him to follow it up with something more in tune with who he was—like pulling a live water moccasin out of his ear.

When it became clear he wasn't going to add anything more to his performance, I made note of his blood pressure on the acute flowchart, placed a blue plastic urinal on his side table, and labeled all the IVs. Then I made the mistake of touching his exposed feet.

The swift and precisely aimed kick sent my chart into the wall. Two of the guards stood quickly, both reaching for the nightsticks that hung from their thick leather belts.

"Don't ever touch my feet." Every word was growled, his teeth clenched and slightly bared. It was a pretty good Clint Eastwood impersonation.

I gripped the footboard of the bed and leaned over his legs, although I will say I was careful not to touch his feet. "And don't you ever kick at me again, mister, or—"

The middle guard—the one whose hands were so beefy,

they looked as though they could feed a family of five for a week—stepped between me and the bed, blocking my view of the patient.

"You need to do something with his feet?" The guard's tone was calm but threatening, except exactly *who* he was threatening wasn't clear.

"I was trying to feel the pulses in his feet to check how his circulation is, but I don't need to find out bad enough to get kicked."

The guard turned to Max. "Let the nurse do her job, Max. No more kicking."

Max gave me a narrow-eyed, come-on-I-dare-you stare-down and suddenly I was six years old, standing in the Mohawk School playground being taunted by the neighborhood bully, a girl named Bambi. The hell with you, I thought, and without comment, gathered the scattered chart and walked from the room.

At the nurses' station, I put the chart back together, thinking that I had been foolish not to request an assignment change right at the beginning of the shift, even though tight staffing rarely permitted that luxury anymore. Now I would have to keep a constant check on how I acted around Max and take the utmost care that I was unbiased, treating him exactly as I would any other patient.

In reality, I knew it wasn't going to happen.

Each week for three months, one of Max's poems had been printed in every major newspaper in Northern California. It was like one of those radio contests where the listeners tuned in to hear the clues that would lead them to the hidden treasure. Concealed in the lines of his poems, Max gave subtle hints as to his whereabouts. A million readers joined the law in the task of deciphering the cryptic and ingenious verses.

Still and all, it took officials six months before they found the self-proclaimed genius who had one day purchased a shotgun, taken it home, and as his mother watched in horror, blown his brother's brains all over the kitchen walls. Using his finger as a pen and his brother's opened skull as the inkwell, he jotted a brief farewell poem on the white plastic tablecloth, finished off his coffee, then executed his mother in similar fashion.

Max's mother's name was Amanda, and the way I figured it,

at the moment he blew her into the next world, I had just set out the teacups for her and me.

Amanda and I always met at my house, never hers. She told me when we first became friends, some five years before, that her youngest son was extremely antisocial and didn't like having visitors at the house.

This didn't bother me, but I felt sorry for Amanda. Max was her burden in life, as she put it, hinting now and again at his emotional problems and his repeated refusals of professional help. She grew uneasy and somewhat reticent whenever he came up in our conversations, almost as if she were afraid he had a bugging device hidden somewhere on her person. Only once—the time she came limping, bruised, and frightened to my door—did Amanda admit she was scared of Max.

It was because of her consistent reluctance to speak out that I hadn't pried. After her murder, I wished that I had. The hindsightful if-onlys plagued me for a few years; one more thing to add to my Perpetual Guilt/Shame List, which was longer than that of any Jewish person I knew.

Amanda's and my friendship was based on our mutual love of gardening, my Italian recipes, and her ability to sew like a wizard. On that Sunday morning, Amanda and I were meeting at eleven so I could demonstrate my father's recipe for the world's best pizza from scratch and she could show me the tricks of hemming my new pair of slacks, which were so long, they could have been a fashion statement in either pants with trains or built-in shoe covers.

Three hours, ten unanswered phone calls, and one bowl of crusting, overly risen pizza dough later, I decided to drive by her house. When I saw her car in the driveway, I didn't think she was ill or had forgotten about our meeting—I knew that she was dead and that in some way Max was responsible.

Lily-livered coward that I was, I drove to the nearest pay phone and made a brief, anonymous call to the sheriff's office.

It was seven-thirty P.M. and I was eating my salad at the monitor banks. This was against hospital policy. According to one of the hundreds of senseless rules and regulations designed by Redwoods administration to make a nurse's life miserable and affirm she was low man on the totem pole, it was unprofessional to be seen eating while on the job. Although the nature of our job frequently did not allow for meal breaks, it was better in their eyes to look professional and go hungry.

It didn't matter that I hadn't had a bathroom break since three P.M. report, and who gave a damn that I was hypoglycemic? The fact remained there wasn't anyone to relieve me. And from what I could see and hear on the intermediate side, there wouldn't be anyone to relieve me until eleven-fifteen when I reported off.

I had a choice: I could either respect the rules, wet my pants, and pass out from low blood sugar, or I could compromise.

I decided on a compromise. I would eat at the desk, and that way, if I wet my chair, at least I would be conscious to clean it up.

Ginger, a CCU nurse who had burned out and crashed many years before, sat next to me talking on the phone to someone of uncertain gender named BooBoo. By my watch, she had been on the phone with BooBoo for one hour and thirty-two minutes.

I was not fond of working with Ginger, who I felt was lazy and overtly hostile (she called it "forefront assertiveness"). Ginger's basic feeling about nursing was that she hated the job but it paid the rent. She was the only nurse I knew who could coldheartedly walk away from patients in emotional distress, and go read a magazine while they wept.

Her co-workers got even less consideration.

At five P.M., she had been pulled from her patient assignment on the intermediate unit to admit Mr. Wong, a sixty-three-year-old hypertensive acute MI, to bed 4. She made a perfunctory attempt at filling out his assessment sheet, tossed a urinal on his bed, gave him some Lasix and morphine, but left his call bell hanging out of reach. She then settled herself in at the desk and called BooBoo.

Acting as the on-call codependent, I took over Mr. Wong's care, dividing my attention between monitoring Max's blood pressure and rhythm and relieving Mr. Wong's angina and emptying his urinal. It was steady running, but manageable.

At the point where Max's blood pressure again began to deteriorate and Mr. Wong was having his third bout of chest pain unrelieved by morphine, I politely interrupted Ginger, explaining that I needed to be in Max's room and could she please see to her patient?

She responded by waving me away and asking BooBoo to

repeat him/herself, because there was an annoying echo on the line.

At exactly the second I reached over to disconnect the phone cord from the wall, Max had a run of ventricular tachycardia. Adrenaline-charged, I ran into his room and tripped over the legs of the guard with the ten-pound hands, recovering my balance in time to see Max's eyes roll back into his head in that heralding sign of a seizure.

I made a double fist, which I smashed into the middle of his chest. There was a momentary jumble of wave forms on the monitor from the disruption of his lead wires. Waiting for a rhythm to come up on the screen, I held my breath and lightly palpated his carotid artery. The man's neck was cool and wet with perspiration. The first slow beats to appear on the monitor matched the faint pulsations of his artery under my fingers.

Behind me, however, alarmed by the unfamiliar stir of excitement, two of the guards had assumed a crouch position by the door. The one with the ham shank hands stood less than a foot away from me, his gun drawn. I suddenly felt like a mother in charge of a playground full of impetuous boys.

"Oh for God's sake, put that thing away!" I hissed. "This is a hospital, not a shooting range."

Abashed, the guard holstered his toy and stepped back to join the other kids.

I took Max's blood pressure, upped his dopamine drip, and ran to get a lidocaine bolus. Rushing past Ginger, I gave her a look that should have paralyzed her from the neck down, and whispered close to her free ear, "Get off the phone, Ginger, before I stab you with a syringe full of insulin. I need some help stat."

My threat did not move her to action other than to swivel away from me cupping her free hand to her free ear, thus blocking me and the unit out of her auditory consciousness.

Max's rhythm and vital signs were stabilizing when Sandy stuck her head around the door long enough to inform me that I was getting a patient from ER: a fifty-six-year-old man in full-blown delirium tremens who'd had a fresh inferior-wall MI.

I looked over at Max's monitor and the myriad intravenous drugs, then to the pale and diaphoretic Mr. Wong, who was still holding on to his chest and grimacing. My eyes went next to bed 2, which would have to be readied for my admit from hell, and finally rested on Ginger, who had added insult to injury by putting her feet up, propping them against the monitor banks.

I headed over to the intermediate side, jaw and fists clenched. I would revert to early-development tactics: I was going to tell on Ginger.

The blind determination of anger propelled me full throttle through the double doors and into Beth, our newest nurse on swing shift. We smashed hipbones with enough force to make my teeth jar.

"Jesus Christ, have you registered those hips with the police as deadly weapons yet?" Beth asked, bent double and rubbing her left hip.

"No," I groaned. The numbing pain was spreading down from my right hip toward my knee. "But I've been meaning to have them blunted."

We smiled as the light of recognition flickered on in both our attics, illuminating two people of similar mind. In our case, it was likeness of the I'm-an-irreverent-rabble-rouser persuasion. I was willing to bet that between the two of us, there had to be at least six different strong-willed personalities.

Beth was the first to let go of her hip and stand straight. I noticed she wore the blouse of her nursing uniform the way hotshot nurses in New York and Boston did—with the collar up and the sleeves pushed up to the elbow. "When I learn to walk again," she said, "I can come over. My patients are settled for a while and Sandy said you're in need of help."

"Sandy knows very well that I've been in need of help for many years, but for right now, I'd settle for someone to restrain me."

"What's the problem?"

"BooBoo."

There was a slight frown of concern as she looked me over head to toe. "Are you hurt somewhere?"

"No, BooBoo is the party on the other end of the line." I jerked a thumb in Ginger's direction. "The plastic has been pressed against her ear almost long enough for it to be the first phone-ear fusion. I've been taking care of her patient and mine. I've got a new MI in DTs coming up from ER and I can't get the woman to move."

Beth gave a knowing smile. Long and lean, she moved with easy grace toward Ginger. In one well-executed yank, she pulled the phone out of her hand, scoring a few of Ginger's blond hairs in the process.

"Hi, BooBoo?" Beth spoke into the receiver without hesitation. "I'm really sorry, but Ginger has had a very bad accident with the defibrillator and can't return to the phone right now."

There was a short pause. "No, no. Don't call back," she said, "or we'll have to jump-start her all over again."

I was impressed. No sheep in nurse's clothing here. This woman showed promise of becoming one of the inner circle of Nurse Rebels Without Applause. We were hurting for new members; at this point there was only me, Pia, and Nealy, and Nealy had been showing signs of weakening in her crusade for nurse empowerment ever since she became the sole support of her three children.

Ginger regarded Beth's intervention from a completely different point of view than the madly grinning pair of us. "Excuse me," she said, her lip sliding into an antagonistic curl, "but I was on the phone. Who are you, and who gave you the right to—"

"Let me introduce myself," Beth said, pretending to give Mr. Wong's chart scrupulous attention. "I'm Beth Prochaska, your head nurse's sister? I'm going to be working evening shift for a while. Annie felt she was losing touch with the P.M. staff and wanted me to look after it for her—you know, keeping tabs to see if there are any nurses who don't pull their weight. She's also been concerned about some major phone bills originating from this unit."

I plugged my ears, expecting repeated verbal stabbings from Ginger. Instead, her lips went into a hard, thin line. She grabbed Mr. Wong's chart none too gently and slunk toward the nurses' lounge.

Beth tapped her on the shoulder and pointed to Mr. Wong's very full urinal, which was sitting on the edge of his bedside table. "That's a golden shower ready to fall, Ginger. Why don't you save yourself some trouble and empty the vessel? Besides, I'm sure your patient would like to make your acquaintance sometime before the end of shift." Beth squinted at the monitor. "Looks like his ST segments are elevated too. My guess is, he's having some pain. He probably needs some morphine and a new set of vitals, don't you think?"

If looks could kill, Beth would have been dead three times over without any chance of resuscitation.

"Are you really Annie's sister?" I asked a few minutes later as we prepared the room for the new patient.

Beth pushed her coal-black hair back from eyes of the same

color and frowned. "Are you kidding? If I was related to management by family ties, I'd kill myself, I wouldn't go around announcing it."

She clicked on the bedside monitor, set the alarm limits, and straightened out the tangle of lead wires. The nurse projected a hard edge I couldn't place. It was either complete self-assuredness or a wall of defense.

"Believe it or not," she went on, "when I was young and naive, I used to be an assistant nursing administrator of one of the big hospitals in New York. I know the pro-greed, give-the-nurse-the-shaft game firsthand. I gave it up when I realized I didn't have the required lack of conscience."

We turned down the bed and set out the rest of the routine admission supplies: admit information sheet, first-line medications, IV equipment, and electrodes. Beth checked the oxygen by turning it up full so that it blasted out of the humidifier nozzle and into her face. "Some of the things that went on in those management meetings blew my mind," she said, taking several huge breaths of the gas. "The filth of hospital politics would make a great book." She gave me a quick sideways glance. "By the way, did I hear that you wrote a book?"

The blush was instantaneous. I busied myself with checking the wall suction. "Uh huh."

"What's it about?"

This was a question the publisher told me I would be asked frequently, and even though I had been racking my brain for weeks, I still didn't have a suitable answer. It dawned on me to let the answer roll from my gut and see what came out. "It's about what it feels like to walk in the shoes of a nurse every day. You know, the things we see and have to deal with . . . why we burn out. It's about what goes on behind the closed doors of critical care units."

Beth leaned back lazily with her hip tilted out, her body's natural posture. "Are there any really down-and-dirty parts?"

"Well, I suppose if you think about it in normal people's terms, the whole thing is pretty down-and-dirty. I mean, how many books describe cockroaches living in a person's hair, or the experience of removing thirty-two safety pins from some guy's penis?"

My answer seemed to satisfy her, for she smiled a little and nodded.

"And the title?" she asked, a minuscule hint of challenge in her question.

I thought for a second, mirrored her waggish smirk, and answered, "It's called *Satanic Nurses*."

It was circus time, and I was the nurse on the tightrope without a net.

Mr. Hathaway, the new admit, was apparently at the pool, eager to show off his swan dive in the diving competition. Mr. Wong's STs were still slightly elevated, and Max was getting ready for another run of V tach. Ginger was hiding in Mr. Wong's room, curtains drawn, watching TV with her feet up on the side rails while the heavily morphinized Mr. Wong slept fitfully.

Central supply ignored my repeated requests for leather restraints; thus my hallucinating Mr. Hathaway received more IV haloperidol than I had ever given anyone under two hundred pounds in my whole career. Unfortunately, the tranquilizer hadn't made so much as a gnat's spit of difference in his agitation.

Dr. Meyers finally made his appearance, still in golf attire, two hours after my last stat call. From the minute he walked in the door, he was barely in control of himself. Judging by the small piece of grassy divot riding on the brim of his hat, I figured he must have shot way over par and lost some money besides.

"Give him another bolus of lidocaine!" he shouted, jerking a thumb toward Max. "Get a chest X ray! Give him forty milligrams of IV Lasix! Call the lab! Get that lidocaine onboard and up the drip to four milligrams! Set up for an arterial line insertion and have a pulmonary line standby! Why hasn't he gotten his Lasix yet? Turn up that dopamine. Get lab up here stat!" Dr. Meyers snapped his fingers close to my ear. "Come on, come on, move it. I want—"

"Look, Dr. Meyers," I said sharply, injecting the bolus of lidocaine into Max's IV line as quickly as I dared; if the medication was given too fast, it could cause seizures. "What do you want me to do first? I can only do one order at a time. Now, if you'd like to finish giving this bolus, I'll run over to the other side and see if I can get another nurse to take care of the desk while I set up the art line. Otherwi—"

"Hey, fuck you assholes," Max piped up. He was as white as the sheet he lay on. "Why don't you leave me alone? I don't want any of this shit done anyway. Send me back to the joint to die, man."

Dr. Meyers patted the man on the shoulder in a placating, if clueless fashion. "Now, now, Max, we need to get you fixed up and feeling better."

The prisoner turned his icy stare on Meyers, who seemed mesmerized by it. "Why? So I can be a perfect specimen of health when I walk down death row and into the gas chamber? Won't the taxpayers love that at three thousand big ones a day? You spend all this dough to keep me alive so you can turn around and execute me? Shit, man, you people are the ones who are fucking insane."

Personally, I thought Max had a point there.

Dr. Meyers, on the other hand, stumbled through his repertoire of platitudes. "You'll see things differently when you feel better, son." And my personal favorite, "Tomorrow is another day." When he was in the middle of "You should think positively," I left Max's lidocaine drip at three milligrams, upped his dopamine a few drops, and was on my way to see if I could borrow Beth again from the other side.

A flutter of arms in bed 2 caught my eye.

Mr. Hathaway, despite ten milligrams of morphine on top of the arsenal of haloperidol, was balancing on the footboard of his bed in the stance of one getting ready to spring off the end of a diving board. Behind him trailed the monitor wires still miraculously hooked to his chest. A long streak of blood ran across the bed, still dribbling from his disconnected IV.

"Louise?" he yelled, addressing the wall-mounted TV screen. "Louise, watch this double-twist backflip. See if you can catch it on video."

He put out his arms and my legs unfroze. I got to him as he was bending for the push-off. "Stop! Mr. Hathaway, wait a minute."

Mr. Hathaway was pale and diaphoretic. His heart rate was above 120. He glanced at me, exasperated. "Aren't the judges ready?"

"No. The judges want you to go back and lie down until your number is called. You're out of turn. There are other divers in front of you."

"Well for God's sake," Mr. Hathaway wheezed, short of breath, "I never heard of anything so ridiculous. Louise is waiting. Let me go first and get it over with."

Before I could move, the man executed a backflip off the end of the bed and onto his buttocks. He wasn't a heavy man, but the floor and windows shook with the impact.

"What the hell did they do with the water?" he bellowed. "Damned bastards drained the pool when my back was turned. I demand a rematch."

"And we'll make sure you have one as soon as they refill the pool," Beth said, hurrying in to help me lift the man to his feet.

We checked him for broken bones, then got him going in a smooth reverse shuffle toward the bed.

"I felt the floor rock at the other end of the hall. The rest of the staff are over there under the desk, thinking it's another earthquake. I figured it was you."

"LOUISE!" Mr. Hathaway broke free, swinging at us both. "Get your hands off me," he shouted. "Louise, they're trying to disqualify me. Unfair! Cheaters! Call the fire department, Louise. Hurry!"

As with many dedicated and long-term alcoholics, the man's arms and legs were thin, but in his present state of mind they could pack some powerful blows. Beth ducked several punches, but caught a kick to the shinbone. She also had made the mistake of leaving her stethoscope hanging around her neck. Mr. Hathaway grabbed it and jerked her head down. Instead of the bite I thought for sure would follow, he licked the side of her face.

In retaliation Beth tickled his midriff, which rendered him helpless until we could maneuver him onto the bed and tie his hands to the side rails with cotton wrist restraints. I looked up in time to catch Dr. Meyers marching, stiff-necked, out of the unit.

"Can you take care of Mark Spitz for a minute?" I asked. "My other patient is heading down the tubes and Meyers wants a thousand things done immediately. Of course, if he had called me back two hours ago, I could have had most of this stuff done instead of—"

"Where's Ginger?"

"Closeted in her patient's room, watching TV," I answered. "I haven't had a spare minute to load my gun and go ask her how she's doing."

Beth pursed her lips and nodded, then busied herself with the task of restarting Mr. Hathaway's IV.

Dr. Meyers had put Max's chart in Mr. Wong's rack. Of course, he'd also neglected to write the orders for either blood work or X ray, so I was forced to return to square one and have him paged. Unless the orders were coming from ER, the laboratory and radiology wouldn't even look at a patient without a copy of the doctor's written and signed order. Those were rules.

I wrote the order for the chest X ray, indicating it was a verbal order from Dr. Meyers, then set up the machines and equipment for the insertion of an arterial line. Half an hour later, Dr. Meyers strode in like Cleopatra coming into Egypt.

"Okay, so where's the lab work and the chest X ray?" he asked.

"Chest X ray is over on the screen. The lab work hasn't been done."

Dr. Meyers opened his mouth.

I held up a warning hand. "You left without writing any orders. Outside of ER or a code, they haven't done lab work in this hospital without written orders for about thirty years. I paged you three times, and when you didn't answer, I wrote the order for the X ray, and I might have written them for the lab work, too, but I didn't know exactly what you wanted and I wasn't going to chance being written up by you later on for mind reading."

I crossed my arms. To use a well-worn literary phrase, Dr. Meyers's face grew dark and stormy. I could see his jaw working and noticed for the first time that his head appeared to be remarkably large in comparison with his body. Predictably, he flew to the familiar comfort of his arrogance.

"You never paged me!" he retaliated.

"The operator keeps a record of all the page requests." I picked up the phone. "Let's check with her and find out exactly what times I paged you."

He ignored the phone. "When I tell a nurse to order lab work, I expect it to be ordered stat. I got tired of waiting around for you to finish lollygagging in that other patient's room, and went down to ER to check on a new admit."

"But first you spent five minutes fuming because I wasn't at your beck and call. Why didn't you use that time to contact lab yourself?" I picked up his right index finger and looked at it in mock concern. "It doesn't look broken, doc."

He pulled his hand away. "It isn't my place to be ordering my own lab work. That's your job."

"I felt that it was more urgent that I try to keep my DTs patient from jumping off the end of his bed and injuring himself. And it isn't *my* place to be ordering lab work I don't have any orders for. Those are rules."

Dr. Meyers remained sour, unbending.

"Don't you remember? Two years ago, the physicians vetoed the nurses' request to be allowed to order lab or medications they deemed necessary."

The doctor turned eyes on me that were colder than his patient's. "I don't want excuses. I want action. I've had it with the nurses' attitudes in this unit, and I'm going to do something about it."

"Like what, doctor? Commit suicide?"

We both turned to see who had spoken these blasphemous words, and found Beth standing behind us. Hers was an expression of demonic delight.

She smiled broadly at Dr. Meyers and offered the man her hand. Dr. Meyers gave it a quick tug as though it were something contagious.

"Hi, Dr. Meyers, I'm Beth Prochaska, the new CCU nurse here. Do you have a problem?"

"This doesn't concern you," he said curtly.

Beth cocked her head and wagged her finger in a gentle scolding. "It concerns me when I see one of my colleagues being verbally battered by someone who is supposed to be a teammate. It also concerns me when I see a physician trying to cover his own mistake by placing blame on the nurse."

Dr. Meyers ignored her and abruptly addressed me. "I want the lab work drawn and then I need you in there"—he pointed violently to Max's room—"to assist with the line insertion. Let's get on it."

Without warning, my mood took a lighter, teasing path and my mind flipped into wishful thinking. I suddenly wanted Dr. Meyers to laugh, shake hands, and say the age-old wrestling match between our two professions was over. I wanted us to agree we were working for the same end—the health and welfare of the patient—even if it was a patient like Max. Then, after a while, we'd take a break and go down to the evil food machines in the basement and treat each other to candy and gum.

I stood and touched his arm. Under my fingers, his body immediately stiffened and he got that trapped look, as if I were about to read him some Shakespeare or a long section from the Constitution.

"Now see, Dr. Meyers, you just said the key word: 'need.' You need me." I went for the shock-value-question routine. "I mean, tell me the truth—what would you do without nurses?"

I thought I saw a teeny upward curve at the corners of his mouth, as if his brain were trying to recall what muscles were utilized in a smile.

"We would train baboons to do the same job," he said finally.

Indignation, pure and simple, lifted Beth half out of her seat, fists balled. I decided we'd gone enough rounds; the opponents weren't getting anywhere.

I held up my hands and actually managed to keep my smile. "Okay, doc. I'll help you, but I'm going to warn you that the second you stop treating me civilly, I'm going to have to leave the room and see if I can talk one of the other nurses into assisting. That may not be so easy."

"Yes," Beth said sulkily, smoothing back her hair. "Especially since nurses are becoming more human all the time."

The rest of the night proceeded with a few twists and turns.

Max signed the permit for the arterial line insertion without question, and even consented to the IV Valium Dr. Meyers ordered. His docility did not surprise me—it was all part of the schizophrenic's pendulum ride between violets and violence.

Dr. Meyers was astonishingly calm during the insertion of the line into Max's femoral artery. His deft skill made the procedure seem like nothing more complicated than buttering a piece of toast.

Five minutes after Dr. Meyers began, I hooked up the arterial line and the wave form came up loud and clear on the monitor, indicating Max's blood pressure as 90 over 48. While Dr. Meyers was suturing in the line, I complimented him on his efficiency.

"And that's why I'm the doctor and you're just the nurse," he said, carelessly tossing the used needle into the pile of surgical rubble.

I winced at the ignorance of his remark and began cleaning up his mess. Being "just the nurse," it was my job to search carefully through the pile of debris for the other sharps he had used. Every nurse I knew had, at least once, been stuck or cut by scalpel blades or needles that doctors thoughtlessly threw onto the surgical field when they were done.

An hour later, things were as back in control as things ever got on a critical care unit. Max and two of his guards snored noisily while they slept. Mr. Hathaway continued to rave about empty swimming pools and back twists, though the haloperidol had kicked in enough to ensure he wouldn't be a danger to himself or others.

While Beth and I finished taking off orders, we swapped doctor horror stories, kicking around ideas on why some physicians treated nurses the way they did, and why the arrogant attitude was ever-present.

"Well," Beth said matter-of-factly, "it's partly because nurses continue to allow them to, and partly because the holier-than-thou segment of their mentality has been nurtured since medical school. It isn't every day the physician is going to run up against nurses like us, although I believe that time is rapidly approaching.

"You have to look at how these guys were raised—they go through twelve years of higher education and training hating every minute of it. Who can blame them? It's the most abusive kind of education. They're up for thirty-six to forty-eight hours at a time, barely able to function and having to listen to complaints from everybody. Then, every morning, they get reamed by their attendings.

"Physicians are some angry people when they get out of school. The ones who don't readjust to the real world think they've earned the right to be an asshole through suffering."

"Then to top that off," I said, "we live in the one country in the world where the occupation of physician is looked upon as exceptional above all other professions. Playing God is a lot of responsibility, and when that responsibility becomes a burden, the nurses are the perfect scapegoats."

Beth nodded in agreement. "They're so focused on the clinical aspects of medicine," she said, flicking a piece of invisible grunge off one of the monitor screens, "that most of them don't learn how to communicate with either the patients or the staff.

"Poor babies, I think they're afraid to let down with anyone, lest they lose the illusion of power or get—oh, horrors—emotionally *involved*."

"Plus now they're afraid that nurses are trying to step into their arena." I added, "Procedures and responsibilities that used to be strictly theirs are being turned over to the nurse, but instead of feeling relieved, they're feeling threatened, or should I say their pocketbooks are feeling threatened."

Max's monitor alarm sounded briefly as a bigeminal pattern of PVCs crossed the screen and disappeared. Beth stood and smoothed down the skirt that showed off her long, slender legs to advantage. "Docs, hospitals, insurance companies, all know that nurses are the key to lowering healthcare costs," she said. "The only people who don't realize it are the healthcare consumers themselves. You'll be in a perfect position to tell them when you go on your book tour."

I watched the three rhythms on the monitor bank and thought about my years of hands-on, bedside nurturing. I thought about the patients I'd cried with and held, saved and let die. That part of it seemed so far removed from money and the political battles between nurse and doctor, nurse and administration.

Sticking up for myself and the patients with the docs and management was one thing, I thought, but leading a revolution wasn't anything I wanted to stick my boots into. Or, as Simon aptly quipped from time to time, "I didn't used to want to play, and now I still don't."

I have a slow ear for accents. Because of this, I am constantly having to ask people of foreign cultures to repeat themselves, which is a major hassle when one lives and works in the melting pot of San Francisco. Everything from a heavy Southern drawl to a hard-core just-off-the-boat Chinese accent sounds like Greek to me.

As I got older, my retarded ear became more of a problem. I even went back to college to study sign language. Except each time I used basic signs with the heavily accented, they all thought I was deaf and would begin to shout, which made them even more difficult to understand.

Around eleven I was finishing my charting, when Mrs. Shirinian entered the acute unit and inched her way over to the nurses' station in that shy, downcast-eyed manner of older Iranian women.

Unconsciously, I tensed and caved inward in order to make myself look smaller so perhaps she might not see me. It didn't work. She stood before me and said something with an Iranian accent that sounded to my untuned ear exactly like, "Heshian mooish allowa?"

I sighed. This was going to be pitiful. It had been hard enough understanding Mr. Shirinian, my postoperative gallstone/congestive heart failure patient from two days ago, and Mr. Shirinian had been in California for fifteen years. Mrs. Shirinian had only been here for ten and was still unsure of the language.

She thrust an uncovered plastic specimen cup toward me, repeating the unintelligible phrase.

"Pardon?" I asked. I always began the customary ritual with "Pardon?" geared down to a few rounds of "What?" and "Huh?" went on to an "Excuse me" or two, and finally ended up with a shrug and a simple explanation that I was hearing-impaired and mentally ill-equipped to understand what was being said.

She pushed the cup into my hand, smiling. "Shirmira noimom mistalauwa."

I gave in and nodded, smiling back. Perhaps she would go away.

She pointed to the cup in what I interpreted as a gesture of offering. "Stonmia. Stonmia. Frim emhusblarder," she said.

I looked into the cup and was pleasantly surprised to find it filled with chocolate-covered raisins. Ah, I sighed in relief, the mystery was solved; she wanted to give me a treat for taking care of her husband.

Chocolate had never been a vice of mine, but I was starving, and ever since I'd cut my nocturnal sweet tooth at the age of thirty-five, I had a hard time turning down anything sugary after nine P.M.

Thanking her profusely, I poured out a few raisins and popped them into my mouth.

A strange combination of disbelief and horror passed over Mrs. Shirinian's face. Her single thick eyebrow shot up to her hairline like a shade snapping up to its roller.

Whatever major cultural faux pas I had committed I knew had to be really bad, because Mrs. Shirinian clasped her hands to the sides of her head and screamed.

Friday
2:45 A.M.

My teeth still ache, though thank God I didn't chip any of the front ones. Oh well, I suppose I could go down in someone's record book as being the only person who ever ate a handful of Iranian gallstones.

As if I didn't have enough psychologically damaging trauma going on. Tomorrow is Doomsday, and unless I get some sleep I'm going to need an extra tube of Erace to cover the bags under my eyes.

Matthew sent his Aunt Echo a dead spider, a picture of a

fish, and one of his toenail clippings to carry for good luck while on tour. Hell, why not? Anything would help at this point.

FOUR

"Where are the articles praising the myriad nurses giving basic, sensitive care to those who desperately need attention? Who speaks about the bedside nurse?"

OLIVE Y. BURNER, R.N.

THE RED LIGHT ON THE CAMERA went on, driving my respiratory rate up to over forty per minute. I'd been totally in control right up until then. I'd even joked with the cameraman about his promising to get the camera off me if I threw up or fainted.

At that he'd laughed uncertainly, then asked if I was kidding. Only when I watched the videotape of this interview a year later did I understand why he was concerned, for I very much resembled the "before" photo in a Pepto-Bismol ad.

My mind, feeling as though it had just stepped off the observation tower of the Empire State Building, focused on the heat from the lights and the inch of makeup covering my interviewer's face. There was a tiny glob of hair mousse barely visible on his starched collar. Somehow I was able to form the thought that his careless-looking hair had been carefully arranged like that, messy spike by messy spike.

I grasped for an anorexic ray of hope. Perhaps, it being the noon hour, there would be only five, maybe ten people tops, watching the news. The rest of the Bay Area would be doing lunch with each other.

I was answering the first question in a normal tone of voice (although at the time I *did* wonder whose voice it was), when I realized this was probably much like a near-death experience: finding myself floating above, listening to all that goes on. Then something the interviewer was saying caught my disembodied brain's attention.

73

". . . so medicine is a subject close to my own heart. My father is a doctor . . ." (Here there is a confident smile showing a perfect, $10,000 set of cosmetically bright white teeth) ". . . and I'm sure that as a nurse . . ." (The smile is gone and the word "nurse" is said with the same inflection as would be used with "sewer worker.") ". . . you know how important and necessary the physician's guidance is to the existence of your profession." (A crinkle of challenge breaks through the concealer caked around his eyes.)

Incredulous, I wondered if he was purposely baiting me. On the tape, there was a noticeable pause. It was during this pause that my mind returned to my body, a sense of outrage having cut through the numbing layer of stage fright.

"I wouldn't call what the physicians do to nurses 'guidance.' " (On the tape, my foot started tapping out an irritable rhythm. My vacant, all-teeth Barbie doll smile had disappeared altogether.) "Doctors continue to see the nurse in the antiquated role of the bedpan-wielding . . ." (A speck of spit flew from my mouth and landed on the cover of my book, which the interviewer held in his perfectly manicured hand.) ". . . handmaiden instead of collaborative practitioner. Doctors are one of the main stumbling blocks to our advancement as a profession. They view nurses as threats to their . . ." (I had leaned forward and was practically up in the man's face. This was where the camera cut back to the interviewer.)

"Well, I'm sure this book will make interesting reading for any young lady interested in nursing."

"It is *not* a book just for men and women interested in nursing," I cut in. As if taken by surprise, the camera made a quick, jerky shot back at me, then before I could finish, back at the interviewer. "It's for the layperson, too, people who don't have a clue what goes on behind the doors of a hosp—"

On tape, the interviewer was caught making the cut sign with his finger across his throat; he recovered by fixing his tie and smiling. You can see that his lip gloss has almost entirely dried up.

"Yes, thank you. And our guest today was Echo Heron, author of . . . blah blah blah blah blah."

One interview down. Only forty-five more to go.

I was on a plane headed toward Los Angeles, but in my mind, I wasn't really going there, I was going berserk.

Janey, my longtime friend from nursing school, adjusted the overhead light on the idle(addled?)-mind magazine she'd picked up at the airport newsstand and continued to read aloud.

"Carly Simon has had a long-term phobia about performing in front of crowds. Stage fright has been such a problem for this popular songstress, she finally had to hire a hypnotist."

Without looking up from the magazine, Janey reached over and loosened my viselike grip from the armrest. "Ms. Simon," she continued reading, "is currently able to appear in front of small groups . . ."

I stopped listening and returned my concentration to the shaft of yellow sunlight coming through the window. It slid slowly down the wall of the cabin and onto my lap like a stick of melting butter. Meantime, my stomach was trying to make its way up my esophagus.

"I can't do this, Janey," I blurted. "CNN is the worst. Me in a small room with a camera three feet away from my face? Millions of people staring at me, live?"

"You can do it, and you will," Janey said with resolve.

I didn't answer because I was using the air sickness bag. Then, "Can't," I whispered through the bile.

"Can and will," Janey whispered fiercely. "I didn't leave my kids and husband to fly up from L.A. and escort you back down to L.A. so that you can flake out on everybody. You're going to be in that studio tonight." She patted my hand—no, actually she hammered my hand with her fist and broke my grip on the armrest again.

Media escorts are like life-support systems. They keep you going no matter whether your heart and mind are gone. Arranged for by the publisher's publicity department, they must escort either the author or the celebrity from the airport to the hotel and from there to the interviews. I related to almost every one of my media escorts as the sweet and caring mother I never had. She or he makes sure you're on time, fed, and up-to-date on all the local gossip. They are a wealth of information about the political flavor of the city you are currently touring. For instance, they might say something like, "There's a lot of controversy here right now because the nurses at So-and-So Hospital are threatening to strike."

They'll also clue you in on your various interviewers' political and personal views. I've been told everything from, "Your next interviewer ate a physician he had on the show last week for lunch. His mother died a long, slow death in a hospital, and he's angry with the medical system," to, "This interviewer is hard on her women guests. However, she makes all her own clothes, so if you compliment her dress, she won't be so tough."

Media escorts have the ability to make your life a dream or a nightmare, and, as I was soon to discover, the escortees have the same effect on them.

Barbara, my L.A. escort, was young, tall, slender, and pretty, thus blowing my idea that all escorts were going to be middle-aged and matronly. She was wearing shades, white anklets with black patent-leather strap heels, and a very short polka-dot jumper with shoulder pads rivaling the Rams'.

I could tell just by looking at her that I was in L.A.—the land of the Ultrabeautiful, Slender, and Flawless-Bodied People, where even the waitresses are ravishing. La La Land is one place where you can be assured of feeling guilty for ordering anything with calories, or not looking European salon-spa finished.

Barbara extended her hand and introduced herself as I came off the ramp. Immediately I started to cry.

"You're going to hate me," I said.

She looked slightly amused, expectant, and a little fearful. "No," she said slowly. "No I'm not."

"Yes, yes, you really are."

Janey quickly introduced herself as my caretaker, grabbed the back of my neck, and growled, "You can and damn well will!"

Barbara stared at Janey curiously, then back at me. "Why am I going to hate you?"

"I can't do CNN tonight."

Janey reached up (I am seven inches taller than this deceptively small, frail-looking woman who claims to be my friend) and whacked me in the back of the head with the rolled-up movie magazine that had the article about Carly Simon's stage fright.

"Are you ill?" Barbara asked, ignoring Jane's outburst.

I could have made it so much easier on myself if I had just said yes, vomited again, and mentioned something about eating a tainted tofuburger on the plane. Instead, I told the truth. "I'm having a bad case of stage fright. I can't do it. I just can't do it!" My voice was rising.

"Stage fright? Pssssh. No biggie. I'll give you some exercises to get you through. I thought you were going to tell me you were having appendicitis or somethi—"

"I CAN'T DO IT!" I screamed. "I'll do any show you want me to tomorrow. I just can't get through this one."

Janey now changed her tone of voice to syrupy and understanding, although she didn't fool me for a moment. I knew she desperately wanted to hurt me with the magazine, or better yet, the pocketknife she carried on her key chain. "Now, Ec, you've got to think about—"

"I can't do it."

Jane whacked me in the head. Twice.

Barbara pulled Jane away. "It's really not bad," she cooed, putting a comforting arm around my shoulders. "The interview will be over before you know it. The minute you start answering questions, your nervousness disappears. You have to concentr—"

"I said I can't do it. I'm sorry." To prove my point, I gagged and let my legs buckle.

Jane moaned. Barbara sagged at the shoulders.

Together, they led me away.

Janey O'Hara Justice is not a vindictive person. That night, however, she learned the ins and outs of spite. She refused to speak to me all through dinner—wouldn't even pass me the salt substitute. And during my involved and tearful explanation about my long history of stage fright from the time I was just a baby, she yawned with boredom.

I tried to lighten things up by reminiscing about some of the funnier moments we shared in nursing school. I even made jokes about our old nursing instructors, mimicking Miss Telmack's broom-handle walk and Miss Pearson's monotone personality. She looked up from her newspaper long enough to ask the waitress for another scoop of nonfat cottage cheese for her organic fruit salad. Nothing could get her to loosen up the prune-mouth expression.

In our hotel room, I threw myself on my bed and pulled the blanket over my head as a last resort. Totally dispirited by my inability to pull myself out of terminal wimpiness and, too, hoping to evoke some sympathy, I wept.

Over on her bed, Jane read a book of Gary Larson cartoons and roared.

At the appropriate time, Jane switched on *CNN Newsnight* and turned it up full blast. There was the substitute guest, sitting where I should have been sitting, smiling like a madman, having a great old time talking about summertime safety in the home.

"That could have been you!" she brayed with such force, it was clear she had been waiting all night for this moment of triumph. She narrowed her green eyes for the best nasty effect. "You could have been there speaking up for nurses all over the country, making a difference for your profession. You're a coward, and all I can say is, you better shape up by tomorrow or I'll never let you write about me again."

One of the stagehands carried me onto the set of *Hour Magazine* and propped me up on the couch. He hooked a tiny microphone onto my lapel and walked away shaking his head. I figured I was probably his first live carry-on.

The stars of the show were taking a small break, so I had a bit of time to compose myself by repeating over and over that even though the show was national, it was taped.

The audience in the studio, however, was very much alive.

I dared once to glance at the rows of people and saw Jane in the front corner seat. Her head was in her hands. Next to her, Barbara was biting a thumbnail, looking as though she had aged ten years.

On monitor I caught a glimpse of myself, white as a ghost and breathing very fast. If I had seen myself walk into an ER, I would have predicted I was going to have a cardiac arrest. I didn't even find it the least bit humorous that the interview was going to center around how critical care nurses beat stress.

I looked at the camera, then at the audience, and decided the hell with it; *Intensive Care* was going to have to be a word-of-mouth book. Unclamping the mike, I was preparing my legs for an exit, when a dark-haired man sat next to me and introduced himself as a psychiatrist who appeared regularly on the show.

"I understand you're having some stage fright," he said.

"Bad," I managed to croak. "I've gotta get outta here."

He put his arm around me and hugged me close. "I promise you'll do great. The host is a sweet guy. He won't throw you any curves. Forget about the cameras, forget about those people out there. Just concentrate on the questions, and if you start to panic, I'll be right here. I won't let anything bad happen to you."

In the man's eyes I saw a mixture of compassion and mirth,

and agreed to stay put. Okay, I thought, but if I throw up or faint, it's all in your lap, buster.

The show went without a major hitch. Other than visible rapid respirations and flared nostrils (an involuntary reaction when I am in a highly emotional condition), I answered the questions asked of me without sounding too much like a moron.

The best part came after the red light on the camera went out. I was walking out (under my own power), when my couch companion tapped me on the shoulder and asked to speak to me alone in the Green room.

"Why do you still believe the garbage your mother told you about yourself?" he asked before the door was even closed.

My eyes widened so much, I must have looked like a Keene reproduction. "Excuse me?"

"Why do you continue to let your mother sit on your shoulder telling you that you don't deserve to have a successful tour?"

I stared at him in total amazement. "Christ, don't tell me she visits *you*, too?"

The dark-haired man smiled. "Any time anyone is as frightened as you are of presenting themselves and something good that they've done, I can almost guarantee that in the background there is a parent's tape playing over and over, beating them down, telling them they don't deserve success."

I started to cry, and he let me for a while.

"Get some help turning off those shame tapes," he said finally. "Before you fly to New York for the *Today* show get in to see a certified hypnotherapist on an emergency basis." He walked me to the door. "Good luck, and don't forget to tell Mom it's your show, not hers."

I managed to get through the rest of the L.A. tour, which consisted of several radio shows and a newspaper interview. I did one live local TV show, but I was on with two other nurses and let them do most of the talking. Plus, the bulk of the attention from both cameraman and host went to the bosomy (*so* bosomy, I doubt anyone ever noticed her face) redhead who had been a nurse's aide and was currently a private-duty nurse to an older Hollywood studio executive.

In the Green room before the show, she'd talked nonstop for

forty minutes about how private-duty nursing had it all over hospital nursing.

"It's a piece of cake." She nudged me in the ribs and pursed two collagen-filled lips that were so overdone, they looked like they could suck eggs out of a barren chicken. "You get to live the life of a queen, traveling all over and meeting important people. All you have to do is hang out around the pool all day wearing a string bikini, accompany the old fart to dinner showing lots of cleavage, give him his pills on time, and take his blood pressure when he starts looking liverish. When he gets drunk and passes out, all you have to do is roll him onto the nearest flat surface, throw a blanket over him, and turn his head to the side so he doesn't choke if he throws up."

It sounded tempting for about three minutes, until I realized I didn't have the essential credential for the job anyway, since somewhere between the ages of twenty-three and thirty, my cleavage had escaped me.

Janey and Barbara put me on the plane for San Francisco, both, I think, happy to see me go. Jane kissed me on the cheek. "You're going to be fine," she said, always ready with her lousy optimism. "Somebody will hypnotize you, make you sign over all your money, have sex with you, and take care of your stage fright all in one session. You'll be penniless and have VD, but you *will* walk on the *Today* show with complete confidence."

Jane Pauley was shorter than I, and her hands were colder than mine. She also reminded me a lot of Virginia Bradley, a pale, freckle-faced girl I went to grammar school with.

At that point in time, all I knew about Ms. Pauley was that she was married to Garry Trudeau and she was going to interview me. I remember thinking that she looked too young to have been interviewing for any length of time. I hoped she had had enough experience so that when I froze up, she could pick up the thread of conversation and keep going with it until someone offstage could hook me by an ankle and drag me off the couch.

My media escort warned me to be nice to Ms. Pauley. Jane, my escort said, had slept that previous night—the first night of the NBC strike—on the news counter, head to head with Bryant Gumbel, because they had been told not to cross the picket lines.

Not that I believed this outrageous story, but I could see that the members of the skeleton crew left in the studio were stressed. And Ms. Pauley *did* look tired.

One of the crew was clipping my mike onto the collar of my jacket, when I leaned forward and asked Ms. Pauley why her hands were so cold. If she hadn't been recently handling ice, I was going to suggest vitamins C and B, plus perhaps an iron supplement.

To my surprise, she apologized for them and settled herself opposite me. "Are you still nursing?" she asked, chafing her hands.

I noticed her suit was perfect, without a wrinkle, and wondered what she had slept in on the news counter. "Yes. I'm on vacation."

Jane cocked her head and lifted her eyebrows. "You're doing this tour on your vacation time?"

I nodded, contemplating telling her how difficult it was for a critical care nurse to get any time off these days. I doubted she would believe me if I told her that nurses sometimes injured themselves on purpose in order to get time off.

A production person handed Ms. Pauley a copy of my book, and behind her, a man's voice came out of the dark. It said, "Thirty." This, I knew, meant there were thirty seconds until the red light on the top of the camera would go on.

Panic snuck up my temples, into my ears to my mind. The light-headed, get-me-outta-here! feeling was taking over like a rocket out of control. The ringing in my ears was making me deaf, and spots of my vision were missing completely. It was stage fright to the max.

Automatically, my thumb and forefinger made a circle, finger pad pressing finger pad. It was the release signal that the hypnotherapist had programmed into me two days before. As in predeath visions (that is, if you believe in the old my-whole-life-flashed-before-me line), the highlights of my day with the hypnotherapist blazed through my mind.

I had walked into his office a stiff-legged, defensive, hyperventilating mess, and assured him in no uncertain terms that he would never, in a million years, be able to hypnotize me. Three hours later, I slipped behind the wheel of my car feeling like I was floating on the back of a dolphin—exactly as he had suggested.

I was regaining my vision and hearing, when Jane Pauley adjusted her mike and picked up her notes. "Now, one of the questions I'm going to ask you is why the little sisters from England are coming over to America looking for jobs."

The man behind her was saying, "Ten, nine, eight, seven . . ."

Little sisters? Who or what the hell were the little sisters, and what were the British up to now? Could they have something to do with Mother Teresa? Monty Python?

The subsiding wave of panic rose again. There weren't any little sisters in my book, except maybe in the acknowledgments. Suddenly I was convinced she had the wrong book, or the right book but the wrong author, or since there was a strike on and the network was in chaos, maybe she had the wrong day altogether.

"God forbid, don't ask me about that!" I whispered hurriedly. "I don't know anything about little sisters in England. I'm only speaking for—"

The red light flashed on.

I finished my five minutes with Jane Pauley intact. When she asked me the question about the little sisters from England, I flubbed my way through an answer—not even remotely close to the right answer, mind you, but still an answer.

Outside the studio, I suddenly felt alive. I couldn't wait to get to my next interview. I didn't care what it was, just bring them on.

It was thus that the media monster lurking in the shadows of my spirit was brought out of the closet.

The same week my book hit the shelves, news of a nursing shortage crisis in America made the front page of *The New York Times*. Overnight there was an instant and overwhelming influx of requests for my appearance on shows from *Oprah* to religious radio. Suddenly everybody wanted to know where all the nurses had gone . . . and why.

The interview pattern was always the same whether it was television, radio, or print; approximately thirty seconds were spent on the book, and the rest of the time went to the politics of nursing and healthcare. People, I discovered, were starved for information about what made nurses tick and what we actually did. They wanted to know from an insider what *really* went on behind the closed doors of a hospital. There were hundreds of questions: How did nurses handle all the suffering and death? How did it affect our personal lives? What was the reason behind the age-old doctor-nurse conflicts? Why were administration-nurse politics so vicious? How did it feel to have children die in our arms? What could people do to protect themselves as healthcare consumers? And—the most asked question—how could we bear to do what we did?

I made it my business to answer with the truth. Blowing the Cherry Ames, Subservient Nurse, myth all to hell was my delight, and if I had never done one more thing in this life, that alone would have been enough. If I'd thought before that I wanted to stay out of the political arena, I was wallowing in it now, up to the tops of my Wellingtons. I was blabbing everything from patient rights to nurse revolution and empowerment all over the place and, as my mother used to complain in her disapproving way, spilling my guts onto everyone's shoes.

Everywhere I went, nurses were shedding their sheep's clothing, becoming squeaky wheels in revolt against the systems that had kept them mute for a hundred years. I could only hope that those squeaky wheels would create a roar that would reverberate through every healthcare institution in the nation.

The way the needle came out through the back of my hand made me think of some of Mr. Spielberg's special effects. It also made my switchboard ladies hit the red-alert buttons.

Ever since I fell, wrist first, on a broken milk bottle at the age of three, I have imagined the inside of the mind as a switchboard with a squad of minuscule women (all of whom resemble Lily Tomlin) manning the lines.

As everyone knows, when accidents occur there is a split second in which the mind refuses to believe that the accident has actually happened. It is during this brief interlude that the red-alert alarm goes off, and I expect all those lilliputian women are frantically disconnecting the input lines from the brain switchboard. It is when they disconnect too many that one goes into shock and passes out.

I stared at the sharp tip of the needle and felt the pain charge up my arm and into my shoulder. I imagined the switchboard ladies clucking their tongues over yet another physical mishap, saying things to each other like, "Sheesh. Another red alert? That makes six in one week. What a klutz."

It wasn't until I was at the sink scrubbing the wound that the other disquieting thoughts were put through by the switchboard operators, one thought at a time.

Okay, so I'd brought my hand down, full force, on top of the full sharps box with the one-and-a-half-inch-long intramuscular needle sticking upward, out of the top.

And the patient occupying the room for the last four days was a young man who had come in for chest pains and FUO, or fever of unknown origin.

And the man was gay and an admitted IV drug abuser.

Bingo, and welcome back to the wonderful world of nursing.

The woman bleeding onto the ER floor was drunk. She was handcuffed, and there was a policeman sitting on each side of her. One of them, in an unusual show of kindness, held a gauze dressing over the gash that separated her nose into two distinct halves.

Her yellow polka-dot dress, cut midthigh, exposed long, thin legs dressed in white fishnet stockings that she had probably stored since the mid-sixties. Under the clingy material, her breasts were, to put it mildly, exaggerated. It was clearly a uniform of sex.

She reached up to scratch her scalp with one hand while the other, led by its chain, had no choice but to follow. The short, grotesque red nails dug into ringlets of pink hair. Looking like a big dead cotton candy, the wig slid down over her face in slow motion and landed in the puddle of blood.

She muttered in falsetto and drunkenly kicked at it with her yellow-rhinestoned spiked heel. Airborne, it whirled around several times until it came to rest on the toe of my running shoe. I immediately plucked it off and handed it back to her.

She accepted it graciously, then stuffed it down the neck of her dress. One of the officers shook her arm. "Say thank you to the nurse," he said.

Her well-shaved head wove from side to side as she tried to control her involuntarily wandering bloodshot gaze. She struggled briefly to bring all six feet two of herself to a standing position and carefully placed one cuffed hand on her outturned hip. Keeping time with the haughty, provocative bounce of hips and shoulders that made Mae West so Mae West, she brought her shoulder almost level with her cheekbone and fluttered her extra-long false eyelashes. I was fascinated by the tiny yellow rhinestones which lined her lids. Coordinated shoes and lids—it had to be a San Francisco fashion statement. "So," the transvestite said in a low, sexy tone, "you want me to do Garland or Streisand?"

One of the officers roughly pulled her back down into her seat.

"How about Streisand?" I said, headed back to bed 6 where Sarah stood warming the two syringes meant for me. Clamped in her left armpit she held the tetanus syringe, and gripped in her right was the misery shot from hell—gamma globulin, known in nursing school as Grandma Goblin. It was an unusual but effective technique of warming the medications inside the barrel so they wouldn't hurt as much going into the muscle.

"Okay, kiddo, drop those scrubs and bend over, feet turned inward."

"I don't want to." I crossed my arms over my chest, pouting. I hated getting shots as much as I hated giving them.

Sarah put the syringes down on the side table. "Okay then, you can wait until I get another chance to come back, but be forewarned, it's a full house and I may not show up for another hour. In the meantime you can listen to all these . . ."

From the other side of the curtain boomed a beautiful, well-modulated voice.

"Come to me, my melancholy baby . . ."

It was so Streisand, we could have been in Central Park.

Sarah rolled her eyes. "See what you've started? Now cut out the crap, bend over, and don't forget to report to employee health before work tomorrow for your first series of HIV tests."

I bent over and bit the sheet on the gurney. Gamma globulin wasn't a bee sting kind of shot. It wasn't a shot that was over when the needle was pulled out. I would be limping for days.

"Cuddle up and don't be blue . . ."

Sarah swiftly injected the needle into my hip. "I saw you on *People Are Talking*," she whispered. "I liked the comments about nurses being treated like bedpan-wielding handmaidens and being the healthcare bargain of the century."

I let go of the sheet and picked a piece of lint off my tongue. "Why are you whispering?"

Sarah pulled out the needle. It felt like my muscle had been infiltrated with a cup of hot lead.

"We're not supposed to talk about it at work."

"Talk about what?" I stood and retied the drawstring on my scrub pants.

"Nurse politics." Sarah wiped off my upper arm with an alcohol pad and injected the tetanus. I winced. Never again would I tell patients it was like a bee sting.

"The word from management is that they disapprove of us watching your interviews. The assistant director told Gus she thought it inappropriate and that management considered what you were saying as unprofessional."

My temper flared. "Inappropriate? Jesus, I can't think of anything *more* appropriate for nurses to be watching than people speaking out about wanting to be treated fairly," I said. "And if I'm being unprofessional telling nurses to demand their rights as professionals, I wonder what management does consider professional? I suppose if all two million of us remained in our places as martyred women, they'd be happy. I think a hundred years of being powerless is enough, don't you?"

Sarah put a Band-Aid over the injection site on my arm, which had dribbled a thin stream of blood down to my elbow. "Maybe," she said slowly, "but I think you're going to find nurses are divided on some of those issues. Not everybody is willing to stick their neck out, you know. Some of us have mortgages and mouths to feed."

"*. . . Every cloud must have a silver lining.*"

I couldn't argue with Sarah on that point, recalling the show on which I had been a panel guest for two tedious segments in a row. The host had all she could do to keep her temper under control as the all-nurse audience argued among themselves and with the nurse guests over every issue that came up, from sexual harassment on the job to unionization. Boos and applause erupted simultaneously. It was a rowdy, divided group to be sure.

At one point I was booed for saying that unionization was one of the ways nurses could stand up for their rights without being afraid of losing their jobs. The exasperated host removed her famous horn-rimmed glasses and, with neck veins distended to bursting, asked the audience what the problem was, since unionization seemed to be the best answer to nurses' woes.

After a couple of yea/nay comments, an outspoken member of the audience stood and explained: "I think people aren't going to talk about unions on national TV if they're afraid to talk about it in a hospital sitting together at a dining room table."

I sighed. "Well, Sarah, unless we start agreeing on the major matters, we're going to continue being regarded as the peons of the hospital instead of the backbone, and the cost-of-living wages we get now will be where we stay."

"Yeah, but Ec, we're women doing women's work. Who's going to listen to *us*?"

I put my arm around her. "Everybody and anybody who will ever need a nurse."

". . . Smile my honey dear while I kiss away each tear . . ."

I stuck my head around the door. "Pssssst."

Kathy McCormack, encased from chin to hips in what looked like a giant white baking dish with breasts molded into it, shifted her eyes toward me as far as they would go. "I can't see you, whoever you are," she said.

Realizing my mistake, I moved into her line of vision. "Hi. Do you remember me at all?" I asked.

A smile broke. "Hey, you're the nurse from the emergency room. We looked all over for you. My husband even went down to the nursing office, but they said they'd never heard of you."

How typical, I thought. "Must have been a new secretary. For future reference, you can usually find me in CCU . . . So, how are you?"

"I'm doing good," Kathy answered. Her strawberry hair had been attractively cut to better match the new hair filling in the shaved places. Above the body cast, her eyes were large and bright in the thin face. "I finally got those ice picks taken out of my skull and they took me off that torture bed— the one that flips you back and forth every four hours? My chin and forehead are still sore from where they rubbed against those stupid straps that held me in."

A nurse entered the room, saw me, looked shocked, and excused herself, walking backward out the door. I ran a hand over my face to make sure I didn't have something hanging from it, then offered Kathy a puzzled smile. She raised her eyebrows, which I interpreted as a substitute shrug.

"I've got five more weeks in this cast, then six weeks in a neck brace."

"What's the prognosis for movement?"

Kathy paused. "Well, when I first woke up in ICU, some gem of a doctor that my mother-in-law hired told me the very best I could ever hope for was to spend the rest of my life in a nursing facility strapped into a reclining wheelchair.

"Of course I immediately thought, Son of a bitch can't tell me *my* life is over. I've got two babies at home who need a mother.

"So I ordered him out of my room and asked for Dr. Schupbach again. At least Schupbach lets me have my hope."

I smiled at Kathy's statement. Dr. Peters, one of Redwoods's oncologists, once explained what he told his patients when there was absolutely no hope. "You never take away a patient's hope," he'd said. "Even if you have to commit some sins of omission, remember that hope might be all they have to live on. And, once in a great while, it actually leads them into a remission that wasn't supposed to be possible."

"Five days after I fell, I moved my left big toe," Kathy continued. "Schupbach had me in physical therapy the next day. When they slapped this tank on me a week ago, I could lift my knees a half inch, and my arms three inches. I can even be in a vertical position without passing out.

"How do you like my cleavage?" She lowered her eyes to the molded plaster breasts, complete with erect nipples. "I told the guys who made the cast to make me a size larger."

"You could liven things up around here and have someone color them in for you," I said. I stepped closer to her bed and looked her in the eye. "So, how are you, really?" I tapped her head lightly with my finger. "What's going on inside?"

A vein rose in the middle of her forehead, and she shifted her eyes away from mine.

"You know, when I first realized what was happening, I was one self-pitying bitch. I mean, I hated everyone who could walk and wave. Then, after I'd been here about two weeks, I got a roommate who had both legs amputated. Well, this lady was one of the sorriest human beings I'd ever run across. Physical therapy was up here two hours every day just trying to teach her to swing herself onto her artificial legs. So one night she decided to try it alone and swung herself halfway across the room. All I saw was this torso with flapping arms fly past me and plop onto the floor."

Kathy snickered, which broke through my professional resolve not to react to the mental image. Together, we laughed out loud, fully ashamed of ourselves.

"This lady lay there and cried, moaning about how she was going to be a cripple for the rest of her life, and how hopeless and worthless she was and on and on. At first I felt as sorry for her as I did for myself, but then I realized I had a choice—I could either be crippled and happy or crippled and a miserable, self-sorry bitch. So, I decided I'd compromise and be a crippled, happy bitch."

I laid a hand on her cast. "I've got a feeling that the doctor who told you you'd never move again probably helped more than you know. Anger can be a powerful weapon when entering the ring."

"Yeah, probably," she said. "I was so pissed, I told Schupbach I'd grind that guy's predictions under my heel on my way out of here."

"Well, when you do walk out," I said, "I want to be there."

Mooshie was curled up on my forehead, and the tape recorder rested on my stomach. I was taping to Janey, recounting a funny story Simon had told me about a lawyer and a moose, when the phone rang.

I glanced at my poor imitation of a Rolex watch, and my heart rolled over and skipped a beat. It was one A.M.

Now, every mother of an adolescent knows that when the phone rings after midnight, it's the coroner or the police calling. I began waiting for this call when Simon first began breaking curfew and going out with friends who had driver's licenses.

On the second ring, I sent an entreaty to the powers that arranged fate, and picked up the receiver.

"Yes, this is Simon Heron's mother," I said.

"Jesus. Don't you even say hello first?" asked Beth.

I sighed, and three bones in my neck and shoulders cracked with the release of tension. "Oh, hi. Yeah, well, when he isn't home by this time of night, I'm always convinced his skull is paving the highway somewhere. What's up?"

There was a long exhalation, then a slow and lazy, "Oh, nothin'. Just wanted to talk, is all."

I recognized that particular exhalation, a frequent punctuation for the alcoholic's aimless conversations. I was also familiar with the late-night calls and the ever so slight slur to the ends of specific words.

How many times had the same drunken sounds invaded my bedside, on a thousand midnights of my childhood?

I nodded my head sadly, the sudden disappointment completely unexpected. I hadn't figured Beth as a drinker, but then again, I was one of those people who had a blind spot when it came to detecting that kind of marker.

So out of it was I that I'd once spent six hours in a room full of people who were stoned out of their minds on cocaine, and never suspected a thing; I innocently thought they all had head colds, drank too much coffee, and were very horny, all at the same time.

Friday
1:30 A.M.

I face the left side of the bed, which has been empty for years, and feel the loneliness of that space. When the moon is so bright it hurts the eyes, I want someone I can turn to and say, "Hey, look at that moon, will ya!" In the middle of the night, I want to have a warm hairy leg to rest my ice-cold feet against.

I'm convincing myself it'll never happen. Besides, I'm set in my ways. I like not having to account for my strange behavior patterns.

Oh sure, tell us another one, honey.

Got pulled into a political debate with Beth and Dr. Cramer and Dr. Mahoney. What I found fascinating was Susan's view that even in the physician's realm, female physicians are considered "less than." Then there was Beth's comment that whether you're a woman who is quietly competent or a woman who speaks out, won't make any difference, because you won't get ahead anyway.

I am becoming more and more aware that feminism and nursing are so bound with each other, it becomes difficult to differentiate the two.

Simon has once again broken his curfew, and I am furious that he hasn't called to leave a message as to his whereabouts. And that room of his—it resembles the state of his hormones. I wonder if this is why most parents are in their forties when their children turn into teenagers; we've had that much more time to practice self-control.

When I returned to the unit from ER tonight, Nealy told me about a nurse from oncology B ward who stuck herself with an AIDS patient's needle. On her third series of tests, she came up positive for HIV. Even though the incident was thoroughly documented, the hospital is refusing all responsibility, and has refused to pay for any further testing. The

nurse, who has been here since 1956, was suspended imme-
diately.

The insomnia god is in his glory tonight, and I can't stop
humming "Melancholy Baby."

FIVE

"To nurse is to tend the flow of life ..."

MARIE THERESE CONNELL, R.N.

MAJESTIC DESPITE ITS ARCHITECTURAL CONFUSIONS, Redwoods Memorial Hospital is a monument to the notion that man's architecture does not have to destroy the landscape. Somehow, the main structure and its four outpatient facilities manage to blend into the palm-studded, California-style hill upon which it sits. Surrounding the 247-bed facility, however, are eight designated-parking areas—wherein lies many a rub.

Lots 1 to 3 are large, well-lit parking areas twenty yards from the hospital entrances. These are specifically for emergency vehicles, physicians, and administrative personnel.

Lots 4 to 6 are designated for visitors only. They are unlit, but easily accessible, only seventy-five yards from the entrances.

Lots 7 and 8 are referred to by the female staff as the Lower Forty, Rapist Haven, Killer's Cove, and Derelict Row. These lots are bordered on one side by the road, and on the other by a square mile of marsh and bird sanctuary that is frequently inhabited by human and nonhuman wildlife. From these areas to the hospital is a long hike, and a dark one at that.

Lots 7 and 8 are for the nursing staff, ninety-seven percent of whom are women. The majority of these women walk to and from their cars after dark. Alone.

The administrative and physician staff are ninety-seven percent male. Most of them leave the hospital before eight in the evening. They have to walk twenty yards to and from their cars in well-lit lots. Alone too. Tsk, tsk.

There came a point during my employment at Redwoods when I stopped parking in Rapist Haven. I'm not sure, but I

92

think it had something to do with the two female employees who had been attacked on the way to their cars, one of them shot by a roaming lunatic.

Right after the shooting, I naively circulated a petition among the female staff demanding safe, close parking, especially for the night and P.M. nurses. It was presented to administration, and five weeks later, the official reply was posted:

Recently it has come to the attention of Redwoods Memorial administration that an increasing number of nursing staff are parking their automobiles in the parking areas designated only for physicians and visitors.

The convenience and safety of our visitors and physicians are the priority of this administration. Be advised that nurses who park outside their designated lots will have their automobiles towed at their expense.

I pulled into lot 5, marked "For Visitors ONLY," and checked my watch: 2:56 P.M. Perfect timing. I had four minutes to run up the hill, through the lobby, up nine flights of stairs, and into CCU.

I gathered my bagged dinner and stethoscope and stepped out of the car into the end of a pointed finger.

"Hey. You work here?" asked the uniformed young man who was attached to the finger jabbing my shoulder. His voice was still cracking, barely broken in. He bared his teeth. Through the smooth mounds of mustard-tinged white bread caught in the wires, his braces sparkled like new.

"Yes, I do. Why?"

"Turn around and get back in that car. Then I want you out of here. Park down in the lower lots." He stopped jabbing, but moved his hand to the top of his nightstick.

"The lower lots are full, sonny." The "sonny" popped out before I could stop myself.

A strange light came into his eyes—violence, perhaps. He didn't say anything for a second or two. It was as if I had punched him.

"Then park over by St. Adolphe's. That's where I'm making the other nurses park."

St. Adolphe's Church was a quarter mile down the road, the same road that also bordered Killer's Cove. I calmly locked the car. Partially ignoring Sonny, who had drawn his nightstick fully out of its sheath, I began to walk—backward—up the steps. One thing I learned during antiwar demonstrations in the sixties was, never turn your back on a man in uniform who has a nightstick in his fist.

"Sonny, at midnight, when you're tucked all safe and cozy in your bed, I'll be getting off work and having to walk to my car in the dark by myself. I'm not going to be an assaulted-nurse statistic. The car stays where it is."

Sonny made a threatening move toward me, the veins in his forehead throbbing with rage. He actually raised his nightstick to nipple level. I decided to wait until it went above shoulder level before I started screaming my guts out.

"They told me I could do anything to keep you nurses out of the doctors' and visitors' parking. Don't be surprised if you don't recognize your car when you get off work tonight, lady." Sonny forced a smile, although his forehead veins were still pumping iron.

Now, I'm not into cars the way some other California people are—acting as if their BMW or Mercedes were their only intended soul mate on earth—but when someone directly threatens the Blue Prince either on or off the road, it gives me pause.

I looked on my old Honda Civic hunchback, with its bruises and growing tumors of rust in the faded blue paint, and felt a tenderness for the vehicle I'd never felt before. "Sonny," I said calmly, "you touch one flake of rust on that car's hood, and you're going to be looking for another job."

"You don't even know my name," Sonny said. One of his fingers kept twitching over the handle of the nightstick.

"Don't need to," I said, hurrying on. "How many security guards work here who are under twenty-five, weigh less than two hundred and fifty pounds, and have pimples *and* a mouth full of silver?"

After I crammed my dinner into the wonders-of-science refrigerator, my muscles tensed the same way everybody else's did when they walked into the hall and looked at the assignment board.

There were several reasons for apprehension. The first concern was whether one was floating or not. The second source of consternation centered around whether one's assignment was too heavy and ultimately unsafe. Third potential problem was the people you were working with—were they helpful and pleasant, or were you working with a Ginger? Even worse than the Ginger types were the fledgling management hopefuls who wrote up their co-workers at the drop of an exam glove. Fourth concern for those of us with injured backs was, did we have one or more patients weighing over two hundred pounds?

My neck, back, and ulcer spasmed with joy—I had four patients on the intermediate side. Pia was in charge; Beth, Nealy, and Risen were with me on the floor. Disneyland, here we come.

Whistling up a breeze, I headed for the report room.

Report is basically a concise exchange of info on each patient, given by the off-going nurses to the on-coming ones. There are several different methods for nurses to give and take report. True to form, Redwoods nursing report procedure was the most inefficient and time-consuming of all.

Each on-coming nurse was required to write down the particulars on every patient whether that patient was assigned to her or not. Therefore, it was not unusual to end up with two pages of written information on a patient you would never see.

It had once been a practice at CCU that charge nurses were required to look over each nurse's notes to make sure she or he hadn't been slack in taking down every detail. It was reminiscent of grade school, complete with a red-penciled "OK" or "PAY MORE ATTENTION" written on the top of the report sheet. The remedial report routine ended, however, when the patients began to complain about the nurses being unavailable for so long at shift change.

Report was more often than not a dreary and boring affair, made even more unbearable if the reporting-off nurse was long-winded or the on-coming nurse was inexperienced and asked a lot of useless, nonpertinent questions. ("Does this patient have any cousins named Belinski who were in the meatpacking business in Iowa?")

From the amount of laughter and smiling going on in report, it was clear that for once the patient assignments were evenly distributed. The day shift charge nurse was one of the relaxed, more intelligent souls who didn't believe in antiquated rules or wasting time. She gave each of us a concise report on our patients, while Pia, as on-coming charge nurse, was the only one who had to take report on everyone.

There was a brief show-and-tell after report was over. Risen told us about the latest exhibition of his paintings at Cunningham's Gallery, Beth said she was depressed and wanted to kill herself because of premenstrual bloat, Pia showed us a photo of herself dressed in formal riding habit, accepting an award at a dressage event, Nealy told us about her youngest's chickenpox, and I displayed my most recent photograph of Mooshie, lying on his side with six stuffed toy mice lined up along his belly, apparently at suck.

I laughed until I wheezed. The others simply sat and stared, their expressions full of grave doubt.

Clara Tuttle's long and bony fingers slowly wound themselves around my hand. The coarse and yellowed fingernails didn't seem to belong to the fragile white fingers.

There was an imperceptible pulling at my arm.

"Tell me," I whispered, leaning down, my arm grazing the tent her legs made under the covers. Her head twisted on the sweat-drenched pillow, the sound of her distress coming closer to my ear. She stopped writhing long enough to look at me—or through me. She was too much bone, the rest all eyes and hair. Her anguish made the pit of my stomach contract.

With the advance of her liver cancer, her dark yellow skin was tight to her skull, her face already a death mask of yellow clay. A single tear rolled down the hollow of her cheek in slow motion.

"Help me," she said in a voice that was barely a sigh. "Please get something for the pain." It cost her to breathe. Her body twisted in a spasm of pain as her bluish lips distorted into a silent cry.

The sob became audible behind me. I turned around to locate the source of the sound and found Ruth, Mrs. Tuttle's daughter, withdrawn into her father's arms, crying.

I took the dying woman's vital signs: BP 180 over 70, heart rate 110 and irregular, respiratory rate 44, oral temp 102.5. Furious with the floor nurses for not adequately medicating the woman before she was transferred to CCU, I searched the med sheet for the time and amount of her last dose of pain medication, and found nothing.

"What the hell . . . ?" I glanced over at Mr. Tuttle and his daughter and excused myself from the room. At the nursing station, I scrutinized the chart again, page by page. Zippo. Not one standing pain medication order had been written for the entire seven days she had been in the hospital. Not only that, but Dr. York had purposely canceled the CCU standing orders for morphine and Demerol. I skimmed through the pain assessment columns in the nursing notes.

"Pt. requesting pain medication. Called Dr. York for order. Order refused."

"Pt. appears to be in severe generalized pain. States 'it hurts all over.' At daughter's insistence, Dr. York called for pain order. Request for IM morphine refused. Oral acetaminophen with codeine ordered. Pt. unable to swallow tablets due to ulcerated throat."

And yet again: "Pt. has continued increasing discomfort in throat, lower abdomen, and low back. Disphoretic, BP 170/100. Requested med order from Dr. York. Dr. states 'the pain is all in her head.' Dr. York refusing at this time to give order for pain medication."

Every day for the first week, the columns had similar remarks, until suddenly there was no reference at all to Dr. York, only that the patient has ongoing and unrelieved pain that centered in her abdomen and ulcerated throat.

I stopped reading and my thoughts at once went to Jan Tobin, the young CCU nurse who died not many years before of Hodgkin's disease. As my mentor and closest friend, she had often confided in me during the final months of her illness that the pain from her ulcerated throat was almost unbearable.

There was a light, fluttery touch at my back. Behind me stood Mrs. Tuttle's tearful daughter. Her too small white cardigan sweater had slipped off one shoulder, revealing a wrinkled pink blouse.

"Please get my mother something for pain," she pleaded. "This can't go on. The person in that bed isn't my mother."

I readjusted her sweater and guided her into the deserted kitchen. Under the bright fluorescent lights, the thick blue veins that marred the backs of her legs were plainly visible. It was easy to imagine her as the night-shift waitress at Bob's Truck Stop.

"I don't understand what's going on," I said, leaning against the refrigerator. "Why isn't your mother receiving any pain medication?"

Ruth Tuttle wrung her hands. Her anxious, tortured expression was one I'd seen a thousand times on the faces of patients and family alike; it was part of the I-can't-stand-what's-going-on-but-I-don't-want-to-rock-the-boat syndrome.

"I don't like to complain," she said, barely above a whisper.

"Complain." I smiled wanly. "This is your mother we're talking about here, plus your parents and their insurance company are paying a bundle for this hospitalization. You have every right in the world to complain."

"If I tell you what's happened, will you promise not to say anything? I mean, do as much as you can, but be"—the woman winced apologetically—"discreet. I don't want anyone to get into trouble because of me."

"What you say isn't going to change how I need to handle this situation," I said. "I'm obligated to question Dr. York as to why your mother has been denied pain medication. That she's been allowed to suffer at all, let alone this long, is a serious error. I can't let this just slip by."

Ruth nodded, letting her arms fall to her sides. "The pain has been horrible. For over two weeks my father and I have pleaded with Dr. York to give her something for it, but he refuses."

"Have you asked him why he's refusing?"

"He says . . ." Ruth's mouth drew tight. "He says he's the doctor and he'll be the one to determine when she really needs drugs. He said that if we start questioning his judgment, we can get ourselves another doctor—if we could find one—to step in and take care of Mom.

"I don't know what to think. Dr. York has been Mom's doctor for twenty years and I guess he feels that he—" Ruth stopped, afraid she had said too much. She shook her head.

"Come on, tell me," I urged. "Get it out."

"Oh, this is probably all wrong," she said after a pause, "but I think he's angry with himself for messing up. See, Mom went to him a couple of years ago because she felt tired all the time. If you knew Mom, you'd know that was really out of character for her—she never liked to complain about anything."

I nodded. Like mother, like daughter—a bequeathment of codependency.

"Dr. York gave her a sample of iron tablets and told her she'd be fine and not to worry."

Ruth stopped to pass a hand over her face, as if she were tormented anew by old painful memories. "Six months later, she couldn't even walk to the bathroom without getting tired, and her liver hurt her all the time. One day my father finally just carried her out to the car and drove her to Dr. York's office, demanding that he find out what was wrong.

"Dad said Dr. York wasn't happy about it, but agreed to take some blood tests. When they left, he told my dad that Mom's problems were all in her head.

"I was so furious when Dad told me what happened, that I called Dr. York myself."

I watched Ruth's fingers work over the sleeve of her sweater. It was stretched out so far, it looked like a bell-bottom cuff.

"I told him he had to be blind not to see how sick Mom was."

Still stinging with indignation, the woman put a hand on her hip. "Do you know what he did?"

Even though I could well imagine, I shook my head.

"He got upset with *me*. He said I needed to see a psychiatrist and find out why I wanted my mother to be sick, because she wasn't and he knew better than I did what was really going on.

"And when my mother's lab tests came back? He said, 'Well, Clara, you've really gotten yourself into a mess this time.' Like it was *her* fault! He never said he was sorry, or mentioned anything about putting her off for so long. It was like we'd never consulted him before.

"When we asked him for some details about what was happening, he told us it was too complicated for us to understand, and that he was the doctor and to leave everything to him."

Sudden outrage caused me to bite a new hole through my tooth guard. "Did he refer your mom to an oncologist or suggest you get another opinion?"

"I asked about a specialist, but Dr. York assured us he could do everything they could. Dad and I felt okay about that until this difficulty with getting Mom medicine for pain."

When I regained some composure, I forced a smile. "For future reference, this—" I had to stop myself from saying "asshole," lest I sound too unprofessional. "This physician is working for you, not vice versa. Your family, and especially your mother, have rights, the first of which is to have every detail of your mother's illness—cause to treatment—explained to you until you understand and can be *part* of the decision-making team about what's best for her. Dr. York is obligated to listen to you and work with you.

"Your mother needs pain medication. The nurses have documented that fact every day since she's been here. It's also documented that Dr. York has consistently refused to write any orders for pain medications.

"Right now my primary concern is making sure Clara is pain-free."

Ruth lowered her eyes, all guilty humility. I would have bet that the caption under her high school yearbook photo read, "Sweet Baby Ruth."

"Tell me," I said, talking more to myself than Ruth, "why is it people allow themselves to be treated so shabbily by some doctors? It's almost as if they just hand over their bodies and go deaf, dumb, and blind."

"I don't know." Ruth shook her head. "Fear, I guess. We aren't trained in medicine—we don't know what's right and what isn't. Most people think that if they don't trust their doctor, they'll be lost."

"But don't people realize that they have more than one choice of doctor?" I asked.

"It's too expensive and complicated to change doctors," answered Ruth. "Plus, the doctor you started out with always makes you feel so *guilty*."

I studied Ruth for a moment. If she continued to be cowed by Dr. York, and allowed her mother to suffer, she would struggle with her anger and guilt long after her mother was dead.

I held the kitchen door open.

"Okay, first of all, I'm going to get your mother medicated with or without York's consent. Second of all, trust your own instincts. Dr. York isn't God, nor is he the only doctor in the sea. There are other competent doctors who will really *hear* what you and your dad have to say."

I studied Ruth's dubious expression and smiled confidently. "Remember, *you're* the ones in charge."

The female voice that came from the other end of the receiver conjured up a mental image of Roseanne Barr playing a humorless anal retentive.

"Dr. Bradley York's medical suites."

I snorted. Dr. York had three tiny rooms in a dingy office building. "Dr. York's medical suites? What, did you acquire another closet or something?"

"May I help you?" The question was curt, the voice frigid, British butler–like.

"This is Redwoods CCU. Is the doc available?"

"Which of *Doctor* York's patients does this regard?"

I had the urge to ask if he actually had more than one, but curbed it. "Mrs. Tuttle."

There was an irritated moan and a weary "Oh, not again," then a click.

I waited, listening to the hollow, soundless void of hold. Dr. York's office wasn't up with the times—most doctors' phone systems now played such great music during their holds that I actually resented it when someone came back on the line.

"This had better not be about pain medication," was how Dr. York answered the phone. It was an old tactic used by some physicians to intimidate the nurse.

"It certainly *is* about pain medication, doctor." This was the nurse's you're-not-dealing-with-a-weak-hoho return. "I'd like an order for morphine. Mrs. Tuttle is in a lot of pain. Her vitals are coming off the ceiling. We need to give this woman some relief."

"You've been talking to the daughter. Don't be taken in by her." Dr. York lowered his voice in a way that gave the impression he was taking me into his confidence. I got the feeling he thought it would help me trust him. "That woman has been trying to get narcotics for her mother since day one. If you ask me, I think she wants her mother out of the way so she can get her hands on the estate."

"I don't believe that's the case, Dr. York. The patient herself has asked for something. She's in acute discomfort."

"Oh come now, let's not exaggerate." He chuckled faintly *at* me. He definitely had his intimidation techniques down pat. "I was there all day, and the patient didn't exhibit any signs of being in pain."

I was astounded by his lie. He must be desperate to protect himself, I thought, desperate enough to keep a dying woman in agony. "Okay, well, I can only tell you what I've observed since I came on at three P.M., and that is that this woman is in severe pain."

"It's probably gas, or hysteria at being moved to the CCU from the floor. It'll pass."

"Excuse me, doctor, but I don't think it's going to pass. This is high-scale distress and I'd like—"

"This is gas," he insisted. "Don't get dramatic."

Not only was he desperate but in denial, too. I decided to try some intimidation myself.

"Dr. Ostermann has seen her briefly," I lied, "and agrees that this pain needs to be treated ASAP."

There was a pause and then a sigh. "Boy, you people really get taken in by these hysterical women, don't you?"

Hysterical women. I'd heard this phrase a million times in my career. There were still doctors who considered all women hysterics, not to be taken seriously. Prescribe some Xanax or a couple of antidepressants, give an encouraging word and a pat on the back, then send them home to a hot-water bottle.

"Clara Tuttle has terminal cancer. She isn't hysterical, except with the pain she's had for weeks. I'd like a morphine order, backed up with a Demerol order, Dr. York."

The man laughed gleefully. "Well, you're not going to get it. You CCU people are spoiled. You give morphine out like it's water. I don't want Mrs. Tuttle snowed."

"The nurses here are concerned about her pain," I said firmly, unable to control the volume of my voice. This caused Pia to peer over the monitors, and Risen to stop in the hall. Nealy finished washing her hands and leaned against the sink to listen. "That's our job, to keep a dying woman pain-free. I want a morphine order from you for this patient, or I'm going to notify my supervisor and then go to the director of the unit."

"Ah, Christ!" he spat into the receiver. "Give her subcutaneous codeine thirty milligrams, one time only."

The connection was broken with a loud click. Pia, Nealy, and Risen waited expectantly.

"SQ codeine thirty milligrams," I said, "one time order."

We all knew that thirty milligrams of codeine might do for a headache, but for Mrs. Tuttle, it was like expecting a fly to carry away Mount McKinley.

Risen was incredulous. "Man, what *is* this weenie's problem?"

"He's an incompetent bastard," I said.

"*Who's* an incompetent bastard?"

Dr. Ostermann, grinning from ear to ear as usual, came in and sat down, waiting for the rest of the joke. I squinted and decided this was his real smile. With him it was hard to tell, since a grin was part of his normal facial expression.

After I'd told him everything that had happened, I asked that the usual CCU standing orders for morphine be reinstated.

Dr. Ostermann raised his shoulders and put out his hands. Instead of a cardiologist, he looked more like a Jewish grocer from the Lower East Side telling me he was out of knishes and gefilte fish. "What do you want me to do? I'm only the consulting doctor. He's the primary."

I groaned and squeezed my hands into hard fists. "Please don't do this, Harry. We need an order for some pain control here."

"I can't do that."

"Why," I asked, sensing his ambivalence, "can't you do what it seems like you want to do?"

"I don't have the right to be ordering drugs for York's patient unless it's for cardiac problems."

I sat down next to him. "Harry, the woman is suffering. Imagine that's your mother or your wife. We can't sit here and let her die like this."

"Okay, okay," he said, finally, "I'll call York." He refused to look at me, but reached for the phone.

I ran to the narcotics cabinet.

Dr. Ostermann tapped his pen against his pepper-and-salt sideburn, while waiting for Dr. York to come on the line.

"Hi Brad, Harry. On this Tuttle woman, the nurses think she needs some pain medication."

My heart sank. I opened my mouth to protest, but Dr. Ostermann held up his hand.

"I don't know about that, Bradley. I just came out of there and I agree she's in quite a bit of pain. How about if I order some MS?"

There was a pause. Dr. Ostermann rested his cheek on his hand, and said, "Uhn huh" a few times.

Ever hopeful, I unlocked the cabinet and signed out a syringe of morphine to Mrs. Tuttle.

"Well, okay," he said, and hung up.

"How much can I start with?" I asked, flicking the air bubbles to the end of the syringe.

"Bradley is a fan of Mrs. Reagan's. He said no to drugs."

Dumbstruck, I gripped the rounded back of the chair and sat down hard. "Jesus Christ, why?"

"He says he doesn't want to confuse matters."

"Confuse matters!" My voice was headed upward. "Confuse *what* matters?"

"I don't know—something about wanting to make sure her mentation is clear, because he thinks she might have metastasis to the brain." Dr. Ostermann heaved a sigh and rubbed his temples. "I don't know what the hell he was talking about."

"Brain metastasis?" I screamed. "This woman has brain metastasis like Queen Elizabeth has poverty. Harry, she's been like this for two weeks!"

My temper was blinding me, getting in the way of my judgment. I looked to Pia for help.

"Hey, Ec, do what you gotta do," Pia said. "Go for broke."

I picked up the phone Dr. Ostermann had just set down. It was still warm from his hand. "Nurses have certain protocols to follow in order to protect their patients, Harry. If I can't get a pain order for my patient, I'll call the supervisor and the medical director at home and explain what's happened."

I punched two numbers, waiting a long time between punches, giving him time to think about it. "You can save me some time and yourself some questions by ordering the MS now instead of having the chief of medicine do it for you."

I punched two more numbers.

"Okay, okay already." Dr. Ostermann scowled. "But give the subcutaneous codeine first. Wait a few minutes—then she can have up to fifteen milligrams of IV MS an hour until her pain is relieved."

I hugged him and gave him a quick kiss on the back of the neck.

Dr. Ostermann fought to retain his scowl. "Oh yeah, sure, *now* you're nice. Where were the hugs when I was facing Brad babe? . . . York is going to blow his top. You can bet he's going to cancel this order as soon as he comes in, so give the MS as quickly as you can without killing the woman."

I sailed past Ruth and Mr. Tuttle, gave the codeine, counted to three and injected four milligrams of IV MS. Within ten minutes, Mrs. Tuttle's body relaxed, the pain held at bay. Her BP went down to 150 over 60, her heart rate slowed to 100, but her respirations stayed high at 36 per minute.

Ruth and I each held one of the spindly hands. Mr. Tuttle sat at the end of her bed massaging his wife's feet. Clara's breathing made a light, dry noise, like autumn leaves blowing around a sidewalk.

I wiped away the sweat from her pale forehead, and her eyes fluttered open.

"God bless you," she whispered. Her voice seemed to leak into the air. She was so weak, there didn't seem to be enough of her left to still be alive.

I gave her another four milligrams of MS an hour later, and when I was certain Mrs. Tuttle was completely pain-free, gently rolled her to each side of the bed while I changed the sweat-drenched sheets one side at a time.

Ruth and her father helped me bathe the skeletal body. Ruth

deftly sponged her mother with the warm, soapy water and Mr. Tuttle dried and powdered. They paid attention to the small details: taking care that their hands were warm, not rubbing too hard at the paper-thin skin, and was this the brand of powder she liked so much?

Mr. Tuttle, flushed and bent like an old red maple, touched my shoulder after we finished our tender chores. His gnarled hand was spotted with old bruises and badly chapped. "We will never forget you for this," he said kindly. "No sir. Never forget what you did here."

I blushed, not knowing what to say. Nothing great or unusual had been done; Mrs. Tuttle had simply been given what was rightfully hers—freedom from pain.

When the door opened and someone came in, I didn't even have to turn around to know who it was. Dr. York's presence was so heavy with hostility, it filled the room instantaneously. He wore a dour expression with a full-lipped pout. The look was so exaggerated, his lips resembled two hot dogs pressed together.

Ignoring the three of us, he leaned over Mrs. Tuttle. "Clara!" he shouted, and roughly jiggled her arm. Mrs. Tuttle moaned and stubbornly pulled away from his grasp like a child not wanting to get up for school.

He turned to me, his face full of injured pride. "Well, I see you've managed to snow her. You purposefully went over my authority to get that morphine order." He glared at me as though I were a street person caught peddling drugs to innocent children.

Before I could answer, his accusing eyes shifted to Ruth. "Is this how you want your mother to be when she dies? A doped-up dummy?"

Ruth shrank back from the man and sat down on the edge of her mother's bed, hidden from his view by me.

"It beats being in agony, Dr. York," I said. "Mrs. Tuttle's vitals are a lot more stable now, and she's comfortable. I think the morphine could have been safely administered several weeks ago."

Dr. York's color deepened. "She didn't need that stuff weeks ago, just as it wasn't warranted today."

"Now that's not true!" Ruth stood, getting right up in the man's face. "My mother has been in the worst pain I've ever seen. Dad and I have watched her suffer for months. You don't know what we've been through . . ." Ruth faltered, lowered her voice. "You just don't know."

Dr. York seemed lost, and when he spoke, anybody could tell the fire was out. "You were determined to question my judgment, weren't you?"

The room went quiet. Dr. York was using his last bit of power by challenging her. I didn't dare look at Ruth, but in my mind, I begged her not to back down.

"I think Dr. Ostermann's direction to give my mother morphine was the best thing to do." Ruth spoke in a small voice, but it was a voice.

Dr. York stiffened as though she'd slapped him. There was a pause; he looked at me, then over at Mr. Tuttle, and finally back at Ruth. He snorted in disgust. We were the conspirators. Against the three of us, he wasn't going to win and he knew it.

His leather shoes squeaked as he walked to the door. "Fine," he said. His voice was harsh, but his face was impassive. "If that's the way you want it, I'm taking myself off this case and signing your mother over to Dr. Ostermann." He threw me a withering glance. "Let strangers take care of your mother."

For a second Ruth looked like she was going to crumple. She began to say something apologetic, then changed her mind.

"Twenty years," Dr. York mumbled, so we could all just barely hear him. Hanging his head, he searched the floor as if he were looking for a lost ticket. He then glanced once more at his sleeping patient and left the room.

Ruth was miserable with remorse. "I shouldn't have done that," she said.

"Yes you should have," said Mr. Tuttle, shuffling to his wife's bedside. "You did the right thing, Ruthie. The fellow didn't know what he was doing. . . . Clara?"

She opened her eyes and smiled up at his familiar face. Their hands met and clasped on top of the covers.

"Clara? We fired Dr. York. What do you think about that?"

Clara closed her eyes. "Oh good," she murmured weakly. "He was such an ass."

Osbert was his real name. Most people called him Oz, but those of us in CCU knew him as Risen.

The nickname came about on one particularly slow night

shift around three-thirty A.M., when Osbert decided to sneak into a vacant bed for a quick snooze.

Dozing on the job, even when one had nothing to do, was a major infraction of the nursing rules and regulations. Thus, to ensure himself fifteen minutes of undisturbed sleep without being caught, Osbert pulled the curtains all the way around the room and covered himself from head to toe with a sheet.

Earlier in the shift, a patient had expired on the intermediate side, and it wasn't until 3:35 A.M. that the overworked night orderly remembered he had a morgue pickup in CCU. Not wanting to draw attention to his slackness, the tardy orderly didn't check with the nurses as to where the departed soul lay, but located the body on his own. Without making a sound, he pulled the sleeping Osbert onto the morgue wagon with such gentle respect, the nurse's slumber was not disturbed.

Osbert figured he would have spent the rest of the night in the cold file had it not been for a dream he was having about being trapped in an elevator that was falling. He jerked himself awake and sat up with a gasp.

"It was a real trip," he related to us later, "to come out of this deep sleep and find myself actually in the elevator of my dream, and not only that, but lying on the morgue wagon with the orderly pressed against the doors screaming, 'He is risen! He is risen!' "

I thought of this story while eating my final salad of the day in the nurses' lounge. Because I usually ate salad three times a day, I sometimes coped with mealtime boredom by pretending I was a cow or some other bovine creature grazing on pieces of endive or romaine. Risen's presence had given me something other than cows to think about.

The thought of the orderly's face as Risen rose, brought forth a burst of laughter which caused a piece of endive to fly out of my mouth and land on Risen's scrub top.

He looked down, saw the wild piece of lettuce on his shirt, flicked it off without so much as a glance at me, and went back to devouring the gray hockey puck of a hamburger that smelled like a by-product from one of Pia's horses.

"Prices in this cafeteria are outrageous," he whined. "This burger, twenty prefrozen fries, and a cup of tepid tea cost me six-fifty. Can you believe that? It really puts my knickers in a twist."

"Don't most hospital cafeterias give their employees

a discount on meals?" I asked, knowing full well that Redwoods was one of the only hospitals in the area that didn't.

Risen was quick to jump on the complaint department bandwagon. "This hospital eats kitty litter. They're such cheapskates. Last week when the unit was slow, I requested a day off—begged was more like it—but they turned me down, then floated me out to ICU.

"Then ICU gives me two total-isolation patients with raging serratia infections, plus a fresh craniotomy. I complained first of all that I didn't think it was too swift an idea to be mixing contagious patients with fresh postoperative ones.

"They told me if my isolation techniques were good, nothing would get transferred. Right?

"Okay, then I told them that I didn't feel comfortable caring for the serratia patients, because I was on steroids for some out-of-control allergies and was too immunosuppressed to be taking chances with such a contagious bacterial infection.

"They said, and I quote the exact words used by the charge nurse, 'Tough shit, Ozzie.' " Risen's nostrils flared in indignation.

"Six hours into the shift, after I'm up to my eyeballs in serratia, the supervisor comes in to tell me CCU got three admits and they're pulling me out of ICU.

"I told them to stick it. I said if the nursing office would let CCU staff the shifts with a little bit of margin, they wouldn't have to be running around the hospital pulling back CCU nurses from hither and yon."

I nodded in agreement and we were both quiet for a while. Risen leaned his chair so far back, my knees got weak just from watching. After a moment, an expression came over his face that was a strange combination of amusement, embarrassment, wonder, and smug disapproval.

"Some of the nurses and a couple of the docs were talking about your book last week," he said.

Boom.

I refused to give in and ask the obvious question. Risen was one of the worst gossips in the hospital, so I waited, knowing there would be more to come. I took another bite of salad and chewed, bovine-faced.

"They think they need to be careful around you or they'll end up in a book or being discussed on radio or TV." Risen laughed and got to his feet. "God, if I were in your shoes, I'd be blowing people's covers left and right."

I remained impassive and grazing, making believe I was a Guernsey cow; I was hoping he would go on to name names. Instead, he stood at the mirror and began combing his thinning reddish hair with one of those black pocket combs that only men use. I could see he wasn't looking where he was combing, but rather studying me in the mirror, measuring me up for his next question.

"Do you know Beth very well?"

"Why?" I asked. "Do you want to ask her out?"

This was a joke—everyone knew Risen was gay.

The tall, thin nurse rolled his eyes, turned out his hip, and executed a limp-wrist wave. "Tsk, not *really*, dahling. It's just that you two seemed so chummy, I thought you might know what was going on."

"What do you mean?" Risen had won my full attention; I stopped grazing.

"Tonight I helped her turn Mr. Elgin, and the smell of alcohol—I believe it was Jack Daniel's—almost knocked me over. I know it wasn't Mr. Elgin, because he's one of those Vedanta Society purists.

"And then, did you see her out at the desk? Right in front of God and everybody, she's sitting there squirting Binaca every five minutes like it's gourmet cuisine or something. Honestly, I thought I'd drop."

I looked away, faking indifference for fear he would see my distress. "Oh Risen, maybe she had a beer at lunch or something. You know how one beer can stay on people's breath for hours."

"Believe me, this was more than beer. Besides, it isn't the first time I've smelled it on her. The other night she was positively bleary-eyed." He patted the hair down over his bald spot and checked his teeth for burger bits. "I think I'll say something to her if I notice it again."

Risen came to the table and began emptying his pockets of the usual leftovers nurses always carry with them—pens, alcohol wipes, germicidal pads, paper clips, foil packets of this or that skin barrier, sealed syringes, rubber bands, Band-Aids, gauze pads, rubber gloves. The pile was familiar. Like most nurses, I too had a basketful of this odd pocket loot at home.

"Did you know Mattie over on four south?" He idly chose a few items to return to his pockets.

"What do you mean, *did* I know her?" I asked, immediately alert to disaster. Had Killer Cove claimed another victim?

"She's been fired."

"What?" I sat up. Mattie was an institution at Redwoods. She'd been a nurse on the medical floors since the days of white support hose and nursing caps.

Risen heaved a dramatic sigh and fluttered his eyes, overjoyed to be able to tell the story—probably for the sixth time that evening. "You know how nurses are forever bringing home all this garbage?" Risen indicated his pile of nurse leavings. "Well, she decided a hundred pens and five pounds of alcohol wipes were a bit much, so she put all of it in a paper bag and brought it back to the hospital.

"There she was in the elevator headed to four south, when Heidi, the day supervisor who happens to be riding up with her, asks what's in the bag. Thinking she would get some Brownie points, Mattie told her what was in it and what she was doing with it."

In a typical Risen move, he held up a finger, twirled around into the bathroom, urinated, and came out with a length of toilet paper hanging from his shirt pocket.

"The next day, they fired her for pilfering," he said, picking up where he left off. "Not only that, but they waited until she got to work to fire her in a major show of public humiliation."

I must have gone scarlet with rage, because Risen gave my back a pat and laughed.

"Now, now, don't get your knickers all in a twist, Ec. Mattie's no doormat. She's taking Redwoods to court. My guess is, she'll not only win but be rewarded damages for the public humiliation."

"What is wrong with these people?" I asked, wondering at management's stupidity. "Why do they continue to try and beat us down?"

"Hey, *you're* the one who said it, Ec—power, control, and money. It's the name of the game."

It was eight P.M. when the announcement came over the public address system that visiting hours were over on all nursing units. Thank you and good night.

Mr. Knapp, my forty-seven-year-old postarrest patient, walked his wife and young daughter to the double exit doors.

I looked on from the other side of the monitor banks, where I was relieving Pia for dinner.

With one hand on the door, Mrs. Knapp, a svelte blonde in her late thirties, leaned over and kissed her husband lightly on the mouth. She pulled back a little and smiled at him; it was a smile of seduction and promise.

I hoped the nurse educator had told them they had to take it easy his first week at home. However, when Mr. Knapp pulled his wife against him and returned a long and passionate kiss, I guessed that that part of the educational program had been overlooked.

"I love you," Mr. Knapp said earnestly, holding her eyes.

My throat swelled and I had to look away before I began to cry. *That* is what I want for my life, I thought. A friend and lover who would hold me with his eyes.

"Tomorrow," she said, still smiling that easy, sensual smile.

"Tomorrow," he said.

He gave his daughter a quick kiss on the top of the head and called her "Pumpkin Sweet." Then he waited until the doors closed behind them. He waved through the porthole windows, watching after them until the last pink frill of Pumpkin Sweet's dress disappeared around the corner.

He turned and swaggered to the monitor banks, his joy plainly visible.

"My wife and daughter," he announced proudly.

"They're beautiful."

"Yep." He nodded and looked back toward the doors as if the image of them still lingered there. "It's my birthday tomorrow," he said suddenly.

"Hey, great birthday gift—you get to go home."

"Better than that even. I'm *alive* and I get to go home."

He was right about that. Three weeks before, he had come in after having a cardiac arrest on the tennis courts. He stayed unresponsive and on a respirator for the first week. His heart had sustained enough damage, and his condition had been so unstable, we didn't expect him to live.

But, to paraphrase Buddha, there's never any telling, is there?

"Do you have any questions about your treadmill test tomorrow morning, Mr. Knapp?"

"Nope. I'm going to walk until Dr. Cramer gets tired or the treadmill wears out—whichever comes first. After that, I'm out of here and home to some real private-duty nursing care."

Mr. Knapp wiggled his eyebrows, did a Jackie Gleason "And—away—we—go" deep knee bend, and disappeared from sight behind the counter with a thud.

I giggled at his antics, hoping he hadn't banged his knee too badly. Keeping this guy on his slow-buildup exercise program was going to be a major problem; he was the type who'd probably try to play a vigorous game of tennis his second day home.

My attention was drawn by the red monitor alarms. On the narrow strip of screen representing Mr. Knapp was the jagged, snakelike line of ventricular fibrillation.

Doubtful about what I was seeing, I called his name and checked the wide-angle mirror on the wall. Mr. Knapp, looking like a heap of old laundry, lay motionless under the monitor desk.

At that instant, Beth shot out of room 9, did a double take, and ran toward his crumpled body, grabbing the crash cart on the way. I dialed the emergency operator and informed her there was a code blue in CCU.

Two seconds after I hung up, the PA system came to life. *"Attention all personnel. Code blue, heart unit."*

On my way around the desk, I made a silent prayer that Mrs. Knapp was out of the building. At least she could have another half hour of peace before we shattered her world.

Beth and I turned Mr. Knapp over onto his back and yanked the gown away from his chest. Out of habit I felt for a pulse, although I knew there would be none. Beth gave the precordial thump while I forced the green plastic airway into his mouth. With the mask of the bag–valve device firmly in place, I tilted back his head and forced oxygen into his lungs.

Risen and Pia ran to assist. Risen attached the cart monitor's electrodes to Mr. Knapp's chest; Pia had straddled him and was doing chest compressions in synch with the forced respirations. Every so often she would stop and stare first at him, then at the monitor, searching for signs of life. Nealy immediately greased the defibrillator paddles and charged the machine.

We were waiting the eternity of three seconds for the defibrillator to charge to 360 watts when the double doors burst open and the rest of the code team rushed in.

All of us gave our best, working to save a life that had already eluded us. We did everything possible there was to do. And yet, when it was over, all of us were somber and guilty, straining our minds to think of that one thing we could have done to save him.

When I helped lift his body to the morgue wagon, I forced myself to remember that it wasn't part of our job to worry about what we could have done to change the outcome after the fact. Our job was only to do our best until the decision was made for us.

Dr. Ostermann made the call to Mrs. Knapp. While we listened in on the tragedy unfolding over the phone, we pretended to be busy: Beth and I restocked the cart and cleaned away the mess; Risen and Nealy charted; Pia watched monitors and filled out the staffing request for night shift.

He asked her first if someone was there with her.

Her sister. Good.

Then he told her right out in one long, rushed, unpunctuated sentence: "We've had some trouble here after you left we did everything we could to save your husband but I'm afraid he was gone before we ..."

We heard the confusion and then the scream—a high, thin wail—come from the earpiece.

"I'm so sorry, I'm so sorry, I'm so sorry," Dr. Ostermann said slowly over and over in a low, almost inaudible tone.

But we knew no one was listening except us.

At 10:45 P.M., Mrs. Tuttle's heart sped up, slowed down, did an irregular bump-and-grind routine, then stopped.

Thanks to Dr. Ostermann, she had been made a no-code patient, which meant we were to let her go in peace. No useless heroics. Nothing to be disappointed over later.

I called Dr. Ostermann at home to tell him. He was quiet for a long time. I could feel his depression through the phone.

"Let me call the family," I said softly. "I think the daughter would like to hear it from me. You go to bed. I'll have the ER doc pronounce her."

"You're a good kid," he said, and hung up.

Without warning, I began to cry. Risen stopped charting and put his arm around me. Beth did the same from the other side. Nealy leaned against Beth, and after a minute, Pia came out from behind the monitors and put her long arms around us all.

That was how night shift found us—our heads all resting together in mourning for those we could not save.

* * *

Wednesday
1:30 A.M.

One more day to go and then I have three days off in a row. I am so exhausted, I can't even think straight, and if this migraine doesn't kill me, my backache will.

I wonder what Mrs. Knapp is doing right now. How will she tell Pumpkin Sweet? Instead of making love tonight, she will be planning a funeral. She has lost her passionate, smiling hero. How many times have I seen the spouses limp away, the walking wounded? Yes, I know—her pain of today will be softened slowly, slowly until it becomes only the memory of pain.

Okay, I think I see what is to be learned here: Live for today, moment to moment. Expectations always disappoint you.

I wrote an incident report on Dr. York and put it on file in Annie's office. Let's see how far this gets. There are seven witnesses, including one physician and two Normal People. It's sad to know that if the nurses were the only witnesses, the incident report wouldn't carry an ounce of weight.

Waiting for night report to be over, I wrote: "Why? What is the answer?" and handed the question to Beth. Her reply was: "Still working on it. Hindered by current equipment and insufficient information. Maybe to continue to make an effort to love."

Beth. What to do. Should I confront her, tell her that people have noticed? My instinct tells me to exercise my patience.

I was going to ground Simon for not meeting curfew again last night, but I felt ridiculous looking up into the face of this man who towers over me and outweighs me by thirty pounds, and telling him to go to his room. Maybe I could take his electric razor away for a week?

Tonight in that circle of arms all I could think of was that we are such a family. I love the security of our understanding of one another. I love these gentle, caring people who see death every day and still laugh. Peer support when the ship is sinking is comforting; you know you won't go down alone.

I'm paranoid after what Risen told me. I have noticed that people seem uneasy around me in the unit. Are they avoiding me, wondering if the writer side of me is storing up derogatory things about them? I thought it was my deodorant failing.

Two questions of the day: Do penguins get barnacles on the bottom of their feet? And is it really fair for deaf people to play charades with the hearing?

Oh yes—happy birthday, Mr. Knapp.

SIX

> *"What sets the critical care nurse apart is the ability to size up the situation within thirty-two seconds and take care of it before anyone else even knows what's happened."*
>
> LINDA STONE, R.N.

IT WAS ONE OF THOSE "OFF" DAYS where everybody I saw walked with a limp or had purple hair. Even the old-timers hanging around downtown were out in force, wearing their phosphorescent lime-green polyesters and natty brown wing tips.

Simon wasn't quite himself either. His asthma, which we all thought he'd outgrown, had come back for a visit, and not only that—I found him watching a rerun of *The Price is Right* at ten A.M., utterly entranced. True, his choice might have been influenced by the young woman contestant who—enthusiastically heeding the command of "Come on down!"—bounced down the steps, revealing all to a cheering TV audience as her tank top slid down around her waist.

Even though this incident gave new meaning to the term "boob tube," I still thought it was a strange choice of programs for an adolescent who *never* watched television except when Jimi Hendrix or Woodstock specials were aired.

Nor had Mooshie escaped the strangeness of the day. On my way to the mailbox, I discovered him in sitting position, back leaning against the Honda's rear tire, with a well-chewed stalk of fresh catnip half hidden under his stocky Burmese body. He was drooling.

Among the bills were three letters forwarded by my publisher from people who had read *Intensive Care* and were writing to say they had applied to nursing school.

There was another letter from a reader, which was sent to my actual address. (God only knows how she managed to get *that*. In certain postal circles, I'm known as Echo Salinger.) It was from a woman who claimed to have God's mouth at her ear. She wrote to say she had read the book and liked it, but advised me to pray *real* hard to Jesus for forgiveness and divine guidance. If I did that, she went on, He *might* forgive me for writing such blatantly sinful and Satan-loving blasphemy.

To the people who had applied to nursing school, I wrote to suggest perhaps they should read the book again, paying special attention to the parts about the rigors of nursing school and the ulcer-causing effects of same. If they still wanted to join up after rereading those parts, well, hell, welcome aboard, you crazy fools.

I sealed up the letter from the woman who admonished me for being Satan's tool, and crossed out my address with a flame-red Magic Marker. Next to that, I printed: "RETURN TO SENDER. ADDRESSEE GONE TO HELL."

When I walked into employee health services, Miss Milks, Redwoods's nurses' nurse, looked over the top of her bifocals, which had been focused on a very disorganized-looking desk piled high with papers, odd rolls of tape, and boxes of syringes.

"Heron, you were supposed to get your butt in here yesterday for that HIV test," she growled.

I shrugged. "Sorry, I forgot. HIV tests aren't something one looks forward to, Miss Milks."

Miss Milks, R.N., was a relic left over from World War II. She had, in fact, been a WAC. When I closed my eyes, I could imagine her, bobbed red hair all flyaway under her officer's cap as she did the lindy hop in some crowded USO club.

The tough old bird was sucking on a cigarette—a constant companion from the look of her nicotine-stained teeth and the smell of her office.

"Yeah, well, the next time you want to miss an appointment, think about the fact that AIDS ain't no picnic either, Heron."

"Neither is lung cancer, Miss Milks."

Tortoiselike, Miss Milks snapped her jaws open. For a split second she looked like she was going to ram the half-finished coffin nail down my throat. Instead, she hacked with a smile; this, I assumed, was laughter.

"Damned straight," she sputtered in her cigarette-rough

voice. "Can't shake the goddamned things. Don't know what the hell I'm going to do when they make it a law that I can't smoke in here."

Miss Milks hacked again, only without the smile; this was her emphysema.

"Roll up your sleeve and let me see those ropes."

I did as I was told, exposing not ropes but threads for veins.

"Pitiful." Miss Milks sighed, tightening the tourniquet. "Is that the best you've got, Heron?"

"I'm afraid so."

Her misshapen, yellow-stained fingers, with knuckles the size of marbles, briefly felt around, then slipped the needle into my vein as clean as a hot knife going through butter. The old battle-ax still had the touch.

"Do you do IV drugs, Heron?" She released the tourniquet, squinting one eye to keep the cigarette smoke out.

"Of course not. All you have to do is look at my veins to know that I—"

"Do you practice safe sex?"

An entire book of possible answers to this straight question of the ages opened in my mind. So as not to miss the beat, I gave the standard reply. "I'm a born-again virgin on the brink of atrophy."

Miss Milks hacked and snorted. All the same, she didn't jiggle the needle one bit.

I looked away from the cerise blood filling the laboratory tube. I didn't want to think about the results of the test. I didn't want to imagine Miss Milks saying, "I'm sorry, Heron, but you've tested positive. Now, now. Chin up. Take it like a soldier."

There were, in fact, a number of healthcare workers who had been infected with the virus. According to the Surgeon General, our kind of work could be dangerous to one's health.

I began to sweat. What *would* I do—for real?

Without thinking, I spoke aloud. "Christ, if I turned up positive, I'd just *die*."

Miss Milks stared at me strangely. "You sure would, Heron, no doubt about that."

Miss Milks sent me away with three appointment cards for the HIV test series that were to be drawn over the span of nine months' time. She also gave me orders to call her office in a week for the results of the first one.

As I was walking up the stairs to CCU, a nightmarish image of hands and arms glistening with blood came to me, triggering an unpleasant memory of an incident that had taken place only six months before.

Pia had answered the call bell of a patient who had had a cardiac catheterization done earlier that afternoon. The patient complained of feeling "wet" under his buttocks. Knowing what she would find when she pulled back the covers, Pia should have thought of gloves, except the instinct of the critical care nurse is to *act without delay*.

The culprit was the catheter insertion site in the right femoral artery, which was now literally spurting blood to the beat of the man's heart (*lub dub*, spurt, *lub dub*, spurt). Still acting on blind instinct, she pressed her bare hand against the gusher and held pressure.

I had seen Pia enter the room, but when the call bell wasn't silenced immediately, I grew suspicious enough to have a peek. The sheets were soaked with blood, and Pia was coated with a sticky red film from fingernails to wrists. "Get me towels and call Dr. Meyers stat!" she yelled the moment I appeared in the doorway. "He's lost a lot of blood."

I ran halfway to the nurses' station, yelling at someone to call the Cartel. From room 9/10, I snitched a stack of towels and hurried back to Pia. Hastily snapping on a pair of gloves (I got three fingers stuck in the thumb), I pulled her out of the way and shoved her toward the sink.

"Scrub yourself down, now!"

I folded two towels and covered the stream of blood, bearing down with enough force to knock the wind out of the man.

Pia, hearing my thought in the tone of my voice, did a three-minute scrub with surgical soap. When she finished, she came to me and silently held up her hands for my inspection. Between index finger and thumb on each hand were open cuts actively bleeding. "I was training a new horse today," she said sadly, her eyes somewhere distant. "I forgot my riding gloves."

After the patient's bleeding had stopped, and while we waited for Dr. Meyers to return our call, we looked through the chart and found that the patient was married with two kids, and had never used IV drugs. Hugely relieved, Pia swore she would never so much as take a blood pressure without gloves again.

About eight P.M., as she was trying to convince Mr. DeLong how good his new no-sodium, no-fat, no-sugar, no-nothin' diet could taste, Dr. Meyers called. In the background, I could hear the clubhouse radio blaring Mitch Ryder and the Detroit Wheels' "Devil with a Blue Dress On."

He listened to my account of what had happened and gave me orders for lab work. Then, as if he were adding an incidental order, he casually said, "Oh yeah, do me a favor and write on the chart somewhere that this guy is HIV-positive. His primary doctor called this morning from Stanford to tell me. Thanks."

He hung up.

Numbed, I watched Pia hold up the detailed plastic model of a human heart, pointing to the various chambers, which magically flipped open to give the student/patient an inside view. When she got to the left ventricle—the biggest and most important of the chambers—she flipped it open, and inside was a tiny plastic Mickey Mouse, waving. She laughed her infectious horse whinny of a laugh. Mr. DeLong threw back his head and roared.

From nursing school days, I recalled an effervescent nineteen-year-old Pia announcing to our group that she never wanted to be old, sick, or die in her whole life.

I dialed information for the number to the clubhouse. When Dr. Meyers came on the line, I had to swallow before I could speak.

"Why didn't you let someone know immediately that this guy was HIV-positive?" My voice was thick and shaky. "Do you know that Pia was in there—gloveless—up to her elbows in this guy's blood? She's got cuts the size of the Grand Canyon all over her hands."

There was a pause.

"I'm sorry," Dr. Meyers said, not sounding sorry at all. "I forgot to call in the information earlier. I was very busy this morning. Listen, how do you think *I* felt when I was doing the cath?"

"I think . . ." I was snarling now. "I think you probably felt pretty safe with two sets of gloves on. How do *you* think Pia is going to feel when I tell her that you 'forgot' to let us know this guy has AIDS?"

"I'm sorry."

"I have to write this up, Dr. Meyers. Pia will need to be tested."

He repeated again that he was sorry.

"Sorry isn't good enough," I said and hung up.

When I gave Pia the news, she didn't say a word, but took on the lackluster expression of someone doomed.

Depositing my supper in CCU's dubious refrigerator, I tried to think of the positive side of the story—Pia's first two series of tests had come out negative. When she got a third negative test, we planned on having a wild celebration.

Then, because of the kind of day it was, I gritted my tooth guard before I faced the assignment board:

"TO FLOAT: HERON—3P TO 7P ICU / 7P TO 11:30P ER."

The ICU part gave me pause. I imagined apprehensively the types of patients I might be assigned: fresh postop liver transplants, an infected sternotomy, ricocheted gunshot wounds with a hundred drains, a mesenteric thrombosis or two. These were not problems I dealt with every day, or even every five years.

Oh, give me the coding MIs and fulminating pulmonary edemas, or give me ER. Outside of that—give me the day off.

I was assigned a fifty-six-year-old AIDS patient fighting her way through pneumocystis carinii pneumonia, a forty-eight-year-old man who'd had his right arm torn off at the shoulder when his shirtsleeve caught in the motor of a boat, a nineteen-year-old dying of testicular cancer, and a twenty-three-year-old septic-shock patient with a fresh colostomy.

This assignment didn't sound so bad, considering there weren't any infected sternotomies or ricocheted gunshot wounds. However, as soon as report was over, the thought did cross my mind that I should have called in sick the minute I saw the purple hair and the neon polyesters.

The four patient information cards, known as Rand cards, told me in black and white that each of my patients was moderate acuity. What that meant, in Normal Person's language, was that no one human being could do everything that had to be done for them in four hours. It was a physical impossibility.

On day shift, these same four patients were split between two ICU nurses. But because evening shift nurses earned a differential in pay, the hospital insisted staffing be cut tighter. On nights, these patients *plus* two more with the same acuity or higher would be assigned to one nurse, because night shift nurses were paid the largest differential.

Management's way of looking at it *sounded* practical—after all, the patients slept at night, didn't they? But the fact of the matter was that in critical care, the rotation of night and day meant little to patient or nurse. Dressing changes, suctioning, turning, administering of medications, and constant monitoring of equipment and vital signs went on twenty-four hours a day. It was not unusual for patients staying more than a week in ICU to suffer from sleep deprivation psychosis, euphemistically termed "hospitalitis."

The staffing issues had always been contingent on what management could get away with. I glanced at the phone thinking I should advise the supervisor of the situation and ask to fill out a protest-of-assignment form; that would help cover me in case one of my patients suffered, or died, due to my inability to attend him in time. It would also be another slap on the hand that starved us. If the hospital was reprimanded enough times, the hope was they would someday stop unsafe staffing.

If that didn't work, the nurses speculated they would have to wait until enough patients died before the public could be alerted to what was wrong—and maybe not even then since the owner of the county's main newspaper was on the Redwoods board.

I arranged the Rand cards in front of me and outlined a timetable, filling in the absolute necessities of what had to be done—a dressing change here, skip one there; vital signs every half hour on him, once an hour on her; combine medication times, giving this one a little sooner and that one a little later; suction once every forty minutes instead of every twenty; and pray to the powers that be that no one suffocated on a mucus plug or bled to death.

Reciting my motto, "I only have two arms and legs, I'll do what I can," I prepared myself and walked into the room closest at hand.

I looked like a Robin Cook/Stephen King character in my blue paranoia wrap: shoe covers, gloves, paper gown, mask, and oversized safety goggles with the fancy three-way shutters around the edges.

Mrs. Mazzucci was used to it. Three years after contracting the HIV virus from a blood transfusion, she had been through the gamut of healthcare.

A Normal Person looking on would have automatically assumed that the protective measures were for my benefit, when in fact they were for Mrs. Mazzucci's protection. In practicing what was properly know as reverse isolation, our main concern was to avoid exposing Mrs. Mazzucci to any new germs we might bring in. She already had enough to deal with just trying to survive pneumocystis pneumonia.

"So, how do you like my Paris creation?" I asked, parading and turning like a fashion model on the runway. The blue paper crinkled with each movement.

Mrs. Mazzucci smiled around her endotracheal tube and made the okay sign.

"Le Blue Ragbag by Princess Schmatte."

She shook her head, careful not to trip the respirator, and gave me a scolding look: "Don't make me laugh or I'll choke."

I calibrated her arterial and Swan Ganz lines, checked the oximeter, hung her pentamidine and gentamicin, and wrote her vitals on the flow sheet. The mechanics done, I hastily drew a basin of soapy water; Mrs. Mazzucci had soiled herself. According to the nurse's notes, it was the fourth time that day. The puddle of liquid stool had soaked through to the mattress and had spread from her ankles to the middle of her back. While I worked, I described to her how the hospital had decided to redecorate the front lobby.

"The furniture is a cross between early postmodern . . . or postmortem, and Flintstone. The wall art is a collection of big lips and depressing watercolors of famous people with ill-shaped heads or . . ."

Mrs. Mazzucci had ceased listening and was staring at the discolored nodules on her wasting legs and abdomen. She touched one with her finger, and a look of disgust crossed her face.

"Kaposi's sarcoma," I said.

She nodded sadly, then coughed hard enough to buck the respirator. Pointing to her endotracheal tube, she lifted her shoulders in the attitude of someone taking a deep breath. It was the common sign used by long-term respirator patients to indicate they needed to be suctioned.

I finished with her bath, changed her bed, and did a sterile glove change all in fast motion. Feeling her air hunger, I hastily uncapped the side port of her endotracheal tube and squirted a few drops of sterile saline down the inside to liquefy any thick mucus clinging to the walls of the tube and the upper portion of her lungs. This sent Mrs. Mazzucci immediately into wrenching spasms of coughing, the force of which tripped the machine's alarm. Its shrill wail set my teeth on edge.

I waited until Mrs. Mazzucci sucked in a desperate breath to push in a lungful of pure oxygen. When her air hunger subsided, I threaded the clear suction catheter down the endotracheal tube until I hit resistance. Plugging the suction hole with my thumb, I pulled the catheter back slowly, producing the sound of a vacuum sucking mud off the bottom of a pond. Most Normal People would never be able to understand this, but to a nurse, this vile racket is immensely satisfying.

What came back through the catheter was copious, thick, greenish-yellow mucus tinged with strings of blood. I was so elated, I repeated the procedure twice more before I hooked Mrs. Mazzucci back to the respirator. The process was similar to doing a thorough spring cleaning.

Tears streamed down her face as she gasped, tripping the machine to give her extra breaths. At the same time, she patted my hand, then grasped it firmly and held on until her color returned to normal and she was no longer laboring to get each breath. When she finally looked at me, it was with gratefulness, compassion, forgiveness, and the unmistakable message of "Ain't life a bitch?"

Jonas Yi reminded me of one of those statues you frequently find next to the cash registers in Chinese restaurants—the folklore entities that represent the god of good appetite, or the spirit of good fortune. Rotund and smiling despite the traumatic loss of his right arm, he looked like anything but a Sausalito boat person.

Sausalito boat people were of a different breed—a different era altogether. They were the flower children grown older and wiser, wilting evidenced by graying hair. Artists, writers, musicians; chronic soul-searchers all, living in a tight-knit community whose common bonds were Alan Watts, Krishnamurti, and most of all, San Francisco Bay, its steel-gray beauty constantly held in frame by the graceful art deco lines of the Golden Gate Bridge.

The enormous bulky dressing covering his shoulder did not reduce my peculiar yearning to see the right arm where it should have been. It was a matter of retraining the eye to accept the absence of the limb.

I slipped the thermometer under his tongue. "I'm going to take your arm now," I said.

A nanosecond passed in which I heard the statement I had just made. I willed the floor to open up and swallow me.

Oh God. Another deformity slip—the most excruciating type of embarrassment. My worst deformity slip came vividly to mind: I was a high school student, my first day on the job as a cashier in a bookstore. I was ringing up the purchase of a woman who had six fingers on each hand. Forcing myself to ignore the deformity, I looked directly at her face and said, nice and level, "That'll be five dollars and ninety-six fingers, please."

Mr. Yi looked up at me strangely, no doubt amazed by the dramatic change in color of my face and neck. I turned away to collect myself and wait until the burning stopped. I then began to unwrap the huge, bulky dressing covering his shoulder.

"Do you need any pain medication?" Phantom pain in the amputated limb was frequently a problem, and it was reported to me that he had been complaining of a searing, stinging sensation in the invisible elbow and forearm.

(Bring the wide gauze strip back around the torso twice. Crisscross over the shoulder. Remember to make note that there is some evidence of drainage on the outer layers. Yellow. No odor.)

"I'm okay right now," Mr. Yi said, nervously watching the unwrapping.

"Have you seen the wound site yet?"

(Unwind over the lateral part of the stump. Not really a stump. A place where an arm used to be. Make note the drainage is now an area of about four inches in diameter and light tan in color. Nothing malodorous.)

"Yes. Twice so far."

I smiled. He needed to be drawn out. The Chinese always seemed to need drawing out.

"And what do you think?" I really had wanted to ask, "How do you feel about it?" but this was a Chinese; asking for thoughts rather than feelings seemed safer—less rude somehow.

"It's . . ." He paused, the smile fading from his lips. "It is the price I have paid for my carelessness," he said heavily.

Had he said, "It's ugly," or, "My life is ruined," I would have responded with the nurse's standard pitter-patter about hope and prosthesis. His tenet about having "paid" for his mistake didn't leave a whole lot of room for comments.

"Is this going to affect your job?"

(One more turn of the strip and now for the layer of absor-bent pads. Soaked. But clean—nothing green to be seen. Ha ha.)

Jonas Yi's smile reappeared. Quietly, he said, "I carve."

Ah yes, a carver. I imagined him in the kitchen of a Chinese restaurant, standing behind giant turkeys and slabs of beef with a long saber in each hand. I sighed with relief. Had he said he was a concert pianist, I would have been really bummed. But then the thought came that he was an artist—a carver of wood or stone.

"You mean . . ."

"Yes. For many years I have created medieval figures and scenes in fine woods. Have you seen them?"

I stared at him, mouth agape. Not only had I seen the man's work, I had been in love with it ever since I arrived in San Francisco during the Summer of Love. His "carvings" were exquisite pieces of art—wizards with flowing beards to match their robes, gnarled trees holding flawless birds, damsels in long dresses—all incredibly detailed and alive within the pol-ished woods. His characters had often made guest appearances in my dreams.

"Oh my God," I said, "*You're* the one who does those?"

He nodded, not flattered but with the knowing acceptance of a master craftsman. "Those are my children, yes."

"Mr. Yi, I am so honored to meet you." I put out my right hand, withdrew it quickly, and changed over to my left. His grip was strong. "I love your work. I—I actually own a small wizard of yours. He sits on my mantel. He's—"

Two things dawned on me simultaneously. One, I needed to hurry—pull off the last layer of fluffs and expose the wound—and two, he carved with his *hands*. Plural.

My heart sank like a bleeding stone. There would be no more medieval wonders to delight me whenever I passed by gallery windows. Collectors would go out and pillage every gallery and shop for miles.

(Slowly, carefully, peel away one, two, three, five fluffs and . . .)

We both stared at the swollen wound. It was a red, yellow, and purple hump with a crazy-quilt pattern of suture lines. It was ugly, but it was healing. No smell of staph or some other hospital-borne infection. No suspicious drainage.

Mr. Yi looked worried. "Is it okay? These colors and the swelling—it is not gangrene?"

"No. You're healing very nicely as a matter of fact. It'll take time."

His sigh of relief told me the fear of gangrene had been preying on him. Using the strictest of sterile technique, I began the process of cleansing and redressing his shoulder. The clock at the end of the bed kept drawing my attention, nagging at me that I was behind.

This was the heart of the understaffing problem: If I rushed, it would result in a slipshod job and the patient might suffer, but if I took time to be correct and precise, one or more of my other patients would go without some essential part of their care.

The voice of Tessie, my favorite second-year nursing instructor, went over the address system in my head.

"Remember what I told you, Echo—a job not well done is a job that will come back to haunt you and the patient. You'll both pay for it in the long run.

"Pretend you are doing this dressing on Simon or Janey. Better yet, imagine that you are watching another nurse do a crummy job on one of them. Think about that. Think about it right up until you finish doing this excellent dressing."

Satisfied with the results of my efforts (a Neiman Marcus dressing if ever I saw one), I made ready to put on the speed and see if I could catch up on my next patient. Mr. Yi reached out and tapped the back of my hand.

"Please. Don't worry about my carving."

I looked at him sadly.

"No, no. Don't despair. Good fortune is mine." His smile widened. "You see, I am left-handed."

This 19-year-old Caucasian presented with disseminated choriocarcinoma with metastasis to lungs. Prognosis for this youngster is grim despite orchiectomy and bilateral retrograde lymph node dissection performed 6 months ago w/follow-up abdominal radiation. 2–3 weeks postsurgery, chemotherapy w/cisplatin, Velban, and bleomycin begun.

Pt. today is having significant respiratory distress with ARDS, along with severe pulmonary infection. Chest X ray shows marked increase in pulmonary infiltrates and worsening blood gases. Presently on 100% nonrebreather mask. At this time, I doubt Dr. Cohen's suggestion of pulmonary toxicity caused by bleomycin. Will consider intubation only as last re-

sort, due to prognosis. If pt. continues to complain of pleuritic chest pain, will start morphine drip.

Significant pain also from enlarged breasts secondary to gynecomastia from hormones released by tumors.

Spoke with pt. and family again re: poor prognosis. Decision made to request medical intervention short of cardiac arrest. Morphine drip alternative to ease patient at end as last resort discussed and accepted by all.

Truly a depressing situation.

Elias Peters, M.D.

I placed my hand lightly on my patient's smooth chest and counted his labored respirations. Under my fingers, his rib cage fluttered with the motion of his rapidly beating heart.

"Paul?"

The dark lashes opened slowly and two sweet blue eyes met mine.

"Ma?" he gasped.

"Not Mom. Your nurse, Echo."

He organized his thoughts and tried to sit up but couldn't. "I was having a dream I was at camp." He looked around, shivering. The dark hollows under his eyes didn't seem to belong on so young a face. "Could you give me some more blankets? I'm cold."

I looked over his head. According to the monitor, his blood temp was 103.1. This was another of those small but meaningful choices the caregiver faced every day—whether to be the humane and merciful angel, giving the dying boy a hot blanket that would comfort him but drive his temperature up, or the professional clinician, adding to his present suffering by placing him on a cooling blanket in the hope of lessening his fever and chills. Then there was the knowledge that no matter what I did, he was going to die.

"Do you think you can stand it for a while longer? You've got a fever. How about a few minutes on the cooling blanket?"

He groaned and turned his head away, his teeth chattering. "Not that. Don't do that to me."

I pushed his hair, damp with sweat, off his forehead. He was very pale. "Okay. We won't do the cooling blanket, but I've got to get your fever down. I'll see what other tricks I can pull out of the bag before I throw you in the ice chest."

Mrs. Mazzucci's respirator alarm screamed loudly for a few

seconds, then abruptly stopped with a curt *screeeeep*. The noise was a reminder not to dally.

I looked around the room at the lines and the IV meds, then back at the boy. His eyes pleaded with me to help him. Make him live.

I took his hand in mine. *I am here for you, Paulie. We are only strangers, but I am here to ease your pain and escort you to death if that's what is in store.* I stood, pushing away another shock of hair from his forehead.

He deserves more, Ec. Dying or not, he is suffering, and he's scared. Do the best for him you can. Do your best because it will be his last gift.

I was searching through orders and the med sheets looking for untried escape routes from Paul's fever, when Dr. Peters came in and sat down. "Hey Elias, I was getting ready to call you about the Crowell boy's fever."

Elias let his shoulders slump and his head fall back. I could see the red spots of ingrown neck hairs at the edge of his beard. He'd nicked himself shaving and bled onto his shirt.

"I don't know, Ec," he said slowly, staring at the ceiling. "This is a shitty one. I talked to the kid this morning. He's scared. I could feel him begging me to give him a chance, as if I had the power to pull him out of it. He's depending on me to take away his pain and keep him breathing. He thinks I can make the cancer disappear.

"He asked me not to give up on him. He said if I break, he's going to break. And there I was, trying to make myself give him the options speech: We can put you out of your misery, Paulie, with morphine little by little, or we can snuff you all at once when the pain can't be controlled anymore."

"Jesus, Elias, did you *say* that?"

Dr. Peters pulled his tie down and unbuttoned the collar. "I told him we could hope things would turn around, but I gave him his options, too, in case they didn't." He took the chart from under my arm. "The kid doesn't have a snowball's chance in hell. Where the hell is the cavalry when you need it?"

"Elias, stop. You did what you could."

"I don't know," he said wearily. "Paulie isn't the first and he won't be the last, but nobody ever likes hanging it up on a nineteen-year-old kid."

I nodded, flashing over a collage of all the children and

young people I had watched die. There was always a profusion of valiant, beyond-the-call-of-duty strategies made by the medical community in their reluctance to see people younger than themselves die.

But for now it was time to get on with business; the mourning could be done later.

"Okay, Elias." I turned to the medication chart and smoothed it carefully. "So what are we going to do to get this kid's fever down?"

I washed Paul's face with a cool cloth. The feel of his light peach fuzz brought on thoughts about death and its inconsiderations and how much it had cheated him out of. I prayed that he had made love at least once, and had one best friend whom he could say he loved.

I allowed family and friends to visit all at once, which took a little of his attention away from the pain. Sitting on the bed as close to him as she could get, his girlfriend never let go of his swollen and mottled hand. She seemed greatly bothered by his breathing. I could see her trying to breathe the same way he did: shallow and fast. Whether it was in sympathy or she was trying it on for size, I couldn't tell, but she didn't keep it up for long.

Paul's mother was about my age. I could see by the way her eyes never left him that she was searching for the slightest sign of improvement. Her touch lingered every time she sponged his face or held his hand, as if she wanted to be sure she was close so she could pull him back to life should he start to slip away.

Watching her anguish caused my throat, my heart, my gut to ache in sympathy. Sensing her helplessness, I also felt guilty for being thankful that my son was not the boy lying in that bed.

"When I get home ..." He stopped to suck in more air. Talking was a difficult thing for him. "I am going to ... work out every day."

No way, Paulie, I thought. Aloud I said, "Great. You and Arnold, kid."

He was creating a future for himself, or was he bargaining with his higher power? *If I do this, will you let me live?*

Paul smiled as much as he could, which was really only a twitch in one corner of his mouth. "Nikki ... that's my girlfriend ... is going to flip out when I get home."

*Yes, she will, Paulie. Nikki will mourn for a long time.
Someday, years from now, she will tell her teenage daughter
how she lost her first love to death and she will cry. She will
cry because she will still be in love with the memory of you.*

"Can't wait to get home . . ." His voice was drowsy and he
was looking somewhere else far away. When he came back, he
turned and looked through me. "I'll get home . . . won't I?"

I nodded. "Yes." Never take away their hope. "You will,
yes."

"God, I'm so tired," he said, and closed his eyes.

It's true, I thought, one picture *is* worth a thousand words.
Thunderstruck, I studied my patient's presurgical abdominal
X ray. Through the shadowy grays and soft whites, the dark
outlines of two distinctly familiar objects seemed as out of
place as Ronald Reagan at a Mensa meeting.

Groucho Marx waggled his eyebrows and flicked his cigar
on *You Bet Your Life.* "Say the secret word and win a hundred
dollars. It's a common word, something you hear around the
house every day."

"A vase and a clothes hanger?" I said aloud.

No plucked duck dropped from the ceiling, but that's exactly
what I saw.

I flipped to the admitting notes and doggedly (from across
the hall, I could hear that Mrs. Mazzucci needed suctioning
badly; Mr. Yi's light was on for pain meds) struggled through
Dr. Seitz's scrawl. He had obviously studied, and studied hard,
The Physician's Guide to Achieving Unreadable Handwriting—
either that, or he had taken to writing with his dumb hand.

My patient, a twenty-three-year-old model/actor visiting from
L.A., had been partying with his girlfriend in San Francisco
(the "Anything Goes" city). Apparently the drugs were pure,
and the parties wild, because the patient found himself one evening with an embarrassingly large vase trapped in his rectum.

If he had surrendered himself to an emergency room at that
point, he might have been okay. But the fear of humiliation being a strong human influence, he decided to extract the offending vessel himself, with—I kid you not—a rusty coat hanger.

I paused in my deciphering, a pun having slithered into the
sick mind to which I belonged. I supposed, if you really
wanted to get technical about it, the patient had tried to perform a sort of self-vase-ectomy.

The end results were gruesome. He had perforated his colon

so badly (finally getting the hanger itself caught) that there was nothing left to be done except a colostomy. Considering rusty coat hangers and perforated colons, it was not surprising that the patient ended up in septic shock, complete with collapse of his cardiovascular system and kidney failure. Initially no one thought he would make it out of the hospital in anything other than a morgue bag. Except his will to survive had managed to do its magic turnaround number on his body.

I went into my mechanic's routine: calibrated arterial and pulmonary artery lines, recalculated the dopamine drip rate, spiked a new antibiotic bag—a task that always proved as difficult as opening one of those utensil bags you get with airline meal trays—and hung it along with a new maintenance IV, emptied the half-full colostomy and urine-collection bags, gave more medications, and changed the pull sheet. The patient had been weaned off the respirator and extubated on day shift—a blessing for us both.

I finally looked at the patient himself. George. Gorgeous George was closer to the truth. The man was so handsome, he didn't look real. He looked like a photo in a men's fashion magazine and if I just turned the page, he would disappear.

"My arm hurts," he croaked. His vocal cords would take days to recover from the unpleasant presence of the endotracheal tube. I unwrapped the overly elaborate dressing from around his IV site and saw that the IV was infiltrated.

"Your IV catheter has broken through the wall of your vein and leaked fluid into your tissue," I told him wearily. "I'm going to have to restart it."

It was six o'clock. Not enough time to restart the IV, suction Mrs. Mazzucci, hand out all five and six P.M. meds, medicate Mr. Yi and Paulie for pain, check vitals, chart, check all lab results and . . .

Dr. Seitz, Dr. Bell, Dr. Peters, and Dr. Cohen entered the double doors of the unit.

. . . and give reports to Dr. Peters about Paul, to Dr. Bell and Dr. Seitz about George and Mr. Yi, and to Dr. Cohen about Mrs. Mazzucci and Paul.

I turned up the speed to hypernursing. I divided the lab result slips by patient and handed them to the appropriate doctors, suctioned Mrs. Mazzucci, restarted IVs, did a dressing change, emptied more urine, gave Paul a kiss while he slept, delivered meds—praying I gave them to the right patients in the right doses—checked a BP here, a temperature there.

And at the end, I did the kind of nurse's charting that makes a malpractice lawyer's dreams come true.

It was 7:35 when I finished giving the most jumbled, and probably most inaccurate, report I'd given that year. I was surprised the on-duty nurse didn't ask to check my nursing license. Between 7:04 and 7:35, ER called ICU four times asking when the hell I was going to arrive for duty; they *needed* me and they needed me *now*.

My stomach growled, my feet and back ached, and I felt light-headed. How I was going to make it through another four hours was anybody's guess.

I did not, however, break my tradition of saying goodbye to each patient. I was waving (left-handed—a sympathy wave) to Mr. Yi and was ready to enter George's room, when a man holding a long narrow box with a white bow on the top approached me.

"Are you Echo Heron?"

"That depends on whether you're a process server or not."

The man handed me the box without smiling. I was sure he'd heard that and similar lines about as often as I'd heard the dozen or so puns about my name. I hadn't been fair; at least he hadn't said, "Hey, is there an echo in here? Ha ha."

The greeting card was attached to the bow by a purple ribbon.

Dear Nurse Heron,

We will never forget what you did for Mom and will keep you in our prayers every day. Dad and I both wish you and she could have gotten to know each other. You would have been the best of friends.

She would have wanted you to have something nice for your trouble. We thought these suited you. Thank you so much for being there for all of us.

God bless you,
Ruth and Albert Tuttle

Inside were one dozen long-stemmed white roses.

My hunger and the light-headedness evaporated into thin air. My feet and back suddenly didn't hurt so much.

George, who had watched the scene unfold, crooked his finger.

I stepped closer to the bed. There was a faint smile on his pale face.

"Hey, nurse," he whispered hoarsely. "Need a vase?"

The second the pneumatic doors hissed open, I knew something was wrong. The atmosphere was as heavy as lead weights. Ileta, usually an upbeat, funny lady, shuffled papers around her desk, averting her eyes as soon as she saw me.

"What's going on?" I whispered.

She shook her head and waved a thumb in the direction of the trauma room.

Through the small window in the trauma room door, I saw Dr. Mahoney leaning against the far wall, arms folded over her chest. Her mouth moved continuously, obviously delivering some kind of report to one of the other people in the room. Dr. Packard, a pediatrician, stood with his back to me, blocking the head and upper body of the patient. Don was at the head of the gurney, ventilating the patient with the bag. He paused to wipe the sweat away from his face with his forearm, then brushed his drooping handlebar mustache against his shoulder.

Sarah was on the other side of the gurney, apparently helping the laboratory tech search for a vein, while a respiratory tech stood by Don preparing a strip of adhesive tape as an anchor for the endotracheal tube. A supervisor nurse sat in the corner, filling out one of the red-edged facility-transfer forms. They all looked, for want of a better description, severely depressed.

Only the float nurse was animated, quickly going from one side of the room to the other, putting things in order. She set a white plastic bag on the counter at the end of the gurney and into it placed a badly torn T-shirt with an airbrushed picture of New Kids on the Block that was almost completely concealed by bloodstains, a pair of blood-soaked jeans, and beat-up black Air Jordan high tops.

The items were the familiar uniform of a typical nine- or ten-year-old boy. Simon had lived in an outfit exactly like it during most of his preteen years, except instead of New Kids on the Block, it had been Independent Skateboard Trucks. T-shirt logos, I supposed, would one day be simple but accurate measures of what progressive generations were into.

Dr. Packard shifted his position, giving me a clear view of

the boy on the gurney. The thinness of his body coupled with the paleness of his skin made it appear that the child had already bled to death or was quickly heading in that direction. The small white body was disfigured with four or five ugly purple-and-red gouges I recognized as stab wounds. A nearly empty unit of blood was hanging from the IV pole next to Sarah. It was certain they had been pouring the packed cells into him as fast as they would go.

The respiratory tech prepared the battered face for the adhesive tape, wiping away the dried blood that had crusted around the boy's mouth. Another nurse entered the room from the side door connecting X ray to the ER and handed a fresh unit of blood to Sarah. As Sarah replaced the empty bag, she noticed me in the window, and gave me the wait-there sign.

I pulled back from the window and swallowed hard.

I don't want to do this anymore, I thought. I don't want to see these things. I want to be a Normal Person.

Sarah came out and handed the red-edged transfer form to Ileta. "Ileta, get this on the grill and find out why the hell that transfer unit isn't here yet. We've got to get this kid over to Mercy stat or he's not going to make it."

Sarah turned to face me. I could tell she was in a lousy mood by the slight tone of defeat in her voice.

"He isn't going to make it anyway, but we can always give him the benefit of the doubt, can't we? By the way, it's nice of you to show up, Ec." Her pinched and worn expression said she didn't want any excuses.

"What's been going on around here?" I asked.

Wearily, Sarah waved the question away and greeted the two San Rafael policemen who appeared in the main room. She pulled them off to the side, away from the view of the patients.

Don emerged from the trauma room limbering his shoulders. He ran his hands through his dark hair and down his face. Standing silent with his eyes closed, he took one long, deep breath, let it out slowly, and reentered the trauma room. Dr. Mahoney came out next, followed by the supervisor and the float nurse.

I stopped the float nurse, whose name tag read, "Jean, R.N."

"Will somebody please tell me what's going on in there?"

She moved to the sink to wash her hands. "Ten-year-old's father beat him up, then stabbed him with a kitchen knife because the mother ran off with her boyfriend. The kid is in bad shape, but Packard thinks he might have a better chance in the pedi surgical ICU at Mercy."

"Where's the father?"

"Jail."

"The mother?"

She shook her head. "Don't know. Ileta said one of the neighbors called about an hour ago, asking about the boy. They said they'd scout around for her in the local bars, maybe call the boyfriend." The nurse shivered and hugged herself. "Poor little guy. Jesus, why—?" She stopped and walked away. "Never mind."

Why isn't really the question, nurse. It's, what is the lesson to be learned? Never ask why, because the answer could be dangerous to your mental health and your attitude about your fellowman.

Less than two minutes later, the pneumatic door hissed open to admit the advanced cardiac life-support paramedics and all their intrafacility-transfer paraphernalia. Within seven minutes, their wounded cargo was loaded, along with Dr. Packard and the float nurse, and heading toward the Golden Gate.

For a while no one spoke except to ask pertinent questions—"Did you give bed four his DT shot yet?" "Is the suture tray set up?" "Is the lab work back yet on bed three?"

Later, when the feelings of frustration and depression started to ease, those involved began taking care of each other.

At 8:43 I made a quick exit from the malodorous utility room, where I had just checked a urine and stool sample for occult blood, and noticed a short, overweight woman standing by the side door of the ER attempting to light a cigarette.

I reached her at the same time the flame of the Bic lighter touched the end of her cigarette.

"I don't think you want to be lighting up in here," I said, grabbing the Bic out of her hand.

Delayed reaction caused by surprise and gin kept the woman's lighting hand in the same position. She flicked the absent Bic and inhaled. Pulling the cigarette from her lips, she stared at the unlit end in dumb confusion.

"Hey, why'd you do *that*, huh?" She looked at me with accusing, bloodshot eyes.

"No smoking in the hospital," I said, and dropped the lighter into the scuffed white purse she wore slung over her shoulder. "Besides, it's bad for your health."

The woman grunted and drifted unsteadily toward the main room, her flip-flops slapping the bottoms of her grimy heels. A goodly portion of her Pillsbury Doughboy thighs was exposed by short denim cutoffs. The heavy bones of her posterior creaked as she lowered the mass of her body onto the face of an orange wheelchair. A tuft of dark pubic hair escaped the inside cuff of her shorts. Sylphlike she was not.

"Where's my kid?" she asked in the deep gravel voice of a dedicated smoker. It was not at all unlike Miss Milks's voice.

"What kid?"

The woman raised up on one haunch and pulled at the shorts where they were cutting into her crotch. I took a step back when the sour smell of her perspiration hit my nostrils like a noxious gas.

"One of them nosy neighbors told me to come here 'cause Vic got sick. What's the little shit's problem now, or is this one of his old man's tricks to get me down here so he can beat the crap outta me again?"

The realization who the woman was snuck through the back door of my brain. The switchboard ladies sent a little thrill of panic through me as I further realized she didn't have a clue as to what had happened.

"You sit right there for one sec while I find out what's going on with Vic, okay?"

She nodded without interest, the activities of the main room having caught her attention. Removing the plastic headband from her straggly hair, she scratched her scalp with zeal. A flake of yellowish dandruff fell onto the front of the black tank top stretched tight across her ample breasts.

I found Sarah in the casting corner of the surgical room, making a wrist splint for an elderly man who reeked of old urine and bourbon.

"Was that little boy's name Victor?"

Sarah swung around to face me. "Yes, Victor Boyd. Why? Did they call? Is he . . . ?"

"No—well, I mean, I don't know, but his mother is here. She doesn't know anything about anything." I pointed out Mrs. Boyd, who had migrated from the wheelchair to the door. She was antsy; an unfortunate who desperately wanted a cigarette.

Halfway across the room Sarah asked me to stay with her, and I readily agreed. Telling a mother that her child had been stabbed by his father and was probably dying was not something you wanted to tackle alone.

Mrs. Boyd must have interpreted our solemn expressions as aggressively disciplinary, for as we drew near she held out her hands in a defensive gesture. "Hey, I didn't smoke no cigarettes. Besides, I didn't see no sign says you can't smoke in here."

Sarah gently touched her arm. "Why don't we go to another room where you can have a cigarette, Mrs. Boyd?"

"Call me Babe," she said, happy to be going somewhere where she could smoke. "I don't go by that prick's name no more."

As usual, the Quiet Room was deserted. I noticed that the ugly pineapple lamp and the wallpaper photo of a sunny forest were exactly the same as they had been on a day a long time ago when I had told another woman her child was dead.

Mrs. Boyd plopped down on the love seat and promptly lit up. "So where's Vic?" she asked, lazily picking a stray piece of tobacco off the tip of her tongue.

"I've got some bad news for you, Mrs. Bo—Babe," Sarah said. Her voice was tight.

Babe took another drag, eyeing Sarah suspiciously. There was a hint of hostile mistrust to her gaze. "Yeah?"

"Your son has been hurt very badly. He was taken to Mercy's surgical pediatric unit about an hour ago. He's been—"

"I'll bet the little shit said I abandoned him, right?" Babe said defiantly. She flushed and pulled her bulky frame to the edge of the cushion. "The old man did that, you know. Turned him against me, telling him a bunch of dirty no-good lies. He ain't got respect for me no more, but it don't matter. Far as I care, they can both go piss up a rope."

"Mrs. Boyd, you don't understand. Your son is in serious condition. He may not survive. Do you have any friends or relatives that we can call to be with you?"

From the deep drags Babe was sucking out of her cigarette, I thought perhaps the seriousness of the situation had managed to filter through.

"I got my boyfriend, Lloyd. He's waiting on me in the lobby." Suddenly the woman giggled. "Ooooh man, he's gonna be fit to be tied when he finds out we gotta drive all the way over to Mercy to see the brat. That son-of-a-bitchin' car of his ain't worth a cup of coffee and a good shit."

Sarah and I looked at each other.

"Your son has been stabbed, Mrs.—Babe," Sarah said flatly.

"Your husband stabbed him and we don't know if the child is going to survive. Your husband has been taken into custody in—"

"Where's the crapper around here?" Babe asked, hoisting herself out of the love seat with some effort. "I gotta piss like a racehorse."

I saw Sarah check out. Her eyes went vacant and I could tell her switchboard ladies were shutting down circuits left and right.

"Babe, do you understand what Sarah is telling you?" I asked.

"I—I don't know." The woman rummaged blindly in her purse for the pack of cigarettes. When she found them, she lit one from the end of the one she was still smoking even though it was barely half gone. The only thing that indicated to me she understood what was going on was that her hands were shaking more violently than before.

"I gotta piss first." Some emotion crept into her voice—it sounded like a cross between anger and panic. "Just show me the crapper, then I want to get the fuck out of here. I need to think."

I walked her to the rest room, only a little taken aback that she had her shorts pulled down over her hips before we were even halfway there. Then I went to find Lloyd, praying that he might be more able to deal with the situation.

Lloyd wasn't hard to spot. He was as I pictured him: tall and skinny, wearing a wide-brimmed black cowboy hat and highly tooled pointy-toed boots—one of those leathery, weather-beaten cowboys you see in movies. He was passed out in the corner of the couch, snoring louder than the TV was blasting. I sat next to him and shook him awake.

"Lloyd?"

The middle-aged man grunted, wiped his mouth against the sleeve of his fringed suede jacket, and opened two bloodshot eyes. "Uhn, yeah?"

"There's been trouble. Babe's boy is hurt really bad. He's over in Mercy Hospital. Do you think you can get her over there and stay with her, or do you know if she has some relative we can call?"

"Golly, that's too bad," he said slowly, rubbing the back of his neck. He pulled a pack of Camels from his shirt pocket and lit one.

He seemed to have forgotten my question, so I repeated it.

Lloyd sat up more. The cigarette was like a long white chimney in the steeple of his fingers. "Hell, I don't rightly know," he drawled. "I don't know Babe that good. We only just met up a couple a weeks ago."

I leaned back into my chair feeling very tired. More than anything, I wanted to get up and go home or maybe lay my head back and go to sleep.

"Well, do you think you could drive her over to Mercy Hospital?"

Lloyd debated that for a while, massaging the tops of his knees and then smoothing back his graying hair with his cowboy hat. He coughed a wet, rattling smoker's cough and tugged at the black bolo tie tipped with two caps of silver.

"Suppose I could," he said finally, as Babe came swaggering around the corner exhaling a stream of smoke. Making a bee line for Lloyd, she reminded me of a steam engine barreling down on an innocent victim tied to the tracks.

"Gotta get me over to Mercy, Lloyd. The son of a bitch took a goddamned knife to the brat, can you believe it? The cocksucker's trying to get back at me 'cause I got a life and he don't."

Lloyd stood and ran his hand across his mouth. The top of his hat hit the bottom of the wall-mounted TV. I had the distinct feeling he was struggling to keep himself from laughing.

"Ah, okay. Hope the old Chevy makes it, is all."

"If it don't," said Babe, giggling, "we gonna find ourselves a good ol' bar and get goddamned drunk as skunks in a wine barrel."

Lloyd guffawed, noticed my expression, and stopped his laughter abruptly. Under the wide brim of his black cowboy hat, he rearranged his expression in a pretty good imitation of someone who'd been given mildly disturbing news.

My stomach hurt so much by nine P.M. that I zipped up to CCU and grabbed a pint carton of milk and a couple of graham crackers. I ate on the run, a chew per step and a sip of milk at the end of each flight of stairs. I was back in ER by 9:07, dinner completed.

Sarah was assisting Dr. Mahoney with a combo laceration/burn of a woman's left leg and ankle, while Don buzzed in and out of the orifice room carrying things like a hammer, Vaseline, and ice cubes. Elmo, one of Redwoods's engineers, a dear man who very much resembled Boris Karloff, buzzed in and out right behind him. Ileta had a phone to each ear, having simultaneous conversations, while she logged in several new charts.

I stacked the three charts that had discharge orders (one flu, one broken middle finger, one bladder infection) and issued medications and instructions, making it all policy-friendly by gathering signatures in the appropriate places.

Taking four new charts (an upper esophagus constricted around a large vitamin C pill, a sprained ankle, a nine-year-old who had dislocated his jaw on a jawbreaker the size of Mooshie's head, and an upper eyelid lacerated by the dried stalk of a Jerusalem artichoke), I admitted the patients to the three newly vacated gurneys.

After popping one of the minute nitroglycerine pills under the constricted-esophagus patient's tongue, I applied a cold compress to the sprained ankle, gave moral support to the nine-year-old, and did a vision check on the lacerated eyelid. When I came out from behind the curtains of bed 2, the engineer, Don, Dr. Mahoney, and Sarah, en masse, entered the orifice room and closed the door.

"Ileta, what's going on in there?"

"Honey," she said, "you don't want to know."

Really curious now, I went over to the two-way mirror cut into the door. Standing on tippytoes, I peered into the room and got a full view of the back of Dr. Mahoney's newly permed ash-brown hair, which surrounded her head like a stiff tutu.

I tapped the glass once.

Susan turned instantly and opened the door a crack. "What?" She almost bit me. "What do you want, Reverb?"

"I—I just wanted you to know that . . ." What the hell *did* I want her to know? "That you have more patients."

"Ha! That's what you think. I don't have any patience left at all. Now go do something useful." She slammed the door shut, then opened it again. "And tell Ileta to get that damned bottle man on the phone stat."

Bottle man?

When I relayed the message, Ileta frowned and put her hand over the mouthpiece. "You go tell that fool I'm getting the man at his home right now," she muttered. "Got the poor man out of bed and everything. His wife isn't very happy either. Oh. Hello? Mr. Dycek? Yes, please hold for Dr. Mahoney."

Susan Mahoney and Sarah exited the orifice room, and Ileta handed over the phone.

"Mr. Dycek? I'm sorry to bother you again, but I need to ask another question about the seams. If we hit them with a mallet . . ."

Dr. Mahoney paused, nodded, and took notes.

"Oh, uh huh. How big? . . . Oh, uh huh. In the exact middle or more toward the top? . . . Ah, yeah, okay. That's great. Thank you, Mr. Dycek. Go back to bed. I promise I won't bother you anymore tonight. Thank you."

Before I could ask what was going on, Dr. Mahoney disappeared into the orifice room. Two seconds later, the engineer jogged out the pneumatic doors. I headed for Sarah, who was washing her hands at the staff sink.

"What is going on in there?" I asked in a whisper.

"Oh, it's this guy who—" Sarah started to laugh, which was surprising, since it wasn't something she did very often except at the ER Christmas parties after one or two cups of Dr. Biggin's red bug punch.

Sarah straightened. "This poor old man thought that because he has—" She went off again in a peal of laughter, only this time it had a distinctly hysterical ring. Sarah slapped the sink, inhaled and snorted. That set both of us off; then Ileta began to chuckle, and I saw beds 2 and 4 peek around their curtains and laugh at what must have been a ridiculous scene—two nurses in scrubs and a respectable-looking older woman all bent at the waist, snorting and slapping chairs, walls, and one another with floppy hands. Each time someone snorted, we would all go off again, only harder. We sounded like cackling hens having severe asthma attacks and orgasms at the same time.

Sarah crossed her legs and tried to run to the staff bathroom, but her legs were laugh-crazy and wouldn't carry her straight. I was on my knees beating the seat of an empty roller chair, calculating which of us would wet first.

The phone rang, but no one could answer. Ileta could barely get her breath.

The patient from bed 2, the artichoke eyelid trauma, got off her gurney and answered for us. She took a message and told the caller there had been a temporary lapse of sanity and we'd return the call as soon as possible.

* * *

Elmo ran back through the main room, saw Sarah, who was now panting over the sink, and held up two rubber mallets, smiling in triumph. That set her off again.

Ileta had fully recovered and was back to answering phones, the attack of insanity having passed for her. I was holding my sore stomach, realizing that I didn't even know what was so funny. Refusing to look at Sarah, I splashed cold water on my face and took some deep breaths, blocking out her laughter with sobering thoughts of little boys with stab wounds.

By the time Sarah came out of the bathroom, I was attending to the sprained ankle. Sarah admitted a woman whose finger was being painfully constricted by a too tight ring. She instructed the woman to hold her hand over her head and point at the ceiling. In the "odd instruments" cabinet, she hunted diligently for the ring string: a thin string used for winding tightly around the swollen digit, forcing the blood away from the ring and into the tip of the finger.

"Okay, now tell me what is in the orifice room," I said sternly.

"Oh God," Sarah sighed, picking through a box filled with strange things like a bottle of Adolph's meat tenderizer, a salad server set, wire, pliers, candles, matches, and three spools of twine. "He's a sixty-six-year-old guy who lost his wife about a year ago and decided that he wanted to join the swinging singles crowd. But first"—Sarah held up a finger and giggled—"he thought he should prepare himself for all those wild women out there, and not being very well endowed, he thought he would enlarge himself by doing a daily stretch."

She bit her lip. "So he found a soda bottle he liked and proceeded to stuff himself into the bottle and pull so as to make himself bigger. The problem is, he became so engorged, he couldn't get out."

It didn't seem likely that I could have a vase and now a bottle in one shift. I searched Sarah's face for a sign that she was kidding, and found none.

"You mean he's stuck in the bottle? A *soda* bottle with the teeny little openings that you can't even stick your tongue all the way into?"

Sarah nodded and I could see the impression of her teeth still in her lip. "We tried everything . . . ice, oil, Vaseline, tapping, rubbing. We called the engineer, but the only thing he could think of was to use a glass cutter. Dr. Mahoney thought that was too risky and wanted to check with an expert, so she called the bottling plant and got the home number of the foreman.

"When he finally believed it wasn't a crank call, he said a glass cutter wouldn't work. The only thing we can do without shattering the glass is to pop the bottle open by hitting both seams at the same time with mallets."

"Well, there *is* one good thing about this," I said, not daring to look at Sarah. "This guy may have found a new hobby."

Sarah cocked her head.

"Sounds like he'd be awfully good at building ships in bottles."

Even before Sarah could open her mouth, behind me Ileta snorted into the phone and began to cackle.

An hour later, a very relieved Mr. Goodwin shuffled out the door with instructions to stay out of small places. He didn't look anything like a bottle abuser. He looked like a nice white-haired grandfather who spent most of his time sweeping leaves off the front walk and tinkering around a home workshop building birdhouses.

Before we went home, Don called Mercy's pediatric surgical ICU. Vic was still on the critical list, and his mother had never shown up.

Monday
1:30 A.M.

I built a fire when I got home, and Simon came out to sit with me for a while. It was one of those rare occasions when he really talked from his gut. It reminded me of those evenings when he was a youngster and would make me drive aimlessly for hours just so we could talk undisturbed.

He shared all his fears about the world today—the pollution and the wars—and told me his dreams of wanting to make a better, saner way of life. He was so proud of himself over the success of his skateboard ramp design. My honest praise won me enough of his confidence for him to show me the chemical-free, energy-conserving waste-disposal design idea he has been working on for the last two weeks. I savored every moment and every bit of laughter with him, and as I watched his face while he talked, I felt so very rich.

Later, after Simon had gone back to bed, my thoughts went naturally to Paul. I remembered that when his family came in to visit, they brought one of his young nephews. The child perched himself on the end of his uncle's bed investigating each of his toys, checking out its mechanics—its value—and I noticed that every set of eyes was on him in fascination—even Paul's.

How innocence draws people. Do we keep it only for as long as we remain unhurt?

Went over my schedule of speaking engagements tonight. Next week I am guest speaker at the pinning ceremony of Buchanan's graduating nursing class. I'm nervous, not only because it is my alma mater, but because the new ones are so idealistic and fragile. How can I tell them, the hopefuls, what they are up against? I must keep in mind how it feels to be so full of that driving need to help.

I went by Cunningham's Gallery on my way to the hospital and took a look at Risen's work. What a talent. Each painting generates a million different feelings.

I have always regarded Risen as a silly kind of man, but now that I've walked around inside him, I think I've seen the inner person he does not show us. Next time I see him, I know I will feel a little embarrassed, a little awed. How else should you feel about someone that you don't know well, but intimately?

There was one small painting of a cabin in the middle of a desolate plain on the edge of a small copse of winter trees. And the moon, which is full, has thrown a sort of moonglade on the snow. I was so taken into the scene that I could feel the cold air on my face and the melancholy of that place.

Maybe it's because it is summer, but loneliness is haunting me like a restless spirit. I have been alone for five years and sometimes it feels like such a waste. My love life is like an EKG—it started out in normal sinus rhythm, went into a few episodes of fibrillation, and has finally died after a prolonged period of asystole.

Janey called to say she's started writing a biography. She's titling it: Michael Jackson: A Hormonal Mystery.

I think I might be able to sleep tonight. Then again, maybe not. I'm almost too exhausted to sleep. I try to calm my mind with meditation, though outside thoughts continu-

ally bombard the small gains I make toward some kind of peace.

Tomorrow morning before I sit down to write, I will go up to the mountain and gather berries ... although now that I think about it, I suppose the berries really gather us each summer.

SEVEN

"There are many wordless places in nursing care, and these wordless places are some of our finest moments, and they will remain hidden. And that is all right because those moments do not have to be rewarded by others; they are reward enough in themselves."

PATRICIA BENNER, R.N.

THE SIGHT OF RED ROSEBUDS fastened to white uniform lapels triggered memories of my own pinning ceremony. Buchanan College auditorium still smelled of upholstery glue, greenhouses, and old newspapers, and sounded of relief and applause. In fact, most everything seemed to be the same as it had been then, complete with young children pointing and excitedly yelling, "That's *my* mom! She's gonna win a prize!"

One of the new grads was at the podium welcoming the audience to the kickoff celebration for their new lives, when I felt a sharp tap. I turned enough to catch a glimpse of Miss Telmack, one of the second-year instructors and my old nemesis, sitting behind me.

A steel grip on my shoulder stopped me from turning around fully. "Leave out the politics, Heron," she hissed. "We don't want to turn these kids off before they're even out of the chute."

I managed to strain my eyes to the far sides of their sockets. Illuminated by the dim light of the stage, Miss Telmack's face reminded me of a ferret. For one second, I was the student again, intimidated by that venomous voice. In the next, my outrage came up and out of my gut like so much vomit from Linda Blair's possessed body.

"I write my own speeches, Miss Telmack—I'll tell the truth

147

and no less. I'm not in the business of lying. It's my experience that these 'kids' want it straight, so I give it to them straight."

The steel grip on my shoulder relaxed, but her voice stayed sharp. "They'll find out the truth soon enough. Ignorance is bliss. Let them form their own opinions."

I turned all the way around in my seat and faced her squarely. "Ignorance can be painful." I whispered; people in nearby seats were beginning to notice something going on. "Don't you think it would be nicer if you prepared these people for what's waiting for them by giving them tools to fight with instead of feeding them a bunch of happy horseshit?"

A man sitting behind Miss Telmack put his fingers to his lips and glared at me.

"If you taught them empowerment instead of how to keep their eyes and mouth shut, they'd be a whole lot better off. Did you really expect that I would censor the truth because you . . ."

My switchboard ladies set off a few alarm lights. Sensing a tense stillness, I blinked and looked around. People for two rows up and down were staring. How could they not? Miss Telmack and I sat straining in our seats, eyes flashing like two wombats ready to do battle to the death.

At the podium, the student had been replaced by the director of the nursing school, who was going on about a student who had sat on that very stage many years before, blah blah blah, and would you please welcome Echo Heron.

I blanked Miss Telmack out, stood, and walked up the steps to the stage, thinking about my speech. Talons of self-doubt replaced Miss Telmack's grip. It is true that some of the more conservative nurses had labeled me a card-carrying member of the lunatic fringe. Maybe the new grads *were* too tender to hear such hard politics. By the time I reached the podium, I had mentally deleted four and a half pages of the five-page speech. I'd say hello, wish them luck, and make my exit.

Then I saw Miss Telmack's disapproving face over the footlights and scanned the faces of the new grads, and the self-doubt faded. I glanced down at the first paragraph and back at the audience. Judging by the looks of their proper go-to-meetin' clothes, and the number of children present, I did think it best to skip the joke about my premenstrual cynicism and go on to the second paragraph.

Waiting for my internal cue, I listened for that subtle, thrilling hush of anticipation that only a large audience can emit, and at the right moment, began.

I started with the story of the afternoon Mr. Brachman coded in the hallway, and four of the CCU nurses successfully resuscitated and stabilized him without the aid of a physician—only to hear Mr. Brachman, five hours later, thank Dr. Meyers for the miracle of saving his life.

Of course, Dr. Meyers took the credit like an innocent schoolgirl, with a lot of blushing and scuffing of feet. But when he came out to the desk, the four of us were waiting for him.

"Hey Dr. Meyers, you really did perform some kind of miracle there," Nealy said, and patted his back roughly enough to knock him off balance.

"Yeah," I chimed in. "It sure was some kind of miracle—saving old Mr. Brachman's life from the golf course across town."

The point I went on to make was that nurses were the backbone of the hospital. We were the voice of the patients as well as their protectors—it was our primary duty not to cater to the system, but rather to care for our patients in the best way we knew how.

I didn't look in Miss Telmack's direction when I touched on the feminist issues that surround nursing. Starting with the premise that nursing is, and always has been, considered "women's work" and continues to be reimbursed as such in low wages, I progressed into a narrative about how, as women working in a predominantly male field, nurses are often deprived of autonomy and respect.

Making a lighthearted analogy, I described an administrator's office I'd once seen—an elaborate twelve-hundred-square-foot room done in "masculine" colors of tan, black, and forest green, complete with tiled shower in the bathroom, airconditioning, stereo system, stationary bike, plush carpets, hand-carved wooden ducks from Gump's, rich leather furniture and designer lighting.

Next door, the nursing administrator's office was a dark, ten-by-twelve room without windows or proper ventilation, containing an institutional-gray metal desk, a cheap vase, an office chair, and a four-drawer filing cabinet.

From there I slid into some of the down-side facts and horror stories (I addressed this portion directly to Miss Telmack, who sat sucking lemons, her rose limp at the neck), then surged upward through the themes of fulfillment, solidarity, and the need for humor. I ended forty minutes later with a plea that was not written anywhere in my notes:

"The next time you're working, look into the face of another nurse who is doing CPR, or comforting a frightened patient, or lending herself to the walking wounded known as the family, or giving everything she has to keep one step ahead of pain and death—and know that you are looking into the face of human compassion.

"Then know, that that is your face too.

"Be proud of that, because despite all the hardships and stress, despite all the political unrest, you are a part of the most incredible profession in the world."

What amazed me was that when I said, "Thank you," I knew with absolute certainty that I loved nursing. There *wasn't* any profession like it in the world, and we *were* a family—all two million of us, because we were bonded to one another in the best way possible—through our caring for others.

In the question-and-answer period that routinely follows my speeches, I am inevitably asked what my co-workers think of me. In what must seem like a direct contradiction to my message of solidarity and nursely bonding love, I must admit that I am not an easy person to work with.

Any one of my co-workers would tell you that and more. If you asked, they would be quick to say that at work I am usually stubborn, sometimes irascible, and always outspoken. To put the record straight, Mother Teresa I ain't.

In one newspaper interview, the misguided journalist described me as "saintly." That was good for a few belly laughs around the hospital. Someone tacked the article to the CCU nursing lounge bulletin board and put red asterisks beside the adjective. Over to the side was written, "Must be a typo. Probably meant 'satanly.' "

Okay, okay, but in my own defense, I will say that I make my co-workers laugh a lot (whether at me or with me doesn't matter—what counts is that they're laughing), and I don't think I have ever let another nurse down.

I think most of my fellow nurses would go along with me on that, even the ones who cross themselves or hiss when I enter the unit.

Dr. Cramer was on the landing between the third and fourth floors, busily making an entry in the infamous black book. He was so intensely involved he hadn't heard me come up the stairs behind him.

The golden opportunity was upon me like a cat on a sunny rug, and before I had a chance to question the wisdom of my actions, I peeped over his shoulder.

Showing was a page vertically divided. In the first column was a list of names with dollar amounts written after each one. In the other, written in his precise, tight hand, I read:

> *. . . when the wad of Beemans gum got stuck to the bottom of her penny loafer.*
> *He knew she was Italian from the start, but being a more passionate man (it was rumored he was half German, half human), he did not foresee the problem that would eventually drive a barber's hot razor through the middle of their love—the constant tangling of their mustaches with every tormenting kiss.*
> *Only Admiral Jack could—*

"Yeeeeuck!" Dr. Cramer slammed the black book shut on his pen and turned on me. "Spying doesn't become you, Heron, especially when you smell like you've been soaked in pickle brine."

I sniffed. The redolence of vinegar caused me to look to my lunch bag for the betraying bottle of vinegar-basil dressing that was leaking down the side of my scrub pants and onto the floor.

"I wasn't spying," I insisted defiantly. "I was satisfying my sick and overpowering curiosity."

An evil grin slipped around the corners of Joe's mouth. "And what did you see, Heron?"

I bit my lip. "Oh, nothing . . . much. You write too small, like you're repressing something vital."

Joe threw me a doubtful glance then shrugged. "That's okay, Heron, you're going to be punished. Wait until you see your assignment."

My face dropped as my mind raced through all the nasty possibilities. I imagined the horrors that only a nurse can know: four patients on balloon pumps and lines and every drip possible; six DTs patients in heart block; slimy denture detail; seven sick, excitable, non-English-speaking patients whose families have been allowed to camp out in the room. Whatever it was, by the gleam in Dr. Cramer's eyes I could be sure it wasn't going to be nice.

He descended the same stairs I had just ascended, quite pleased with himself. But before the top of his head disappeared from my view, I forced a laugh of pure disdain, and yelled so that the railings rang with my voice, *"The constant tangling of their mustaches with every tormenting kiss . . .?"*

The photos were hung in rainbow formation on the wall over my patient's head. They were the traditional American wedding-day-memories pictures familiar to each of us—the bride and groom stuffing messy pieces of white frosted cake into each other's mouths, the bridesmaids linking arms, relatives dancing to the tunes played by the hired band, someone's favorite uncle kissing someone else's maiden aunt, a preschool ring bearer holding hands with an older, mortified flower girl, a crowd of young men eagerly awaiting the blue-satin-and-white-lace garter, and the circle of hopeful women jumping for the bouquet.

One photo drew my attention more than the others, and I squeezed myself in between the head of the bed and the wall for a closer look.

Concentrated on the thin, pale face of her bridegroom, her eyes were huge, long-lashed and intense with love. The shining newness of the gold band was the focal point of the photograph, appearing almost too wide for her slender finger. If I hadn't been so intent on observing the less obvious, I would have missed how gently her fingers rested on his jaw.

I pushed wisps of blond bangs out of my patient's eyes, and compared the photo with the real woman who lay in the bed before me. Nothing much was different on the surface; the creamy skin had perhaps taken on a bit of a pallid hue, and the glow was gone, but there were the same long lashes, and the same mole under her right eye, the same gold band. It was the nonphysical change that was obvious, the absence of her spirit, or her essence, or whatever it was that made her who she was.

That photo is three days old, I thought, taken only minutes or maybe an hour before she . . . what?

Before she became the corpse in bed 4, attached to a respirator and a couple of IVs.

On my way into the unit, I'd noticed the handsome man in the waiting room, lean, paler still than his wedding photo. He sat, elbows on knees, the palms of his hands covering his eyes. A younger man, bearing a strong familial resemblance, had his arm around the weeping man's shoulder.

The smell and sound of grief filled the hallway. Normal People wouldn't know that grief really does have a subtle odor and sound. But it is there; you only need be around it enough years to recognize the faint waxy smell like church candles, and hear the particular dusty silence that fills the cracks around the sound of tears.

I wondered if Chris, the day shift nurse rattling off report, was aware of how much she looked like the patient in bed 4. It was such a close resemblance, it was eerie.

"She liked to be called Willy, not Millicent," Chris said in a monotone of discouragement. Her use of the past tense did not escape my notice. "Willy was what her kid brother called her from the time he was two. The name stuck."

A monitor alarm went off, bleeping at a rate of about 100. At the same time, the phone rang. Phoebe, our monitor tech and clerk for the evening, rolled her chair between the two machines, stretched her arms wide in opposite directions, and took care of both noises at the same time.

"She was twenty-three," Chris went on, "an occupational therapist for the handicapped, in excellent health, social drinker only, nonsmoker, took no medications except a daily vitamin supplement.

"She was married on Saturday, and at some point toward the end of the festivities, she apparently choked on an hors d'oeuvre. Instead of bringing attention to herself, she went into an empty room, and obviously, wasn't successful at dislodging whatever it was from her airway. The groom found her completely unresponsive about ten minutes later. When the paramedics got there, her pupils were fixed and dilated."

Chris shook her head, not taking her eyes off the Rand card. "Rob Naylor from Rescue Unit Twenty said she was actually blue. She was in V fib, but they shocked her out of it with one defibrillation. Heart's been perfect ever since.

"Her EEG is showing zero activity. All other systems including her kidneys are in great shape. Initially Cramer had her on low-dose dopamine, but that was stopped yesterday."

Wearily, Chris pushed open the chart and scrutinized the top sheet. She had yet to look at me. "The husband and family contacted the transplant-donor network as soon as brain death was verified. Apparently she had discussed this with her family a long time ago, plus there's an organ donor sticker on her driver's license." Chris worked her knuckles for a moment. "They said she was that kind of person." She looked at me finally, wearing a plaintive smile. "You know the type," she said. "One of those terminal caretakers."

I knew the type well. I reflected on the evening several weeks back when all the nurses on duty had compared driver's license photos to determine if anyone was peculiar-looking enough to actually resemble their picture. What drew our attention was that six out of the seven licenses bore the small pink circle that designated the driver as a potential organ donor in case of death.

From the inside pocket of the chart, Chris removed a folder of papers. "Anyway, here's the donor manual. There's an official organ-procurement coordinator named Mary who's been assigned to Willy. She's the R.N. in charge of the whole operation. Dr. Cramer gave her carte blanche to write orders for whatever she needs to keep the body in optimal condition. She's already taken care of getting the consent signed by the husband and verifying exactly what they want to donate, which, by the way, is everything, including tissue.

"Talk about dedication—the woman was here all day evaluating the results of the lab work and serological studies." Chris squinted. "On Sunday she put in sixteen hours gathering and researching all Willy's medical/social history. She even tracked down her pediatrician.

"Go over this stuff." Chris tapped the manila folder. "It's fascinating. Like, did you know that each recipient hospital has a separate surgical team for each organ?"

I shook my head. "Sounds like the OR could get pretty crowded."

"Yeah, that's what Mary said. The solid-organ guys get to go first, followed by the tissue guys."

I moved a little closer to Chris and lowered my voice. "I've always wanted to know if they really carry the organs . . ."

Chris anticipated the question. "In coolers? Yes. Igloo or Playmate, she didn't specify." She laughed. "I asked the same thing. Anyway, she's on her pager. We're supposed to call her if anything happens. The number is plastered all over the place."

I could see for myself that the red-and-white oval stickers were in abundance—two on the Rand, four on the outside of the chart, and a dozen or more stuck to various pages on the inside. I guessed they were really serious about procuring some organs.

Chris finally met my eyes. She looked worn out.

"The husband is a basket case. The mother and father are taking it pretty well, for now anyway. We were receiving so many calls from friends that we had to put a hold on them at the switchboard."

The call bell went off for bed 3 and Chris ran to answer it. When she returned to the desk, she fell heavily into the chair and groaned.

"The family has specified that they'll release her at eleven o'clock tonight to the operating room." The nurse cocked her head. "I know she's going to benefit a lot of people, but I'm sorry—I overheard the coordinator on the phone saying she was going on a harvest tonight, and I couldn't help thinking it sounded like they're going to rototill the vegetable garden.

"Ah, man." She motioned toward the room with the curtains pulled all the way around, and her eyes became flinty. "It's all such a goddamned depressing shame."

Esther Rau was rushed into the waiting space of bed 1. Using the pull sheet, Gus pushed while Pia and I pulled her off the ER gurney and onto the bed. Pia removed the woman's clothes and detached her from the ER portable monitor as soon as we had her hooked onto ours. Safety net to safety net.

Gus, sounding more southern than the cast of *Tobacco Road*, gave additional report while she packed up the monitor and wheeled the gurney out of our way.

"This sweet lady was having herself a nice little dinner of bacon, sardines, and crackers, when her left arm and jaw began to ache. Isn't that right, Mrs. Rau?" Gus pronounced Rau like Roo.

The seventy-four-year-old widow nodded in a way that said she couldn't have cared less what the hell Gus was saying.

"About an hour later, she felt like there was a tight band around her chest and called nine-one-one."

Mrs. Rau clutched at her chest, the furrows between her eyes growing deeper. The electrode on her left shoulder fell off, and as I pressed a new one into its place, I noticed that her skin was cold and wet from perspiration.

"BP was still in the high one-fifty range before we left," Gus added as I hit the auto button on the automatic blood pressure cuff. "Dr. Ostermann is still in the doom room looking at her admission blood pressures and her EKG strips. Said he'd be up in fifteen minutes to put in the art line and start the TPA. Poor little thing (pronounced "thang") doesn't have any family in the area, so she's going to have to sign her own consent."

"I've got to sit up!" Mrs. Rau gasped, struggling upward.

Pia held her down by the shoulders. "Shhhh. I'll put up the head of the bed. Don't you do anything except concentrate on relaxing."

Panting, Mrs. Rau lay back, giving herself up to the strangers who moved quickly around her bed. She whimpered, "I'm frightened."

I wiped the sweat away from her face, and she groped for my hand, holding it so tightly it hurt. "Don't be afraid," I said, "we won't let anything happen to you. We're going to get rid of your pain first, then we'll take care of everything else. Slow your breathing down. Deep, easy breaths for now."

Mrs. Rau wet her lips and nodded, exhaling, then taking in a long, shaky breath and letting it out through pursed lips. I studied the rhythm on the monitor screen; it was limping badly with a lot of PVCs.

"Did Dr. Ostermann talk to you about what he wants to do?"

She nodded. "He told me he wanted to give me a medicine in my veins."

"That's right, but I'm going to explain it to you a little better and then you'll need to sign a paper giving Dr. Ostermann permission to do that, okay?"

Before she could answer, the blood pressure alarm tore through the room. Mrs. Rau's eyes flew open so wide, my eyeballs ached for her.

"Wha—?"

"It's only the blood pressure machine."

Pia flicked the alarm silencer and checked the screen. "One seventy-four over ninety-four," she mouthed silently.

"First Dr. Ostermann is going to insert a short wire into your groin, right here." I pressed a finger over her femoral artery. "It's called an arterial line and it tells us what your blood pressure is at all times. Otherwise, this machine would be squeezing your arm every ten minutes."

"I don't like that thing." Mrs. Rau pouted. "It hurts."

"Well, as soon as the line is in, Dr. Ostermann is going to inject some blood-thinning medicine through your IV line called tissue plasminogen activator, or TPA for short. That'll dissolve the clot in the artery around your heart so the blood can then get through to give that part of your heart muscle the oxygen it needs. Your pain should go away quickly after that."

Mrs. Rau looked doubtful. "Dr. Ostermann said there might be a problem with bleeding?"

"True. Your blood won't be able to clot normally for a while, so we have to be very careful with you. We'll draw all your blood through a line that's already inserted into your vein, and we'll be making sure you don't bruise yourself or . . ."

As usual, I had to weigh whether to tell her *all* the possible risks, saw her shiver, and decided not to.

I took the soft gauze eye pads off Willy's eyes and squirted in the artificial tears. (Next-to-new corneas for sale. Not a scratch on 'em.)

The very unscientific speculation came to mind as to whether the recipient of her corneas would somehow see the world differently, perhaps a bit like Willy did. I knew it was absurd, but if I were the one to receive those eyes, I would be watchful for the slightest perception that might not be entirely mine.

Glancing through the curtains, I saw that Dr. Ostermann had not yet arrived in Mrs. Rau's room, and turned my attention back to Willy's body. I washed and massaged the fine skin, which was softer than any Caucasian skin I had ever touched. And as I turned and moved her about, I felt as though I were handling a bolt of precious fabric, getting it ready to be cut and sewn. Eyes, skin, joints, tissues, inner ear, heart, pancreas, liver, kidneys, lungs, long bones. Waste not, want not.

It was eerie waiting for a well person to die before a sick person could live. No matter which way I looked at it, organ transplant seemed, by nature, a perverse thing.

The ST segments on Mrs. Rau's EKG abruptly went down to normal size about fifteen minutes into thrombolytic therapy. It was the sign that the clot had been dissolved.

"How's the pain, Esther?" Dr. Ostermann asked over his shoulder. He kept his eyes glued to the EKG machine, which was running out a constant record piling at his feet. The hill of paper was up to his ankles.

"Gone," she whispered. Her face was still grave, still full of worry.

"Hey," I said, rubbing her arm, "you're doing great. Stop worrying."

"It's not me, it's Dobbie," she said. Her chin trembled. "She hasn't been fed, and there isn't anybody to take her out."

"Dobbie is your dog?"

She nodded. "A golden retriever. I got her after my husband died last year."

"Don't you have any neighbors who could . . ."

Tears slid down the creases in Mrs. Rau's cheeks. "Bill and Ellen are away on vacation, and Marcella is in Houston for the week. There's an elderly woman who lives behind me, but she can't walk."

A seventy-four-year-old calling someone else "elderly" brought a smile to my face. "Okay, where do you live?" I asked, taking a direct course to the inescapable conclusion.

Mooshie was going to throw a fit.

At six forty-five I was still taking off Dr. Ostermann's orders when the intercom buzzed.

"Hi, this is Gladys Ryan, Willy's sister? May I come in to see her?"

I thought for a second, trying to remember who was listed on the Rand card under immediate family members. I couldn't recall seeing anything about a sister—one brother, yes, but no sister.

"Well, okay," I said, too tired to press the matter or search for the Rand card. "Come through the double doors at the end of the hall to your right."

In four seconds, the double doors hissed open and a young woman the color of burnt almonds walked quickly past the desk.

"Whoa! Wait a minute. Are you the person who just called in as Willy's sister?"

She answered with a perfectly straight face. "Yep."

I lowered my glasses. "Well, that's one hell of a tan you got there, sister."

Five minutes later, the intercom buzzed again—two more sisters and a half sister wanted in. Ten minutes later, it was her four brothers.

By seven P.M., fifteen people had paraded by the desk and slipped into Willy's room. They were all colors, all ages, all shapes and sizes—all siblings of a sort.

I waited to hear weeping, but none came. Instead I heard the single note of a pitch pipe, and then a chorus of voices began to sing Jackson Browne's "For a Dancer."

Rolling my chair around to face the glass doors of her room, I searched until I found a gap in the curtains. They had squeezed into a circle all the way around Willy's bed, left arms around the person to the left, right hands touching her. I studied their faces as they stood there loving at her: they were sending their love down through their hands and into her.

I blinked, then moved closer to verify what I beheld with my own eyes. The change was dramatic: Willy's pale skin was glowing. There was none of the ashen death in her face.

All eyes were upon her. Some cried, others were smiling. And they kept singing until they'd said goodbye.

When the initial fuss was over, Mrs. Rau said she couldn't believe how well she felt for someone who'd had a heart attack. It was going to make great conversation for years to come at her flower-arranging meetings.

While Mrs. Rau dictated, I wrote down Dobbie's feeding, pooping, and exercise schedules, what her favorite dog toys were, and where she liked to be rubbed the most.

Next, I sifted through the old-lady contents of Mrs. Rau's purse—Kleenex, hankie, badly worn leather change purse, wintergreen Lifesavers, magnifying glass, travel-size hand lotion, lipstick, pill case, rosary beads, fold-up rain bonnet, old grocery list clipped to a small collection of coupons—until I found the single house key at the bottom.

"How do you feel, Mrs. Rau?" I asked, folding the doggie info card around the key and slipping the package into my breast pocket.

"Call me Esther," she said in her fluttery old-lady's voice. "I'm tired."

I looked more closely at her. She had a gentle face, one that suggested she'd spent some time growing violets and geraniums and preparing meals for the less fortunate.

There was something, though, that bothered me. On the surface she seemed okay—in fact, all body systems were running like a top—but on another level something was missing, and I couldn't quite put my finger on what it was. I was trying to decide if this was my nurse's sixth sense or neurosis, when she found my hand and held it. I could feel her old bones soaking up the warmth of my hand.

"Did you know that Esther is one of my favorite names?" I

asked. "And when you have a name like Echo, that's saying something."

Mrs. Rau made a face. "Never liked Esther. I always wanted to change my name to Esmeralda." She laughed the way older ladies do, in that light, reassuring way. "I had a friend in Oregon named Echo many years ago. I was originally from Portland, until I married. You aren't from Oregon, are you, dear?"

I shook my head. "Originally, up near Schenectady, New York."

"Ah, yes," she said, "home of Charles Steinmetz and the first television broadcast."

I looked at her, amazed. She was probably a hell of a Trivial Pursuit player.

For a short time we sat without speaking, comfortable in our silence.

"How about you? Are *you* all right, dear? You look a bit down in the mouth."

"No, not really," I answered, feeling totally down in the mouth. "Only tired."

"Oh my." Her sigh was a sound like a taffeta comforter slipping off the bed. "You girls work so hard. I wish you'd let me do something."

"Well, we've got a couple of rooms down the hall that need to be cleaned."

Esther lifted herself on her elbows and giggled like a girl. "Get me a duster and a hairnet, and point me in the right direction."

"Just get well," I said, laughing. "That'll be your job."

"God willing"—she sighed again, falling back onto her pillow—"I'll live to bake another lemon meringue for Dobbie."

Mother, father, and little brother were together in the room for the last time. The mother was calm, businesslike, as she efficiently tended to the small chores she imagined her daughter would have wanted: braiding her hair, rubbing oil into her cuticles, daubing perfume on the pillow. In the future, she would remember doing these things and it would lessen the horror. Her tears seemed to be held back by a fragile veil of determination as she washed her daughter's face with a warm washcloth and confided, in a gossipy, over-coffee tone, about Doreen and Alan's new house and the walnut armoire down at

Braverman's that she thought would be perfect for the upstairs master bedroom. Willy?

Her father paced idly around the bed, studying the IV pump and the dials on the respirator, probably thinking about improved designs so as to keep the memories away an hour longer.

He watched closely while I suctioned her, his face only inches from mine. I could see his agony and wondered if, when he looked at her now, he was remembering the way she had turned and kissed him when he gave her to her groom. Or was he thinking of the look on the donor coordinator's face as she'd rated his daughter's body for the harvest of its usable parts?

Her brother, wearing his blue football captain's sweater, sat at the foot of her bed. He laced his fingers together, the muscles in his jaw working overtime.

I moved closer in order to retape her IV and saw the faint white crust old tears had left in his peach fuzz. He never once changed position, afraid he might disturb his sister's sleep.

Without preface, he suddenly announced that he remembered the summer she taught him how to fasten playing cards to the spokes of his bike with clothespins so they would make sounds like a motorbike.

His mother and father and I momentarily stopped what we were doing (washing, pacing, taping) and listened while he described the soft weight of her hair in his hand as he held it away from the bicycle chain, black with grease.

Hey Willy Nilly, where are you?

"Hello?"

Mrs. Rau hesitated in her explanation of exactly what she meant when she said she was beginning to feel "funny," but she didn't respond to the woman standing in her doorway, knocking on the glass.

Without receiving permission, the woman entered the room.

"Ah, excuse me, may I help you?" I was annoyed by the invasion of our privacy. I hadn't taken a dinner break and could feel the hypoglycemic/PMS-shrew part of my personality breaking through.

"I'm Mary Giesen," the petite woman said, offering her hand. "The organ coordinator."

She may have been small, but her grip was that of an over-eager salesman. If she could just jettison off some of the Dale Carnegie enthusiasm, I thought, she would be perfectly likable.

"Ah," I said, working to rescue my hand from being crushed.

"Millicent Ryerson is my region. You're the nurse taking care of her for us?"

Region? Christ, it *did* sound like she was talking about plowing the south forty.

"Mrs. Ryerson is my patient, yes." I was aware of the sharp edge to my voice, and mentally slapped my hand.

"I'd like to talk with you if you have some time . . ."

The donor nurse's voice trailed off as her eyes settled on Mrs. Rau. I imagined she was unconsciously surveying and ranking the woman body part by body part. The image of a vulture came to mind.

Without thought, I stepped in front of her, blocking her view. "I'll be out in a minute, okay?"

"Hope so. There's a lot to be done before twenty-three hundred hours."

When the nurse had gone, Mrs. Rau opened her eyes again and took my hand. "You won't forget about Dobbie, will you, dear?"

"I promise. Don't worry about anything, but I want you to finish telling me how you feel funny, okay?"

The monitor alarm went off again, and Phoebe yelled in for me to please do something about it. For the third time in one hour, I adjusted Mrs. Rau's rate and blood-pressure alarm limits. Her blood pressure was up slightly and her pulse was down.

"I'm too worn out," she said with an effort, and closed her eyes. "I'm going to take a nap now. I'll feel better later."

"Promise?"

Mrs. Rau smiled.

At the desk, I instructed Phoebe to put a call in to Dr. Ostermann and pulled Mrs. Rau's chart. I was going over the progress notes, when I felt someone standing over me.

"Can we talk over what we need to do before we take Millicent down to OR?" Mary asked.

I rolled my chair a foot back so I wouldn't get a kink in my neck from having to look up into the nurse's face. "I can't right now. My other patient isn't doing very well. I have to deal with that before I can even think about anything else."

"Well, do you mind if I take over Mrs. Ryerson's care until you're free?"

"Don't mind at all. Put it on my tab, and I'll owe you a liver or something."

The nurse didn't flinch. "Actually," she said, dead serious, "we have a huge demand for kidneys right now."

Mrs. Rau appeared to be asleep when I entered. I set the chart on her bedside table and casually laid my hand on her chest to feel the depth of her respirations. The damp coolness of her body sent a shock of panic through my temples.

"Esther!" There was no resistance; her body had the loose, clammy feel of death. As her head lolled to the side, a large amount of saliva ran out the side of her mouth and down her shoulder and neck, wetting the front of her gown.

Disbelieving, I twisted to look at the monitor behind me. Her rhythm was slower, the complexes were wider—it looked much like the final pattern of death. I threw back the covers and pushed her gown up to her waist, my fingers going for the femoral pulse.

It was there, weak and thready but palpable. On the monitor, the arterial wave form began to dampen. Accordingly, her blood pressure dropped. I yelled for Phoebe to get Ostermann stat and shook her again, yanking away the pillow. Her head fell onto the bed like a rag doll's.

The end of the story was revealed when I pulled open the woman's eyelids. She was gone—she'd snuck out while I wasn't looking, and we wouldn't get her back no matter what we did. Then I vividly remembered the + mark in the code-status box on the Rand card. Her physical body was slipping away, and I had to act even though what would follow was a travesty of life. We would code her, put her on life-support machines and drugs—keep her body alive for another day, perhaps another week, until her kidneys failed or her heart gave out.

I kicked myself for not paying closer attention to my guts. How the hell could I have missed such an obvious cerebral bleed? Did she need to have a flashing neon sign on her forehead?

The guilt immediately turned to fury. What goddamned right did we have anyway to be pumping a seventy-four-year-old with new-fangled drugs that turned her blood to water? Why couldn't we leave these fragile old souls alone?

Mary was at the door with a question in her eyes. In my moment of anger and irrationality, I again saw her as the vulture sniffing out possibilities. My switchboard ladies featured an instant replay of the scene in *Zorba the Greek* when Anthony Quinn's lover discovers that her deathbed has been surrounded by old crones, impatiently waiting for her last breath so they can pounce on her worldly possessions.

"Out!" I demanded. "Get out of here!"

Lowering the bed, I reached into Mrs. Rau's mouth, pulled out her dentures and inserted the green plastic airway. Before I began my assault, I asked her forgiveness.

"Hey buddy," he said, stroking his wife's face. In the sanctuary of her presence, his voice was soft, respectful of where he was. "I'd hate to think what the guys would say if I went on my honeymoon without my wife." He held Willy's hand, kissed it, and quickly put it to his forehead as if he had suddenly remembered an old pain.

"Will? Can you get it together here? Gotta hurry, kid."

A cold chill went down the back of my neck. I glanced up from the IV I was untangling and recognized the never-say-die look.

Oh my God, I thought, hasn't anybody explained to him what's going on here? ("That's not your wife, sir, that's a 4-H project.") My ulcer awoke and pinched at the sight of the young man praying death away from his beloved.

The weight of him leaning against her bed had pulled her gown down, exposing one of her breasts. Without taking his eyes from her face, he tenderly pulled it up and tied the strings.

"She's cold all the time, you know. We really need to get her another blanket."

"Mr. Ryerson . . ."

He ignored me, kind of half smiling as he cried. It was the weirdest expression of grieving.

"We've got three quilts on the bed and she still has cold feet. I don't want her getting pneumonia or something like that."

With trembling fingers, he undid her braid, picked up the hairbrush on her bedside table, and sat next to her. In the awkward manner of a man who is fascinated by, but does not understand, the nature of a woman's hair, he cautiously began to pull the brush through the blond silk.

"Will? Why don't you wake up, honey? Just like you to pull a surprise on our wedding day. You could have been—"

"Mr. Ryerson?"

"Shhhh."

"Mr. Ryerson, listen, Willy isn't—"

"Shhhh! She can hear you. This is my best friend in the world. You people don't know her like I do. She's the best . . ." The brush stopped halfway down a section of hair.

I walked over and put my hand on his arm, holding it until he looked at me. His misery hit me so hard, I had to take a deep breath.

"She's gone," I whispered.

"No." He hesitated and shook his head slowly. "No. She isn't. Not really. She's the most alive person. She's . . . She's all I've got. She can't be."

He pushed his face against her chest. His head rose with each breath forced into her by the respirator.

"She can't be. She's my best friend. She wouldn't desert me. She wouldn't leave . . ."

"Come on," I said, gently pulling on his arm. "I want you to help me turn her onto her side. She's too heavy for me."

It was a lie, of course. Willy weighed about a hundred pounds. But he needed to be lured away from his pain, if only momentarily. Depression and grief could put people in a trap that was sometimes impossible to escape from. Anyone who has ever experienced that foggy place knows there is something eerie about being there; it sets a person apart from the rest of the world.

I found a fresh pull sheet in one of the linen cupboards and spread it out on the side of the bed where the respirator stood. I wanted him to have as little as possible to do with the machines keeping her alive.

"Roll her toward you," I said, hoisting the thin body with the sheet. He took hold of the edges and pulled his wife's body toward himself. When she was close, he dropped the sheet and slipped his arm behind her back, burying his face in her hair. I don't know how many minutes he stayed that way—probably not as long as it seemed.

"We've been in love with each other since high school," he said, not moving away from her.

I continued rubbing her back, and was silent.

"Don't talk, listen," Tessie told us. *"Let people give voice to their suffering. Let them get as much out as they can so it*

doesn't stay inside and fester and get confused. Listen until you can't listen anymore."

"She loved helping people. That's why I gave permission for them to ... use her organs.... I know she's not coming back." He stood, staring at his love. "I miss her. I miss her so much, I can't stand it."

There was nothing that could be said. My arms folded around his trembling shoulders and I let him cry. He would be intimate with time: his tormentor and, ultimately, his healer. He would learn the crazy dance of grieving—weak and strong, up and down.

I wondered if knowing that part of her would still be living made his pain any easier to bear. And if it did, would he seek out the man who wore her eyes, or the woman in whose chest her heart worked?

I imagined that he probably would.

I was preparing Mrs. Rau for the morgue when Mary came in. I didn't look at her right away, but kept on with the washing of the body.

She moved about the room, clearing away the refuse of a short and useless resuscitation attempt.

"A lot of people don't understand what I do. Even other health professionals, especially the physicians, have a hard time with it. People see donor nurses as vultures."

I flinched, recalling my earlier thought.

"Do you know that my friends still think I go from car wreck to car wreck with cooler in hand?"

I let a smile crack through. "I'm sorry about yelling at you. It's just that taking care of someone as young as Willy is hard enough. When you add the wedding, the family, and the donor thing, it's almost too much, you know?"

The nurse looked at Mrs. Rau. She drew a deep breath and slowly freed it. "Oh, believe me, I know too well. I do this every day. It's the norm for the patient to be young. I'm assigned to a lot of kids, and I mean children from three days old to twenty years. If you think Willy was tough, try dealing with a six- or a sixteen-year-old. Now, *that's* hard."

I tied Mrs. Rau's wrists together with the long strip of gauze from the morgue pack. Mary stood across from me looking pained. For a moment I presumed to understand what a heroic and horrible job she had.

Her gaze found mine. "I have yet to have a donor who I felt

was better off dead. This happened to Willy on her wedding day. I can't tell you all the special, tragic circumstances that surround most of my donors at the time of their deaths." She shook her head. Her eyes went to the window. "It's *always* stuff like the day before a kid leaves for college, or the day after a person's retirement, or a mother who has just delivered a healthy baby. It's almost uncanny."

Together, we pulled the sheet up over Mrs. Rau's body, naked except for the toe tag, the strip of gauze, the art line catheter, an endotracheal tube, and the IV in her right wrist. By law, Mrs. Rau was a postmortem candidate by reason of having died less than twenty-four hours after hospitalization. The idea of having the old woman's body explored seemed absurd.

"We're ready now to bring Willy down. Can you help?" Mary's eyes returned to me.

"Okay," I said, "but I want the family to say goodbye one more time."

The strange thing when they took Willy away was the peacefulness. Usually transfers are noisy and a little confused. I suspected that Mary was the grease that made the wheels spin smoothly. She had worked hard to make absolutely sure all the surgical teams were set up properly and on time, all the forms were filled out and signed, and copies of the chart had been made with nothing overlooked.

Willy's family had said goodbye in private, behind closed curtains. Her husband went in last, kissed her, and whispered something in her ear.

He slipped the wide gold band from her finger and put it on the little finger of his left hand, then placed his band on her index finger.

At the door he hesitated, obviously struggling with himself.

After a brief moment, he decided against turning around for that final look, and walked on.

By one A.M., the acute side was deserted. Phoebe and Mary had long since gone home, and for the moment no one was sick enough to need an acute bed. The harsh fluorescent lights, which invariably gave me migraines, had been dimmed to night-light levels, and the hum of the building lulled me into a place of peace. Early-morning hours in a hospital can be like that sometimes, almost as if during the day the building had soaked up all the peace of sleep and death and was slowly releasing it into the air.

While cleaning the two rooms recently vacated by Esther and Willy, I broke more rules and opened all the huge windows, letting fresh, sweet air rush in on the wind. The stale, sick smells vanished, and for the first time that shift, I felt I had accomplished something really worthwhile.

I was signing off my charts when Beth approached, carrying her jacket and purse, head cocked to one side. She looked as though she'd been ridden hard and put away wet.

"Have you got a minute?" she asked.

"I've got minutes up the whazoo. Sit down and tell me the whole story."

Beth sat down in the chair to my left. The creak was enough to wake the dead. "I . . ." She dropped her gaze from mine and looked toward the open windows. Outside, I could hear the wind playing with the trees.

"You all right?" I asked.

"No." Beth picked up a piece of scrap paper from the desk and cleared her throat. "I've been a recovering alcoholic for three and a half years." She went silent, studying the piece of paper without seeing it. When she spoke again, it was in a steadier voice. "The man I've been living with for the last three years betrayed me. He left me a month ago for someone else.

"Vodka, the old clarity in a bottle, was right there waiting for me to pick up where I left off." She shook her head. "I'm dying, and I don't want to. I've got a sponsor, but I can't bring myself to call her right now. I'm . . . I don't want to hear all that twelve-step rhetoric. I don't want to deal with the heavy-handed stuff from a bunch of twelve-step Nazis."

Beth bowed her head and tears fell on the desk like clear round stones.

"My sponsor has it all—a home, kids, a happy marriage. What does she know about being a lonely person or having a job like this?" She gripped her arms across her chest, as if trying to keep herself together. "I need someone to lean on for a while. I don't have a lot of friends right now." Beth watched me, her eyes needful, waiting.

"What else do you do? I mean, you've got to do something other than"—I spread my hand out to indicate the unit—"work here."

"I dance," Beth said, and I thought I saw her eyes take on

the tiniest bit of life. "There's a studio in the city where you can go and pretend you know what you're doing. Jazz, modern, ballet—whatever you want. It helps. It's an addiction too, but it helps."

I toyed with my glasses, thinking that what Beth was asking me to do was unfair to us both. Unfortunately, the lingering, codependent yeah-but side of me argued that she was down enough to ask for help, and maybe, if I could find the right healing words . . .

Okay, okay. So I wasn't going to turn her down and I knew it.

"I'll do what I can until you work through this initial bad time, but I won't be there for you if you drink. Alcoholics are bad for my health."

"Good," she said with a faint smile, and reached over to hug me. "You're not a *total* codependent, anyway."

"Only after years of intensive training, my dear."

Training. The word echoed through the switchboard ladies' headsets. Training. Training. Heel, Rover.

I sat upright with a jolt and looked at my watch.

"Where do you live?" I asked.

"Novato."

"In an apartment or . . ."

"Right now I'm renting a condo from my father at specially reduced rates for the wretched."

I picked her purse and jacket up off the counter and slung them over my arm. "Come with me, darling. I want to introduce you to Dobbie. You'll love her—you guys have a couple of things in common."

Tuesday
2:45 A.M.

It was shoot-out time at the Not OK Corral tonight. Simon came in an hour after curfew (arrgh—give them an inch and you've lost the game), and I was already angry with him about his room being such a mess. I swear, when I go in there I can hear things breathing *that aren't human. The other day I went in to drop off his mail and I couldn't find the desk. I don't know if he's sold it or if it's really in there. On the way out, I tripped over what I thought was a furry stuffed animal and on closer inspection, found it was actually a cheese sandwich from days of yore.*

His pile of dirty laundry made a move toward me—I don't know if it was begging to be washed or just exercising. I screamed health hazard, but it fell on my dear son's selectively deaf ears. I should have taken Robert Fulghum's advice: "Never, never enter your child's room after puberty."

We—no, I mean I—had the usual discussion about taking responsibility and being a member of the family, blah blah blah. The gender gap–apron string dilemma is causing me to go gray.

Maybe Toughlove has a point—maybe I should get tough. Oh yeah. Excuse me while I roar.

Today Risen told me that the nurses are backing down on the benefits issue. How many buses, trains, and planes have I taken—will I take—in quest of getting them to listen? Inciting the taken-advantage-of to speak up, and the unknowing to learn, isn't easy.

But after all, am I not just as bad? One day I stand in front of a thousand nurses, preaching about pride and hope and what an exhilarating profession it is, and the next I walk into my own hospital steeling myself for the latest horseshit they're going to hand me, or wondering what doctor is going to pull an attitude, or what pro-management nurse is going to write me up because she doesn't like the way I wear my hair. It's schizophrenic.

Went to the paramedic run review this morning and as a featured guest they had a nurse from the special microsurgical unit at Mercy. She showed slides of amputations—before and after shots—including some poor psycho who whacked off his own penis (he said it kept him awake nights with its constant talking).

The part about the medical leeches used in postsurgical cases to keep swelling down made even Menowitz blanch. The nurse explained how they rotate the things, letting them feed until they fall off. She also said the clever devils have to be watched constantly, relating a story about how she left the room of a sleeping postop patient who was having his reattached fingers fed upon one day, and when she returned a few minutes later, the fat bugger was feeding off the guy's carotid artery.

At the end we were told that these slimy certified bloodsuckers are a multimillion-dollar business in England, and a hell of an investment. I wonder if I could raise a batch (litter? gaggle? swarm?) in the creek out back? ("We under-

stand you have an interesting hobby to supplement your income, Ms. Heron . . .")

In the case of Dobbie and Beth, it was love at first sniff. While Beth was gathering up dog food and chew toys, etc., I walked through the house making sure everything was closed up and turned off until Mrs. Rau's niece can get here from Houston.

It was an old lady's house for sure, right down to the cro- cheted doilies covering the overstuffed chairs and the ce- ramic baskets filled with peppermints and hard candies. It even smelled like an old lady—cooking butter, cinnamon, and mothballs.

In the living room was a small round table (yes, it had the cream-colored crocheted tablecloth to match the doilies) holding three dozen or more framed photographs of people who belonged to her life. I found one of a young Mrs. Rau sitting on a dock exposing some knockout gam. Written on the back was, "June 1937—Teeter at the Boardwalk."

This one life has ended, and all the days, all the wisdom, all the emotions and every event that went into that life are over. It seems wondrous and sad at the same time.

Someone just walked onto my porch, then ran off as soon as I got out of bed. God, I hate this single life. I think I pre- fer the trade-offs on the other side of the fence.

Sarah called from ER to tell me that Victor Boyd died yesterday. The nurses at Mercy told her that his mother never once visited him. I hope someone was there to hold him when he died. What a life that child must have had. Was there even one day for him that was happy?

Tired down to my soul. Got to sleep. Mooshie keeps stop- ping my pen with his paw and yawning in my face. His breath is a very powerful thing.

Come on, dreams, the projectionist awaits.

EIGHT

"Even in the worst of times, nursing has a reservoir of joy."

MARY MALLISON, R.N.

IT WOULD SEEM NATURAL for nurses to have one or two fingers in the metaphysical pie. Surely they are around death and are dancing with people's hovering souls enough of the time to have plenty of eerie, supernatural stories. But in fact, there aren't a lot of hazy, beckoning figures or ectoplasmic goings-on. I have seen a few miracles, but outside of an abundance of patients who die and come back full of tales about white lights and tunnels, I can produce only one true ghost story from my whole career.

For seven weeks after a massive stroke, which left him speechless, immobile, and, I think, mad as a hatter, Mr. Cheauvington Seymour Dillworth, the prosperous shipping magnate, lingered on in bed 6. Considering his rapacious disposition, and the tenacity with which he had held on to his millions, it was not surprising he would do the same with life. We all thought he was stalling, making deals with the devil while driving a hard bargain with God, then playing them off against each other to gain more time.

According to the nurses, people who are in the hospital for up to a week are patients, and patients who stay for two to four weeks are considered long-term inmates. The rare unfortunate hospitalized longer than that is considered a fixture. Old Mr. Dillworth was so much a fixture that the nurses began to refer to the room across from the station as the Dillworth room rather than room 5/6. Only in cases of extreme emergency did we ever admit a patient to bed 5 while he occupied bed 6.

Perhaps that was a mistake. Perhaps we should have moved

him around from room to room instead of letting him get so accustomed to, and so much a part of, bed 6. Looking back on it now, I think Mr. Dillworth thought of bed 6 as the only true home he'd ever known. For hours on end, he would stare peacefully out the window at the deer-and-wildflower-studded hillside. So intent was he on the view, we were afraid of the damage he might do to his neck by holding it in one position for so many hours a day.

And God help the poor soul who unknowingly closed his window (which has since become the infamous Dillworth Window). Although it was March and colder than Buffalo in December, he went wild when anyone so much as mentioned closing his precious window. By "wild," I mean to say that his eyes would take on a feral quality, and his whole head would literally tremble with fury. The drool spilled freely as he blinked in time to his forceful, angry grunts. "Ung! Ung! Ung!" (No! No! No!)

Renal failure was the cause of his ultimate demise. Right up to the minute he slipped into the coma from which he was never to return, he would not be denied visual access to his window. As he was beginning to slide, Pia had foolishly blocked his view while she suctioned out his mouth. Within a few seconds, one supposedly powerless foot came out from under the covers and kicked her hard enough to send her flat on her butt.

Three months after Mr. Dillworth died, the trouble with room 5/6 began.

With the big push for cuts in hospital budget, Redwoods charge nurses had it lousy. Their list of duties included coordinating assignments for the nurses; watching monitors; paperwork; diplomatically smoothing all ruffled feathers; answering questions from staff, patients, and their families; answering phones; more paperwork; dealing with the physicians; outwitting the supervisors; reviewing and expediting physicians' orders; planning and requesting, then begging for, staffing for the next shift; turfing patients to other units to make room for new admissions; more paperwork; catching and resolving all crises and political problems that arise; and ... the killer? They still had to tend to their own patient assignments.

In the old days it was more humane—the charge nurse did all those things then, too, except she was never given a patient assignment. In the name of patient safety, that had been the rule.

Patient safety was still an issue, but the simple truth of the matter was that budget took priority in a for-profit healthcare institution.

From the start I was ambivalent about being charge. On one hand, it reminded me too much of working behind the desk of a complaint department, but on the other, it was a chance at making a difference in how smoothly things ran.

The charge nurse is all things to all people. To your fellow nurses you have to be the benevolent mother who knows all the answers to the mysteries of life, yet you also have to be prepared to play wicked stepmother. ("I know you have six patients already, Pia, but you *will* take the next admission and be cordial about it, do you understand?")

To the patients you are the boss, the ultimate protector, and the last word. ("Okay, Mrs. Smith, you can have your bridge club here, but we aren't going to serve cookies or check anybody's varicose veins." Or, "I promise not to let Ginger near you again, Mr. Fisk, but tell me one more time exactly what she threatened to do to you if you put on your call bell?")

To the doctor the charge nurse is the person to whom all grievances are addressed and on whom all burdens can be dumped. ("You have *how* many stat admissions?" Or, "Well, Dr. Meyers, I'm sorry you feel that way about the nurses, but perhaps you could open your own hospital and bring in your own baboons.")

To the supervisor you are the opponent, fighting for everything you can get for your nurses and your patients. ("What do you mean you can't get us more than two nurses for night shift?" Or, "Okay, so show me where it says we can't order out for a patient who is dying of malnutrition from the food here.")

In short, the charge nurse is the glue that keeps the unit from collapsing, the grease that keeps the wheels turning smoothly without accidental deaths or threats of malpractice.

Annie decided I was ready for charge about two years after I'd started working CCU, on the day I promised her I would give up wearing my floor-length black sweater over my scrub dress. You can't imagine what a concession this was, since the CCU is kept quite cool and I am one of those dreary wimpettes who are constantly complaining of being cold, even while sweating in a sauna.

Usually the job was turned over to Sandy or Pia. They enjoyed the push-pull dynamics and the abuse-power aspects of the position more than the rest of us. However, my yearly evaluation was right around the corner, and I had to have at least two weeks of charge duty within thirty days to see if I could be broken.

At the beginning of the shift, the odds were already stacked against me; there were thirteen moderately high-acuity intermediate patients, and two admits waiting in ER, one of which was to go to the acute side and one to intermediate. Beth was on the acute side with three one-on-one patients and could not possibly take the fourth. Pia, Honey, and I were on the intermediate side. This was tight staffing that was an automatic setup for trouble.

Plus, with Honey, we were operating with a handicap.

Beth, Pia, and I were certified critical care nurses with at least ten years of CCU training under our belts. Honey was still a rookie and, well, to put it nicely, didn't always appear to run on a full set of spark plugs.

A true California surfer girl, Honey had the pretty blond and leggy look. She was the type of California woman who lifted weights because she found the smell of workout rooms erotically stimulating.

Honey also gave pet names to her breasts. In her case, it was Whip and Flippy. She was constantly telling anyone who would listen about how Whip was a teeny-weensy bit larger, but Flippy was *so* much more sensitive.

Even though Annie verified it, several of us had trouble believing that Honey had graduated from a very prestigious nursing school with a BSN degree. None of us, however, doubted for a second that she had won five beauty/talent contests with her superb baton-twirling talents.

I took report from ER on the new admit and assigned him to Honey, set monitor alarms, ran four o'clock rhythm strips, checked the charts for possible missed doctors' orders, and pasted in all outstanding lab work, marking the results on my report sheet for the doctors' information. That would hold the charge nurse job for about fifteen minutes while I checked my patients.

Mr. Schiff and Ms. Kelly, both MIs who were five days out, were easy. I did vitals and assessments, cleaned up their rooms, filled orders for snacks and ice water, answered questions about treadmill tests and angiograms, and gave them four and five P.M. medications.

Mr. Williams and Mr. Rose were another story. Both inmates of San Quentin, they had been placed in room 11/12, and even though they were far from being death row types, they shared three guards.

Mr. Rose was our celebrity patient. The sixty-five-year-old entrepreneur's trial had been publicized for its humorous and romantic value. Mr. Rose had a weakness for marrying rich widows, sweet-talking them into signing over their assets, and then pulling a disappearing act. By the time his case went to court, he was married to five women and worth over $4 million. He was also plagued by hypertension caused by clogged arteries—undoubtedly a result of all those rich, candlelit meals in out-of-the-way French restaurants.

Three of his wives called every day to send him messages of love and support. It was understandable: although he resembled a mustached cherub from a baroque painting, he was a charming, funny man. By the time I finished with his assessment, we were laughing and talking as if we had known each other for years. I did, however, draw the line when he suggested I order two dinners from Chez Josephine.

I suppose it's terrible to think of it like this, but we got lucky—Honey's intermediate admission signed himself out against medical advice, and the acute admit that Pia couldn't have taken care of anyway, coded in the elevator and died before he even got to the third floor. Dr. Meyers was, at the moment, in a charitable mood (only two over after eighteen holes) and agreed to transfer one of his more stable patients to the medical floor.

Honey sat close to me, sharing her troubles in a breathy Miss America voice while twisting a lock of her Farrah Fawcett blond-on-blond hair around a finger that had a two-inch-long fire-engine-red nail at the end.

"Wull, I *told* him that I wouldn't walk on his back. I mean, he wanted me to put massage oil on my feet and slip around on him. Oh yeah, the other thing that really bothers me? He keeps staring at Flippy and Whip."

I watched the saber-sharp fingernail go round and round a strand of platinum hair, coming closer to her heavily made-up eye. I speculated on what would do more damage—would the mascara-caked eyelashes crack the nail, or would the nail slice through a few of the eyelashes?

"Have you thought about pulling your zipper up instead of having it down around your navel?" I asked, my glance bouncing off her amazingly well developed cleavage. It looked as though it could support a troupe of trampolinists.

"Oh, but I *hate* crowding the poor things," Honey whined. "It isn't fair to them. They get all sweaty and rashy."

"Honey, please. It sounds like we're talking about cruelty to animals here instead of dress codes. Listen, go put a patient gown over your uniform and tie it around the waist. Then, if the patient still wants it, give him a regular back rub . . . with your hands."

"Wull, okay, but what about the window?"

"What window?"

"You know. Bed six window won't stay shut and the call bell keeps going off by itself. Mr. Emory says it's creepy. He wants to transfer out of bed five to another room."

"Call the engineer. There's probably a short somewhere."

"Okay, but what about the window?"

"Lock it, Honey."

"Oh, yeah." Enlightenment spread over and around the pound of makeup. "Why didn't I think of that?"

I held back the immediate answer to her question by taking a deep breath and holding my lips closed with my fingers.

Honey stood and did a Jane Fonda–approved back-bend, double-twist stretch. Through the thin material of her uniform, I could see "Whip" embroidered in red across the left cup of her bra, "Flippy" across the right, and the word "Front" down the elastic webbing in between.

"Mr. Williams?" I shook the brawny, fortyish man fiercely. I knew he had a pulse, because when I couldn't wake him earlier, I'd gone ahead and done his full assessment, including listening to his lungs around the snoring. His eyes *were* rolled back, however, and I had pinched him so hard, my fingers hurt.

"Williams!" I screamed directly into his ear.

Two of the guards jumped up and leapt toward the bed, hands on their nightsticks. I gave them a withering look over the tops of my glasses, which was enough to send them back to their posts by the door.

Mr. Williams snorted, stirred, farted, and flopped onto his back. Slowly, one bloodshot, pinpoint-pupiled eye rolled front and center and gave me a dazed, nystagmic once-over. "Got 'scruciatin' pain," he mumbled. "Gotta give me morphine." The way he said it, it sounded like "mofeen."

Clinically, the man was close to stuporous. I flipped to the medication chart and was stunned by the amount of morphine he had received on the previous three shifts. In the nurses' notes, it was simply stated that the man complained of severe chest pain every fifteen minutes. His pattern was always the same: He refused to take the sublingual nitroglycerine, demanding morphine instead. He would then continue to complain of 'scruciatin' pain until the maximum dose was reached for that time period.

I narrowed my eyes, studying him. His rhythm was regular, his pulse, blood pressure, and respiratory rate were a little low, his tests were all negative for an MI and pulmonary emboli, his EKG was normal and—it had taken me ten minutes to wake him.

I was willing to bet one of Mooshie's lives that Mr. Williams was the inmate version of a pharmacy freeloader—one of those people who on a regular basis go from ER to ER with some bogus complaint until they find a physician (one terrified of malpractice) who will check them into the hospital.

This is a drug addict's idea of a vacation. Where else could they be pampered while taking a free ride? Once admitted, they'll scream pain and bloody murder until they have been legally drugged into oblivion. This goes on for four or five days, until all the tests are run and no one can find a reason for the pain.

By that time, the nurses will have wised up, noting that although the patient claims to be in excruciating pain, he can be quite relaxed, sleeping, enjoying TV, and eating everything in sight. When the narcotic sheet is pulled up for review, it is usually found that the Demerol, morphine, or Dilaudid stores are being depleted by one patient.

Usually, the minute the drugs are cut off, the pharmacy freeloader will be out the door and looking for another hospital emergency room before you can say, "Get lost."

Freeloader inmates presented a bit of a problem. First of all, we couldn't tell them to hit the road, and second, they had a tendency to scream prisoner discrimination if we didn't give them what they wanted. On the other hand, it rubbed me the wrong way to be shooting up a drug addict simply because he wanted a free ride. What made me even madder was that the nurse on the last shift had continued giving him drugs when it was clear there was no real medical need for it.

I checked the nurse's signature. Right. Ginger once again taking the path of least resistance.

"Where do you have this excruciating pain, Mr. Williams?"

Mr. Williams had nodded off.

I am a true believer in the old adage "Let sleeping dogs lie," but as I was drying my hands, I heard the muffled sound of an alarm clock.

Mr. Williams snorted and sputtered himself awake, reached under his pillow, and pulled out one of those small travel alarms. He fumbled with the thing, cursing until he finally managed to turn it off. His head was bobbing and weaving as he flopped around in the bed to hunt for the call bell. He was so stoned, he didn't even see me put my hand over the bell.

When he pressed my hand instead of the bell, he jumped. "Hey! I got 'scruciatin' pain. Gimme my fix."

My eyes widened. "Your *what*?"

"My . . . my pain shot, man, I need my pain shot real bad. It's time for the morphine and this here pain's 'bout to kill me."

"I'd like you to be a little more specific about your pain, Mr. Williams," I said, amazed at how small his pupils were, "because all your tests are negative for a heart attack, and all your vital signs are pointing to the fact that you shouldn't be having any pain at all."

I waited for a minute to let that sink in. The man struggled not to nod off again. He held his arms up over his head and shook them. The tattoo on the inside of his right arm was a red snake winding itself around a naked, buxom black woman; the one inside his left was a coiled rattlesnake.

"You're overmedicated, Mr. Williams, and in all good conscience, I can't give you more morphine. I'd be glad to give you a nitro tablet, but that's all you're going to get for right now."

That got Alvin Williams's bleary-eyed attention. "Hey now, don't be givin' me no shit," he slurred. "I got pain. You got to give me morphine or you gonna get into trouble wid the doctor. If you ain't gonna give me morphine, I want the Demerol. I got rights, you know."

"Mr. Williams, I'm sorry, but I can't give you any more narcotics. Your blood pressure and breathing rates are too low. You've got pinpoint pupils and you're slurring your words."

This news seemed to shock him. "Hey. What you sayin'? Them other nurses, they been givin' me morphine. What's wrong wid you? Why you gotta go and give me trouble for?"

"If you aren't willing to try the nitroglycerine, I'll call Dr. Ostermann and see if I can get you something else."

"What you gonna ask for?"

"Codeine and Tylenol."

Mr. Williams shook his head and silently chuckled. "You gonna mess up everythin', ain't you? What's your problem? I guess you don't like niggers, huh?"

The well-known two-word phrase was on its way off my tongue with a ball of blazing anger behind it when I bit it off right at the *f*. I had to take a breath and reason with myself. Mr. Williams was a drug addict. He was going to do anything and everything he could to fold, spindle, and manipulate my resolve not to give him drugs.

"Mr. Williams"—I smiled sweetly—"I don't give a damn what color you are. I don't even care if you're a Republican and speak in tongues, you can't bullshit me into giving you more narcotics. I'll talk to Dr. Ostermann, and if he wants me to give you more, I will. Otherwise, we're going to come up with a non-narcotic pain reliever."

"I think"—Mr. Rose had pulled back the curtain that separated their beds—"what this lovely young lady is telling you, pal, is, you're cut off. The gravy train just pulled into its last stop. I know the sound of those brakes."

I yanked the curtain out of Mr. Rose's hand, gave him a dirty look, and turned back to Mr. Williams.

"What's your number, girl?" he demanded.

I almost laughed. As in the prison system, Mr. Williams thought we went by numbers rather than names. It was almost appropriate, considering what the hospital system was like. I spun off the first number that came to mind. "I'm four-two-five-eight. Why?"

Mr. Williams stopped bobbing and weaving long enough to fix me with the evil eye. " 'Cause there's gonna be a funeral real soon at your house and I wanna make sure you gets some flowers."

Honey transferred Mr. Emory out of room 5/6 at his insistence. He said the things that went bump in the night were bouncing him out. He added that he got the feeling the room did not want him there.

Honey swore she locked the window twice, and twice she found it unlocked and open no more than ten minutes later. The engineer found nothing wrong with bed 6's call bell, but took it with him anyway. When bed 6's call bell went off an hour after it had been disconnected, none of us was willing to go in and check it out. We called the engineer instead.

He left the room in a hurry, muttering under his breath about a short somewhere in the system.

From the desk, I could see bed 6's window. It was half open. Without much thought, I marched into the room, turned on all the lights, closed the window, and locked it.

I went back to the desk, found a pen and night-staff request form, and glanced back at bed 6's window.

Inside my chest, a few things shifted and bounced into my throat. The window was wide open.

"What do you need, Mr. Williams?" I asked, knowing that his answer would be the same as the last eight times I'd come running to his call light.

On the bedside table, his dinner tray looked as though it had been ravaged by starving rodents. His mouth was full and he was chewing as though he bore a grudge against the Baked Chicken Surprise. Personally, I could fully understand that.

"Lady, I'm gonna ask you one more time. You gonna give me morphine?"

"Look, Mr. Williams, I can offer you codeine and Tylenol. Dr. Ostermann has left it to my discretion as to what I give you for pain. To be honest, I don't see a man in pain sitting in front of me. I see somebody who likes getting loaded."

"You motherf—" Mr. Williams spit out the half-chewed chicken leg and gave the bedside table a strong shove. The dinner tray clattered to the floor. "I got rights!" he yelled. A guard nonchalantly made his way across the room, as if Mr. Williams's behavior was to be expected. He picked up a fork and coffee cup and set them on the tray, which had come to rest at the foot of Mr. Rose's bed.

"I'm getting the fuck outta here right now. Send me back to the joint. You hear me, bitch? You call that Dr. Otterman and send me back. I gotta get me some drugs for this terrible pain I got in my chest."

Perhaps it was my lack of response to his show of violence, or maybe it was the guard telling him to "knock it the fuck off," but Mr. Williams suddenly changed tactics in midmanipulation.

He grabbed at the middle of his chest and squeezed out some tears. "Oh, why you doin' this to me? I'm a poor ol' nigger that got a bad heart and you makin' me stay in this 'scruciatin' pain. Ain't you got no mercy in you, woman?" He covered his face with his muscular black hands.

I tried not to laugh, but I couldn't stop the switchboard ladies from summoning up clips of old Civil War movies. I giggled out of control, and after a minute, Mr. Williams's shoulders shook as he snorted with laughter over himself.

"Oh my God," I said finally, thumping him on the back, "you deserve the Academy Award, Mr. Williams. You should have auditioned for *Roots*."

He nodded, still chuckling. "Yeah, but . . ." His face went from smiles to a look that said nasty. "I still got this here 'scruciatin' pain."

I also stopped laughing and leveled my gaze. "The only pain you're having is coming down from a two-day high."

Behind me, one of the guards snickered.

"Mr. Williams, you *aren't* going to get more drugs from me, so lie back and try to enjoy your stay without them."

Mr. Williams's eyes narrowed into slits and his nostrils flared.

From the other side of the curtain, Mr. Rose let out a long, warning kind of whistle that sounded like "Uh ohhhhhhhh."

Beth stuck her head around the corner wearing a stricken expression. "Help. Help!" She mimicked the old lady in the TV advertisement. "I've fallen and I can't get up."

Laughing, she leaned against the wall between the two units keeping her eyes glued to the acute monitors.

"Well, Ec, if the truth be known, this is a really unsafe situation over here." She glanced at me out of corners of her eyes. "S'pose there's a chance you could get two nurses over here for nights? My ninety-two-year-old isn't as sick as she is set in her ways, but my other lady in bed four is going to hell in a handbag. Mr. Gould is leaking around his new valve, and Dr. Cohen might take him to surgery tonight, so that's going to mean strict one-on-one when he gets back."

"I'll beg," I said, "but there's probably a better chance of Elvis coming back from the dead and asking you out than there is of you getting another nurse over there."

Beth craned her neck to see into bed 2. "Yeah," she said absently, her mind back on business. "Well, if the King shows up and he's in decent shape, send him over to see me. I'm desperate for a date."

On my high school aptitude-and-skills test, I scored in the ninety-ninth percentile in two categories: entertainment and understanding things mechanical. Other than advising me to become a ventriloquist or a singing mechanic, my counselor was at a loss to place my natural talents. Of course, the mechanical part came in handy more than once while I owned my '57 Chevy. It also helped in a profession inundated with machines. Tinkering with malfunctioning IV pumps, ventilators, computer keyboards, and electrical beds was usually pretty easy for me; that I was being stumped by a window was making me crazy.

There was nothing I could see to make bed 6's window slide open, and the catch bar at the bottom worked perfectly.

I closed the window until I heard the catch bar click into place. Exerting as much pressure as I could, I tried to push the window up without releasing the catch. It did not budge.

Obviously that had been the problem; no one had made sure the catch bar was securely in place. My mechanic's heart satisfied, I turned to go, and was enveloped by a surge of ice-cold air. I whirled around, thinking perhaps the blast had come from the window, but it remained shut.

I sighed in relief.

And then, bed 6's call bell suddenly began to buzz.

"I said, we've got three admits waiting to come up from ER and all of us are stretching our limits as it is. I need you to assign a float nurse to CCU now, and I also need six nurses for nights."

Nan, the most innocent and charitable of our supervisor nurses, took off her black-rimmed bifocals and studied several of the lists she held in her hand. I wondered how long it would be before she forgot her years out on the med–surg floors and turned into an unsympathetic management person.

"Well, Sally is floating right now . . ."

I didn't know who the hell Sally was, and at that point I didn't care. "Great. If she's got four fingers and an opposing thumb per hand, we'll take her."

"But she won't work in CCU."

"Why?"

"She's never worked critical care and she's terrified."

I knew the feeling well. Every time I was floated into the newborn nursery, I felt the same way.

"Send her up anyway—all she has to know is how to read, write, and take vital signs. We'll be nice to her."

Nan put her nose to the lists again and hummed "Row, Row, Row Your Boat." After a minute, she slapped the papers with the back of her hand, straightened, and smiled.

"I can't give you six for nights. You'll be lucky if you get three."

I was quick with the comeback. According to *The Flea Market Frequenter's Guide to Bargaining*, this gave me "transaction power." "If I get less than six, I'm going to warn you right now, Nan, that I will close the unit and call the director. This hospital can put out for more nurses."

"I can't squeeze blood out of a stone."

"And I won't jeopardize the patients' safety."

Mr. Williams's call bell rang again. I directed a baleful glance toward his room and put my stethoscope around my neck. "Six nurses, Nan. Not five or less. Six."

Nan sighed and went back to her lists. Silently, I blessed her heart for still trying, even though I knew she was probably following good-manager training and adding up costs instead of thinking of the patients.

"Can you watch monitors while I go hand out meds and do my eight o'clock assessments?"

Nan nodded absently.

"And while you're there," I whispered, hoping my words would drift in on a subliminal level, "page Sally, get three charts ready for admission, and find six nurses for nights."

At nine P.M. I was running out rhythm strips, signing off orders on the three new charts, and trying to chart on my own patients, when Beth rushed through the double doors.

"Meyers has flipped," she said in a panicked whisper. "He's over there demanding that I get Mrs. Pope ready for the insertion of arterial and Swan lines. He spent thirty minutes trying to talk her into having them put in, but she refused. Then he came out to the desk saying he's going to put them in anyway, whether the old lady wants them or not." Beth winced. "Mrs. Pope won't sign the consent, and I don't know what to do."

"Is she with the program enough to know what's going on?" I asked. "Has she got some family we can call?"

"Well, she's pretty sharp for ninety-two," Beth said thoughtfully. "I mean, she doesn't remember the name of her bridesmaids from 1916, but who would? ... There's one son in Tiburon. I've left three messages on his machine asking him to call immediately."

"Does she actually need the lines?"

Beth gave me a blank stare. I knew what was going through her mind. Traitor.

"I have to ask, Beth. If Meyers is at all justified in doing all this, it makes it harder to interfere."

She tapped the tubular steel leg of my chair with her pen. "This woman has been here for six days, Ec. She isn't in the greatest shape, but she's stable for now. It's my professional opinion this procedure can wait at least until we get permission from the family."

"Have you refused to assist him?" I asked.

"I told him I didn't feel right about doing this without a signed consent. All he said to that was to give her IV Valium."

Reluctantly, I got up from my chair and motioned to Beth to take my seat behind the monitors. The charge nurse in me squared her shoulders and walked into the lion's den.

Dr. Meyers ignored the list of patient rights I held out for his scrutiny. "You can't legally do these procedures without her or someone in her family giving consent. The patient has the right to refuse treatment. It says so right here." I pointed to Patient Right #2.

Dr. Meyers waved the paper away. "She doesn't know what she needs. She's my responsibility and I think she needs lines."

"That may be true, Dr. Meyers, but the issue here is that the patient doesn't want the procedure done and we can't locate the family right now to get permission from them. My nurses don't want to assist you until the consent is signed by somebody."

"Then I'll do it by myself," he said, making his way to the supply cart.

Frankly, I'd expected more of a fight, or at least a little ranting.

My visit to Mrs. Pope was an equally brief encounter.

"Do you fully understand why Dr. Meyers wants to do these procedures?" I asked.

Mrs. Pope nodded. Her white hair fluffed out every which way, like Albert Einstein's. "Don't want 'em. I'm ninety-two years old. I don't want people sticking pins into me trying to get this old flivver moving. Can't you people let anything go to rest?"

I sighed and looked through the glass. At the nurses' desk, Dr. Meyers was poring over his pile of supplies, separating out what he needed. Sadly, I turned back to Mrs. Pope. There wasn't going to be any rest for her and I wished I could explain why.

In the end it was Nan who took on the job of dealing with Dr. Meyers—she simply agreed to assist him.

And as he committed his little crime against the totally bewildered and half-drugged Mrs. Pope, Beth and I could do nothing but watch in appalled silence.

I walked backward to the desk, not taking my eyes off the window for a moment. I sat down, purposely looked away for a few seconds, and quickly glanced distrustfully back at the window.

Ah. Still closed.

The phone chime made me chomp down on my tooth guard.

Kathy McCormack's voice asked for Miss Heron.

"Hey, what's going on in the land of rehabilitation?" I asked, momentarily forgetting about the window, although my eyes returned to it almost at once.

"What're you doing tomorrow morning about eight?" she said, an overtone of joy in the question.

"Sleeping, unless you have better plans for me."

"Want to come and watch the unstoppable McCormack walk out of this place?"

"Wouldn't miss it."

I squinted. Something moved ever so slightly on the top of the window near the lock. I blinked a whole bunch of times, readjusted my glasses, and squinted again.

"Okay then, see you at the main entrance at eight."

Unable to say goodbye due to my jaw being unhinged, I mumbled and hung up by feel.

Slowly, so slowly that I thought my eyes were playing tricks, the lock rotated. I stood, biting the knuckle of my thumb.

Pia, who had just come from the kitchen with a tray of bedtime snacks for her patients, stopped and followed my gaze.

Together, we watched as the window slid open by itself.

Cautiously, we entered the room, clinging to each other. Again the air was icy cold even though I'd turned the thermostat up to 78 earlier. We studied the window thoroughly, to the point of actually sniffing around the edges. Pia protested when I finally got up the nerve to apply the tip of my tongue to one corner for a quick taste.

Even though we couldn't find the gimmick or any explanation for the incorrigible window, I will say we were relieved not to find ectoplasmic goo oozing down the inside, or the face of Jesus reflected on its glass surface.

I started to laugh, imagining how silly we looked smelling and examining a stupid inanimate window as if it were the devil himself.

I was still yucking it up when the door slammed shut with the force of hell itself and the window fell so hard, it cracked into a thousand different spiderweb patterns. Several pieces of glass fell to the floor and shattered at our feet.

Pia and I screamed hard enough to rupture blood vessels in our throats. The snack tray hit the wall, sending orange juice, milk, graham crackers, and bananas in six different directions. Running for the door—each of us trying to get ahead of the other—I slipped in a puddle of orange juice and fell in front of Pia's wildly pumping knees. Still screaming, we didn't bother getting up but scrambled to the door and grappled for the handle. Pia managed to pull the door open. It swung back, revealing a small crowd of mystified people; Honey, Dr. Cramer, the engineer, and Dr. Meyers all peered past us, still on our knees, into the shambles of room 5/6.

Dr. Meyers gave us a disgusted look and muttered something about lunatics at play. The engineer—with call bell in hand—entered bravely, looked around, and came out quickly. A giggling Honey gathered up a couple of bananas and ate one as she surveyed the wreckage. Dr. Cramer casually took out his black book and began to write.

I glanced over the top and saw him write the word "BEDLAM" in capital letters.

Monday
2:27 A.M.

Over their dead bodies, they gave the unit six nurses. The scary part is that Honey is doing a double—as charge nurse—with no regular CCU staff. I've been worrying about it since I gave her report. She kept twirling that damned hair, snapping her gum, asking what she should do when somebody died. She didn't ask if, *she asked* when.

I stayed as long as I could, but still feel like I have abandoned innocent people.

Came home and found Simon watching an old Topper *re-run. It used to be one of my favorite shows, until tonight. I hoped Mr. Emory wasn't watching. Before Pia went off duty, she and I went back in room 5/6 and closed the door. While she repeated, "I cast thee out, Satan-Dillworth, in the name of God," I chanted, "Namu amida Butsu," until Joe Cramer crashed the scene with his black book. He must have written three pages tonight.*

Oh God, I'm so tired of trying to incur short-term memory loss as a method of survival.

Big day tomorrow. Gotta go see Kathy walk, go to the dentist, get the results of my last HIV test, and see if the CCU is still standing. Then I get to go back for another nine hours of forced socialization.

That writers are the masters of procrastination is an understatement. I'll find any excuse once I've sat down in front of the keyboard. This morning I sat down and one sentence later decided the window needed to be washed—I spent thirty minutes doing that. Then I sat down again and wrote two words and decided I needed to make a thermos of tea. That took fifteen minutes. Then I settled down to complete another sentence and remembered that I needed to file my nails. When I found myself getting up to see if I should change the part in my hair to the right instead of the middle, I turned off the word processor and went for a second run.

Okay. Question of the day: When a teenage Eskimo rubs her nose, is that like an American teen practicing kissing on her hand?

Oh, my queendom for someone to lie here next to me and laugh at my jokes.

It seems I have more wishes than I ever did before. Does that mean that I'm failing myself?

NINE

"Caring is the essence of nursing. This does not understate the science of nursing. Rather, nursing has identified the science of caring."

NANCY SHARTS ENGEL, R.N.

KATHY AND HER HUSBAND WERE WAITING in the lobby for Dr. Schupbach along with a nurse from the ortho rehab unit. A large steel cart, made conspicuous by the mountain of Kathy's belongings, was parked next to the front door.

"So? What have you learned?" I knelt next to the wheelchair, holding on to the armrest—not so much to be on the same level as because I was so tired, I couldn't stand without weaving.

Kathy jerked her forearm up and swung it close to my hand. Her fingers were flat against her palm in a permanent curl. "I asked myself that question last night."

"And?"

"First I had to face the fact that the only reason I was up on that scaffold doing that stupid job was so I could buy a full set of silver and china to impress dinner guests. I fell because I'd worked the night before, cleaning offices, and I was so tired I couldn't function." Kathy looked at her husband, and a secret joke passed between them. "I'd even talked Brian into taking a part-time second job because I wanted to have a pool put in and get the house redecorated before the end of the year."

Her leg kicked out in an involuntary spasm. She frowned at it with the same warning expression a mother might give an unruly child who is out of reach. "I spent days thinking about what model BMW I could lease that would be the most conspicuous in the driveway, because the people next door had one and I couldn't be outdone." The redhead emitted a sigh. "I admit it—I was a Yuppie caught up in having the best *things*."

"Yeah," her husband said in mock seriousness. "She even considered hiring F. Lee Bailey to file our bankruptcy so she could say we'd gone down in style."

"Now I could live in a tent," Kathy said. "As long as I've got my family and my health, I swear that's all I'll ever want again. I don't care about anything else."

"Oh, get off it, Kath," Brian chided. "Twenty minutes ago you were wondering if BMW made a 450 SL wheelchair."

Kathy laughed, and with some effort, leaned over and gave his thigh a bite.

It was a congregation of believers in courage and miracles who assembled to watch Kathy walk to the door. Three people from physical therapy, Dr. Schupbach, Brian, two off-duty ortho rehab nurses, and I looked on in silence while she pulled herself out of the wheelchair and up to the walker.

Seven laborious steps later, the three semifunctional fingers of her right hand found, then hooked around, the handle of the door. Kathy paused for a moment, steadied herself, and turned to face us, triumphant.

Over the burst of applause, one of the rehab nurses shouted, "Encore. Encore of a miracle."

The dentist whistled "Begin the Beguine" as he reamed out my root canal. I was glad he was wearing a mask, since he looked like he might be one of those wet-whistler types, the kind that sprayed pints of spit by the stanza. I considered myself lucky—he could have been a personable dentist, one who asked a million questions and seemed offended when you didn't give clear answers through the rubber mouth dam. Besides, personable, talkative dentists didn't jibe with my particular dentistry quirk—forbidden sleep.

Forbidden sleep is that deep, ultimately restful slumber one gets when falling asleep under illegal, nonsleep circumstances, or, to put it simply, it is sneaked sleep taken outside of one's bed and jammies.

Everyone is guilty of this peccadillo to one degree or another at least once in their lives. Illicit slumbering may come on at prohibitive times or places, like during an intimate conversation with friends or at a symphony hall during a piano concert. It can also be as innocent as falling asleep in one's street clothes—the most common of forbidden-sleep offenses.

My particular forbidden-sleep faux pas comes the minute I hit a dentist's chair: without benefit of nitrous oxide, I am out like a light. After my first few dentist's office experiences of conking out, I was sure they were sneaking me the gas through that little suctioning tube (the one that takes care of most—not all—of the drool that has a way of dribbling down your chin without your knowledge because you're numb from the nose down), but when I began snoring even before the assistant finished clipping the drool-and-tooth-nasties napkin onto my collar, it was clear I was suffering from (enjoying?) forbidden-sleep syndrome.

Twisted perhaps, but I can honestly say I was disappointed when my dentist couldn't find anything left to do to my teeth. It felt like years since I'd had a good sleep. But here I was, back in the saddle so to speak, a root canal having come through for me.

The magic of the dental chair, and that singular smell all dental offices have, lulled me into a place of impending oblivion. Falling down the well, I must have had a few monster twitches, because the dentist paused in his whistling and resumed only after feeling my pulse.

The arrival of my mail has always been, I am sad to say, one of the biggest highlights of my day. One would think that I would check my mailbox at work with the same sense of anticipation—but it is not so. Usually I can't force myself to check it more than twice a year. In more recent years, it had been less than that.

Refreshed from my sleep at the dentist's, it seemed like a smart idea to purge the crammed wooden box and relieve it of its contents while I was in a good mood. It yielded three invitations for baby and bridal showers that had taken place so long ago the expected babies were in preschool, and the prospective brides had been married, traumatized, trially separated, legally separated, and divorced.

There were no fewer than thirteen announcements for mandatory classes and seven announcements of mandatory staff meetings, none of which I attended. The rest consisted of four advertisements from the Redwoods credit union, a notice that I had been one of thirty-six CCU staff members whose names had been drawn to receive a single grapefruit, from a case of the same—the Cardiology Cartel's gift to the CCU nurses every blessed Christmas, a letter from a university asking me to speak at a conference that had taken place six months before, five announcements for bake sales, and a sealed envelope with Redwoods Memorial administration insignia at the top left corner. The date on this one was recent.

Had I been fired or put on probation? It would be just like them to have me continue working without telling me I shouldn't be there.

The salutation read: "Hail, colleagues!" I checked the signature and laughed—it was from our director of nurses. Colleagues, my foot. My guess was that ninety percent of the nurses employed by Redwoods Memorial wouldn't know their own director of nurses if they fell over her. No one ever saw her on the units, and the only time one could speak with her was by appointment. It had probably been years since she'd even been near a sick person or worked eight hours in a row, let alone sixteen. She *was*, however, awfully good at wearing expensive suits and pouring coffee for the doctors at their monthly meetings.

I went on with the letter, suspicion poking its serpent head out of its dark hole, ready to search out loopholes.

Would you like to give more quality, hands-on time to your patients? Are you tired of having to perform non-nursing duties?

Enclosed you will find a questionnaire exploring how many hours a shift you spend on those tiresome, noncritical nursing duties. There is also a section for you to tell us where you might like to have assistance. For instance, if you find that most of your time is spent doing bed baths, feeding, calibrating machinery, and administering medications, give us your comments on how you think trained personnel could take over these menial tasks for you.

I am deeply concerned about your welfare and job satisfaction. I am familiar with the frustrations of today's modern nurse. The growing technology of medicine requires nurses to spend more of their time away from the patient than ever before. Let us help you return to the true essence of nursing—caring for those who need you.

Shaking my head, I crumpled the letter and made a dunk shot into the wastecan across the room. Wow. This was management's finest training at work. It was like the junk mail fliers everyone receives: "CONGRATULATIONS, [your name here]! YOU HAVE WON A MILLION DOLLARS!"

I wondered how many nurses had read or would read between the lines of this free-gift letter and recognize the Greeks' offering of a wooden horse.

Whatever horrors the unit had gone through the previous night, it had survived and was still standing. Really, the only things that were noticeably different were that bed 6's window had been replaced, and both window latch and call bell were behaving themselves. Other than that, the shift was almost a carbon copy of the night before. The unit had the exact same staff, although the chaos and patient population were elevated. Pia's assignment was another two patients heavier, and Beth was going crazy with a new MI she barely had enough time to medicate. Honey, who had been promised the evening shift off for working the night shift double, was called after five hours of sleep and cajoled, pressed, and manipulated into showing up for work.

The one bit of news that gave the evening a promise of excitement was that when Mrs. Pope's son was told of his mother's medical rape, he came unglued and hit the roof. I think anyone would have had the same reaction—even if he weren't one of the most acclaimed medical malpractice attorneys in San Francisco.

The story, according to Mrs. Pope's day nurse, was that between the time Dr. Meyers walked into the unit and the time he entered Mrs. Pope's room to meet her son, he was told who he was facing and the solicitor's state of mind.

Chris said Dr. Meyers shook the man's hand wearing a tragic, apologetic expression, then blurted out that the unconscionable crime committed against his mother the night before had been almost entirely the fault of the nurses.

From the other end of the phone came sounds like a dog coughing up a full-grown, long-haired cat.

"Heron?"

"Yes, Miss Milks?"

"No."

"This isn't Miss Milks?"

"Yes, this is Milks, you idiot. Who else would it be?"

So many wonderful, sarcastic answers came to mind that I was overwhelmed into silence.

"Did you hear me? I said no."

"No?"

"Right."

"Do you mean no as in yes or no, or do you mean know as in I'm supposed to know what this is about?"

"I don't mean yes or no. I mean a flat no. What's wrong with you? Are you deaf?"

As much as I would have enjoyed a "Who's on First" conversation with Miss Milks, I didn't have the time. I had to nip it in the bud. "No, I'm not deaf, but I don't know what the hell you're talking about, Miss Milks."

"Goddamn it, Heron. You aren't going to die. Your final HIV test is negative. No on proposition AIDS."

"Oh," I said, feeling a brief ripple of relief, although I had already fooled myself into believing there could be no other result.

"Yes, no. That's what I said." Miss Milks went into a spasm of dry, hacking coughs brought on by exasperation.

"No, I said oh, not no."

"Yes, it is no. Clean the wax out of those ears, soldier."

"Yes sir, Miss Milks."

By the time I finished checking the charts, taking care of errors in orders, researching missing charting, and running out P.M. rhythm strips, I was grinding my tooth guard so hard it squeaked. I managed to steer Honey (attired in a white nursing uniform cut tight enough to be squeezing Whip and Flippy right out of their pens) away from her male patients in beds 9 and 10, who were occupying most of her time by dropping things off the sides of their beds and asking her to pick them up. Unaware of their ulterior motives, and more than likely too tired to care, Honey was relieved when I left her sitting at the desk while I checked my patients.

Mrs. Greene, my triple-bypass patient, had developed an ugly infection in the incision site of her right leg where the vein had been harvested for her bypass graft. I was in the middle of the dressing change—no more than six minutes after I left the desk to Honey—when the sounds of the constantly ringing call bells and phones filtered through to my brain. What was most disturbing was the sound of the red-alert monitor alarm, which meant someone had lost his lead wires, was brushing his teeth, or was having asystole or ventricular fibrillation.

Keeping my sterile gloves up and away from myself, I slipped over to the door and watched the Keystone Kops scene going down at the nurses' station: Honey was frantically hitting monitor buttons left and right with the eraser tip of a pencil (so as not to chip one of her red-and-gold-striped talons) while answering phones and yelling out to Pia which patients to check to make sure they were okay.

Dr. Cramer stood over her, giving orders that weren't being heard. Beth was standing between the two units, pointing at the clock and complaining to Dr. Cramer that Dr. Meyers hadn't called her back on an important lab result. Pia was pointing to Mr. Williams's room and saying something about 'scruciatin' pain.

Maybe it was wrong, but I closed the door to Mrs. Greene's room, smiled at the instant peace, and went back to what I was doing.

Unlike Mr. Galante, who scratched and bit the nurses during his course of the DTs, Mr. Lingle, a.k.a. Confusion King, was lovely in his disorientation. When I walked into his room, I found him reciting a constant stream of original poetry into his telemetry battery pack, pausing intermittently to thank his invisible audience for their warm applause. The poems were so engrossing, I forgot about everything, including the chaos going on on the other side of the door—that is, until Honey burst in to say that Mr. Williams was going ape.

Mr. Williams's chart lay open in my trembling hands as my astonishment turned into dismay. Ginger had once again drugged Mr. Williams into oblivion with a total of eighty milligrams of IV morphine in one eight-hour shift. She had done this without documenting the quality or whereabouts of his pain. She ignored the memos (written in red) on both the Rand card and the outside of the chart, which stated that the patient was not to get morphine except as a last resort after all other pain medications had been given.

Calling an off-duty staff nurse at home was not something one did lightly. Unless there was a reason tantamount to accusing someone of murder, a nurse's home was considered her "safety zone." So, when I called and got Ginger's answering machine, I was glad to be able to leave my message without a direct confrontation that was destined to end up in a verbal fistfight.

Mr. Williams's call bell was as relentless as his cries of " 'scruciatin' pain" and "I got my rights to drugs." Stuffing sterile cotton into the mechanism of the bell, I knew, was only putting off the inevitable unpleasant confrontation, but it did give me some time to take care of Dr. Cramer, Mr. Cooney, and Mr. Pope.

Dr. Cramer was upset. He'd ordered a lung perfusion scan on one of his patients and it had never been done because the day shift nurse hadn't taken off the order. It was clear from the dried oatmeal scab on his new silk tie and the circles under his eyes that he was going to be touchy.

"What's going on around here?" His neck was flushed. "Why can't we have nurses who know what they're doing?"

"Oh, come on, Joe!" I said. Unfortunately, I said it with enough vehemence to spit my tooth guard clear across the counter. Joe caught the device before it slid onto the floor, and held it up to the light. He stared at the ugly gadget as though it were an artifact from Mars. Snatching it out of his hand, I snapped it back over my lower teeth.

"This isn't a case of a nurse not knowing what she's doing. The nurse who overlooked your scan order is an excellent nurse, but the fact of the matter is, she had four patients to care for today, plus be in charge of the unit. That's a setup for making oversights on details. Why do you always make it the nurses' fault? We consistently do the best we can with whatever we're handed. It's what's loaded on us that's the problem."

Although it was clear he was still upset, Joe didn't say anything. I didn't even try to guess what might be going on in his mind, eclectic and steel-trap kind of place that it was. Presently he stood to go, stopped, and came back to the desk.

"For a woman so bitter in her public opinions against physicians, I find it interesting that you can't take even the slightest bit of criticism about your own profession."

I pulled back to look at him. What I read in his eyes was anger and a sense of having been betrayed. I was surprised not only by his reaction, but at the realization that although Joe and I had been friends for over ten years, he had never before shared with me his thoughts about my politics.

"My physician politics bother you?" I croaked.

"What do you think?" He looked down at me, incredulous at my apparent lack of acumen.

I started feeling warm at the nape of my neck, under my braid. Damn! The confrontation beast had sprung upon me before I knew it.

"But when I speak about physicians, I always make it clear that I'm not talking about all doctors. I specify that most docs are a fair, hardworking lot but there are some—"

"Doesn't matter. If the community hears people like you talk negatively about any of the doctors, they stop trusting all of them. That hurts us as a profession, as businessmen, and ultimately, it hurts the patient."

The man turned his gaze to the counter and shook his head. "It makes me sad that you're so bitter about the physicians and the administration. I'm really sorry you feel that way, but the fact remains that I find most of what you say about physicians incredibly offensive."

Self-doubt immediately marched over the dead bodies of my inner strength and resolve. Maybe Joe was right, I thought, maybe I hadn't been fair to the docs. Perhaps someone hadn't sought a physician's help when they really needed it because of something I'd said. Maybe I wasn't—

Hey, wait just a minute! I snapped out of my shame attack and did a fast but thorough reality check. Granted, I probably did need to tone down the anger that sometimes surfaced, but the truth remained at the bottom of what I said. Plus, hadn't my views been validated time and time again by hundreds of nurses and laypersons from Maine to Hawaii?

The weight of doubt lifted and I faced Joe. "And *I'm* sorry you feel the way *you* do. I agree about the bitterness and I'll try to muzzle some of that negativity, but the facts of the matter are that the majority of physicians *do* need to work on their attitudes toward the patients and the nurses. The public is wising up. We're finally entering an age of healthcare consumers, patient rights, alternative and preventative medicine, medical teamwork, and all that. People want more for their healthcare dollar than to be treated poorly or ignored by an M.D. The days of people believing that the doctor is the only one capable of running the show are numbered. Doctors have to come down from those ivory towers, stop handing down edicts, and start communicating with the rest of us like equals.

"Physicians who play God roles just don't go over well with anybody anymore, Joe, including the nurses."

I paused to reset a couple of alarms on the monitors, and resumed in a calmer tone.

"And as for the way I deal out my views? Other nurses can stir up the muck by debating with the doctors and administrators nicey-nice over a conference table—if that gets docs and management to consider things from a more realistic perspective and begin the change, great. I just happen to do it in a much more direct and public manner, because that's the opportunity I've been given."

Joe and I stared at each other for a few seconds before we both smiled. Joe shrugged. I shrugged. He left the unit, and I went back to work.

Our debate could have gone on for hours, just in the listing of all the issues and arguments, but the views and opinions wouldn't change on either side, at least not any time soon.

Mr. Cooney is a fixture at Redwoods Memorial. He is not unique to Redwoods Memorial, however. Every hospital in the nation has a Mr. Cooney. Anyone who has ever worked in a hospital or been a patient or a frequent visitor knows him as the man who runs the carpet cleaner and the floor polisher all day, every day.

When I think I have figured out his work blueprint—that is, beginning at the corner of the basement floor and polishing and scrubbing his way up to the opposite corner of the fifth floor—he changes it. One day I might find him scrubbing the carpets in the southernmost corner of the west wing on the second floor, and the next night (his shifts were as unpredictable as his cleaning patterns) I might find him down in the cafeteria, polishing the linoleum.

Whatever floor plan he followed, the fact of the matter was that he and his machines created lots of problems throughout the hospital. How many personnel had gotten tangled in his machine cords and gone sprawling flat on their faces as they tried to sprint past him to a code? And how many thousands of patients had complained that the noise from those industrial-sized machines kept them awake and made them nervous? Many of the nurses, myself included, were highly allergic to the cleaning and polishing agents he used and could not be in the same vicinity as his machines. But whenever the nurses tried to intervene, he would keep polishing, bellowing over the din that we had to regard it as road work—keeping the highways of the hospital clean. Onward Christian soldiers, and the mail must go through!

Tonight, in his never ending quest for fresh carpets, his carpet cleaner was causing all the TV screens on the unit to blink and snow. Patients might not have been so upset had it not been for the fact that *The Wizard of Oz* was airing. My job was to tell Mr. Cooney he had to shut down operations and go elsewhere—at least until after the Wicked Witch melted down.

Mr. Cooney hung his pendulous belly over the handle of the carpet cleaner and searched in his shirt pocket while he guided the machine back and forth over the rug with his abdomen. The rhythm of cleaning had not been interrupted for so much as a fraction of an instant.

Grimly, he handed me a piece of paper that was so worn, it felt like soft cotton, and pointed to a line at the middle of the page. It indicated that the CCU main-hall carpet was to be cleaned on this particular date at this particular time. He said something to the effect that the cleaning must go on, come hell or high water.

I protested some more, until the cleanser finally choked me into silence and I had to go in search of reinforcements. Pia, for all her sweetness, could be pretty devious when she put her mind to it, so it was to her I divulged my dilemma. She finished rubbing down her twenty-five-year-old pericarditis patient, while her mind wheels wobbled and twisted. Washing her hands, she pushed a stray blond hair behind her ear. "Follow my lead," she said, and headed toward Mr. Cooney.

As she passed him, Pia gasped and gripped his arm. "Oh my God!" she shouted, getting herself right up into his face. "What's wrong, Mr. Cooney? Are you having chest pain?"

Mr. Cooney gave Pia a wary glance, but slowed down just the same.

Pia pried Mr. Cooney's hands off the handlebars of the cleaner and yelled for a wheelchair to be brought stat. "It's okay, Mr. Cooney, try to relax. We won't let anything happen to you, don't worry."

Mr. Cooney hesitated, confused. "What's wrong? Why are you saying these things? Do I . . . Do I look sick?"

"Why Mr. Cooney, you're positively gray. I want you to sit down before you—" Pia slipped her arm around his waist and pulled him toward the wheelchair—"go hypotensive and pass out."

Beginning to look a bit pallid, Mr. Cooney wiped his face. "But I—I don't feel very sick. I'm never sick."

I went to his other side and gently pushed him toward the wheelchair. "You don't need to be stoic, Mr. Cooney," I said. "You haven't looked well all night. I know how much you like doing an excellent job, but you mustn't push yourself when you're this ill. It isn't good. After all, we still need you to clean the floors, not be a cardiac arrest victim on one of them."

Pia patted his shoulder and avoided looking at me. One snort would set us both off and ruin the whole plan.

Mr. Cooney let himself be pushed into the wheelchair. "You know, now that you mention it, I *have* felt a bit off tonight. I thought it was gas, but I—I think I'm feeling dizzy. Maybe I should go lie down after I finish the hallway here."

"No, no, no," Pia insisted, reaching over and pulling the plug on the machine. The release of tension was instantaneous as TVs everywhere snapped back into shape. The Lollipop Guild could be heard singing in the background. "You shouldn't strain yourself anymore tonight. You should go down to your office or wherever it is you go—"

"The cleaning machine garage," Mr. Cooney interjected dolefully.

"Okay, go to the cleaning machine garage, get some rest, and then go home to bed. Maybe you'll feel better tomorrow."

When Pia wheeled him away, Mr. Cooney was perspiring and his skin was an ashen color. Yes, we had turned a perfectly healthy man into a freaked-out hypochondriac inside of three minutes, but the rest of the patients—save Mr. Williams—were happy, transported, via the yellow brick road, away from their illnesses and into the Land of Oz.

"Psssst." Beth stuck her head around the double door. "He's here."

I raised my eyebrows in question.

"Douglas Pope, attorney-at-law."

Through the crack in the double doors, I studied the man, surprised to find him younger than I had imagined, and exceedingly handsome. Either Mrs. Pope, the old minx, must have been a very late-life mother, or the attorney had had some fine plastic surgery.

I had grave misgivings about the good-looking part; it put me at a disadvantage since I usually went tripping-over-my-own-feet shy and stuttery in the presence of a man I found attractive.

Mrs. Pope didn't seem all that much the worse for wear, although from the way she kept flicking the art line tubing away from her, it was clear she was most displeased with her current state of affairs.

I was glad she was angry and had not gone the way of depression, as older people sometimes do when their bodies have been assaulted by invasive medical procedures.

An annoyed, brooding look in his eyes, Mrs. Pope's son stood at the end of the bed.

I thought of a few fabricated, perfectly plausible explanations I could give him, then of my mother in her saner moments telling me to remember that honesty was usually the best policy and oh, what a tangled web we weave, when first we . . . etc., etc. Recalling whose ass I was covering and how he had laid the blame on the nurses gave me enough steam to propel me out from behind the doors and into Mrs. Pope's room.

I would have given my eyeteeth to stop perspiring, as it was the only thing that betrayed my nervousness. Taking the attractive lawyer by the horns, I gripped his hand and said in a clear, strong voice, "How do you do? My name is Miss Heron and I've been the nurse in charge of CCU for the last couple of evenings. I understand you're upset about the events of last night, and I'd like to explain exactly what happened."

I don't know what I expected—I guess I thought he would soften and give in on the spot with an "Oh, don't worry about it. Let bygones be bygones." Instead, he fixed me with steely, intense eyes and said, "Please do—if you can."

Immediately I was on the stand, undergoing interrogation by the prosecutor who wanted to send me away for a life sentence. In actuality, I have been on the stand only once. I was so nervous that when the judge asked me to state my name, I couldn't remember what it was.

Mr. Pope waited, searching my face for the slightest quiver that would prove the nurses guilty as charged. It was now or never, so I drew myself up, got a grip, and told him exactly what happened, word for word, misdeed by gross misdeed.

At the end, he nodded thoughtfully, the way he'd learned in the Perry Mason school of lawyerly mannerisms. "I know it wasn't the nurses," he said grimly. "I deal with physicians all the time, so I'm well versed in what they're capable of doing. Meyers is a bad liar besides."

"But he *is* a good cardiologist," I gushed. Call it a moment of weakness. "I'm not defending what he did, Mr. Pope, but I believe *he* thought he was acting in your mother's best interests."

"I know that," said Mr. Pope, stone-faced. He walked to the sink and turned, holding up his finger. It was a classic courtroom pose. "However, that doesn't excuse the fact he still acted without consent at the time he performed the procedures on my mother against her will."

"Oh for God's sake, enough of this, Douglas!" Mrs. Pope declared irritably. "The man acted abominably, yes, but let's not make a federal case out of it. Slap the man's hand and be done with it."

Mr. Pope dropped his counselor facade and smiled beautifully.

My toes curled at the sight.

"Does this mean the judge has passed sentence on the defendant?" Douglas asked his mother.

Mrs. Pope clucked her tongue. "Yes, yes. Just let him know he shouldn't do that again . . . to anybody."

"So be it," Douglas said, and turned to me. "Thank you for your testimony, nurse."

"Echo Heron," I said, and moved toward the door. Perhaps in some rare, lonely moment he might remember my name.

I tripped at the door, recovered, and walked head-on into Dr. Meyers, who glared at me. His eyes fairly screamed, "Tattletale! Squealer! Snitch!"

All feelings of remorse and allegiance vanished. Whatever Mr. Pope came up with as a just punishment wasn't going to be enough.

"Hey you! Hey you! Hey you!" Mr. Williams bellowed again, louder than before. I supposed it was his hospital version of banging a tin cup against the bars of his cell.

I'd put him off as long as I dared. Turning the desk over to Pia, I loaded myself down with stethoscope, Tylenol with codeine, his chart (should I need to prove something), nitroglycerine tablets, and resolve.

Mr. Williams was watching Dorothy dance with the Cowardly Lion. His eyes lit up for a moment with delight at some antic of the Scarecrow's and he chuckled. Still smiling, he began to yell again. "Hey you! Hey you! Hey—"

"That's enough, Williams," I said. "We've got sick people here who don't need to hear your noise."

At the sound of my voice, Mr. Williams snapped around and pointed at me.

"You done it now, bitch," he said. His eyes narrowed and he gave me a look I had not encountered since the night I got lost riding the subway in Harlem. "You makin' me wait to get that morphine for my anginal pain?" He leveled a finger at my face. "I'm gonna find out where you live, then I'm gonna get you taken care of for sure."

Mr. Williams settled back on the bed, giving me a lazy and hostile once-over. I noticed his nostrils were flared as though he were smelling something rotten. He took a toothpick off the side table and began to clean between his teeth.

"I bet you livin' in one of them big houses over in Tiburon, ain't you, white girl? Easy livin' and a heart like stone. I bet you even got a nigger woman to clean your house and a . . ."

I turned to the guards at the door. "Gentlemen, take Mr. Rose for his walk, would you? And close the door on your way out."

The shorter of the two guards rubbed the back of his neck uneasily. "We can't do that, ma'am. Can't leave a prisoner alone, especially with the nurses. Can we help you out with something?"

"Not really. Mr. Williams and I need to get a few things straightened out. It'll be fine. Leave the other guard outside the door and take Mr. Rose for his walk."

Dubious, the guard shook his head, still hesitant to leave me alone with Mr. Williams.

"Look," I said, "the only way out of here is through the window, and there isn't even a ledge for him to hold on to. He'd have to jump, and that's a very long way down." I went up to the guard, pleading. "Just give me five minutes alone with him. I promise I won't hurt him badly."

The guard helping Mr. Rose into his robe snickered.

"Don't you leave me alone wid this cold bitch," Mr. Williams yelled. "Get me back to the joint. Prison is better than dealing wid this broad, man."

The guard, reassured by this speech, winked at me. "Okay. Five minutes. We'll be right outside if you need us." He tapped Mr. Rose's bald spot. "Let's shuffle, lover boy."

Mr. Williams punched his pillow. His alarm clock went off.

The door closed behind us, and we were left face-to-face. I crossed my arms. "First, I need to take your blood pressure and listen to your heart and lungs."

"I don't care what you need, you ain't doing nothin' to me. You ain't gonna touch me till I get morphine." He laid a cold, defiant stare on me.

I returned the stare and went one better by going two steps closer to him. "I can't give you anything before I take your pressure and listen to your heart and lungs."

"You lyin'! That other nurse, she give me morphine and didn't do shit 'bout no pressure and lungs. Give me my morphine, or you can get out right now and let me be."

"I apologize to you for that other nurse, Mr. Williams. She made a mistake. She wasn't supposed to give you those drugs, and I guarantee you it won't happen again unless you really have pain."

I took the cuff from the basket on the wall and pulled the Velcro apart. I waited for his arm.

Mr. Williams shook his head. "You withholdin' medicine from a sick man. You gonna burn wid the rest of the nigger haters."

My body did not move, but my temper was being forced up the fuse at a mile a minute. In the light of the bedside lamp, Mr. Williams glared, challenging me.

"You think you're brave, white girl? Wait till my friend come round your house to take care of you. They won't find nothin' 'cept pieces of your white ass."

I held the man's eyes and said nothing, though I ground my tooth guard a new hole. Mr. Williams looked away, sneering. "What it gonna be, honkie? You gonna give me some morphine, or do I gotta call one of my—"

I didn't like this line of thought or conversation. I tried to take Mr. Williams's threats with objectivity and failed. The words "honkie" and "your white ass" preceding a threat against my life hit the stack like a stick of dynamite.

"Are you done?" I yelled so loud that Mr. Williams jumped. "Who the hell do you think you're talking to, mister? You think I'm Miss Honkie America living in the lap of luxury with maids and driving around in a Mercedes Benz? Shit, use your head, man—I'm a nurse! I get paid less than a grocery checker."

I paused and lowered my voice. "You think listening to your

bellyaching is easy? Man, talk about 'scruciatin' pain! You're one major pain in the ass, mister.

"You think you've got the corner on being tough because you're a convict?" I slowly circled the bed, regarding him with narrowed eyes. "Let me tell you something, pal." (Suddenly I developed a heavy Brooklyn accent.) "When you were stealing candy from the corner mom-and-pop store, I was working the streets of New York."

(Okay, okay, so one of the times I ran away from home, I went to the city and walked from West 107th Street to West 12th Street—in the middle of December, that was work.)

"By '66 I was riding the boxcars, scrambling to stay alive."

(Well, I did ride the rails for a short time, and I did almost do myself in once scrambling to hop a moving boxcar.)

Mr. Williams was feigning indifference to my drama queen speech, but his eyes were wider than usual.

"I'm not proud of it, but I've done time selling shit too."

(Once, at a garage sale, it took me two days and a lot of hard sell to fob off a fifty-pound bag of prehistoric chicken manure for two bucks. It wasn't worth two cents, but I was hard up at the time.)

"The only difference between me and you is that I knew when to get out."

(True. I packed up and left before the guy could try to return the manure and get his money back.)

"I've gone through enough drugs to make you look like a pansy, mister . . ."

(During a rush of acute angina patients, I could sign out two or three boxes of morphine and Demerol in one week.)

"So don't try to con me. I know every druggie trick and story in the book.

"Get it straight for the last time, Alvin—you can shuck and jive all you want, but you ain't coppin' no fixes offa this white broad. And if you don't stop with the yelling and the call bell, I'm transferring you out to ward seven."

"What's that ward seven?"

"Labor and delivery."

Mr. Williams studied me with skepticism.

"You really hop cars?"

"Yep. Mostly in Tennessee and Kentucky."

"Shit, man, that's somethin'," he murmured. "Trains scary to me. Too big, too noisy. You ain't 'fraid you gonna get sucked under them wheels?"

"Nope. I was raised around trains. My dad and my grandfather were railroad men. It's in the blood."

The man shook his head slowly. Above him, the Wicked Witch was engaged in skywriting "SURRENDER DOROTHY" with her broom.

I punched the man lightly on his tattoo. "No more bullshit, okay? Let me do what I gotta do here."

"Oh Lord," he sighed, and held out his arm. "Why did I gotta go and get Miz Honkie Cinderella for a nurse?"

"Wull, I still don't get it," Honey said, twisting that same strand of sun-bleached hair.

Pia sighed. Beth, in her spot by the double doors, kept her eyes glued to the acute monitors, but groaned. I held my breath, hoping that Honey would start giggling and say she was only kidding and she fully understood the transparent stratagem of the administration. She could be so sharp sometimes when it came to understanding medicine and her patients, I'd started to think the dumb-blond-surfer act was just a pretense.

Pia disagreed. She thought Honey was more like an idiot savant.

"It never crossed your mind . . ." Pia hesitated, studied Honey's vacant look through the blue mascara, and corrected her phraseology. "Didn't something make you suspicious about that letter from the director of nurses?"

Honey shook her head. "I thought she was being nice. She sounded like she really wanted to help us."

"When was the last time the director of nurses tried to help us, Honey?" Beth asked.

The blonde puckered her high-gloss lips and thought hard. After a second, she wrinkled her brow and shook her head. "I can't remember."

"You can't remember, Honey, because there wasn't a last time. The letter is a subterfuge," I said.

"A subterfudge?" Honey stopped twisting and smiled brightly. "Sounds like low-cal chocolate. Gosh, I love chocolate. This super foxy guy I dated once was a photographer, you know, and I'd get nude and he'd cover me all over with chocolate fudge sauce and then he'd put his—"

Beth cleared her throat and excused herself. She wished Pia and me good luck in our instruction of the intellectually departed.

"Honey, a subterfuge is a ruse, a plot," I said. "The administration was hoping that all the nurses would fill out the form saying they wanted to hire help to do the busywork. That way, they could hire people who have been trained for a few weeks in how to take blood pressures and give baths, then pay them minimum wage, right?"

Honey nodded. "So good, so far," she said cheerily.

"Right," said Pia. "But then one day, as you're getting ready to come to work, they call you up and tell you not to bother to come in because they don't need you that day. Then they call me and Echo and tell us the same thing."

"Must not have very many patients in the hospital." Honey frowned.

"No, that's not it, Honey," I said. "As a matter of fact, the unit is full and they have Beth in charge on the intermediate side and Risen in charge on the acute side, but taking care of the bulk of the patients are these people who have had nine weeks of training."

"That's silly," said Honey. "They can't do that. They wouldn't know when something serious was happening with the patients. They wouldn't even be able to read the monitors."

"That's right." I smiled, gratified that the light was able to penetrate the fog. "But their wages are one quarter of ours, and administration would rather pay a little bit for one of them than three times as much for an R.N."

"Besides that," continued Pia, "Beth and Risen would be ultimately responsible for all the patients' safety. If one of those helpers made a mistake or didn't tell Beth that somebody's pressure was really low or that a patient was having chest pain and someone was hurt or died, Beth's license would be on the line."

"You mean one of us would be responsible for everything they did? Even if they did bad?"

Pia and I nodded in agreement, pleased to have educated with success.

Honey thought for a few minutes, twisting vigorously. Finally she tossed back the mane of hair and stood. "I think you're being mean and thoughtless," she said indignantly. "What you're talking about is communism."

Pia and I gave each other unsure, sideways glances.

"Our director of nurses is trying to make it nice for us, and you're saying unkind things about her. She's a good American—she'd never let untrained people take care of the patients."

Honey fluffed up her cleavage by pulling Flippy and Whip partway out of their home cups and stormed away as fast as her tight skirt would allow.

After a few moments of silence, Pia and I looked at each other. "If I had a flag, I'd wave it," she said.

Instead, we stood, placed our hands over our hearts, and sang "America" for all we were worth.

At ten, I began pulling report from the nurses, made final rounds on both sides of the unit, checked staffing, and made assignments for nights. I'd used my thirty-minute leeway option for medication distribution to give my nine and ten P.M. meds at nine thirty, so all I had left to worry about was eleven o'clock meds and a dressing change. Honey refused to even look at me, and Pia was busy admitting a chest pain/syncope/hypertension patient to our last bed. It was going to mean overtime for us both, but I suppose it served us right, since the patient was Mr. Cooney.

I finally got Beth to roll a chair and bedside table over to the double doors and watch both sets of monitors while trying to chart.

With five minutes left before I had to give report to night shift, I entered Mr. Rose and Mr. Williams's room. A look passed between them. Mr. Rose smiled sweetly when I handed him his sleeping pill. "Al's got something to ask you," he said.

"No drugs except a sleeping pill," I warned.

"Naw," Mr. Rose said. "It's something nice, isn't it, Al?"

Mr. Williams smiled and hung his head. He resembled a shy schoolboy.

"So, you've got something to ask?" I prompted.

Mr. Williams looked to Mr. Rose for encouragement, then to me. "I'm gettin' paroled in six months. I wanna take you out to dinner wid me."

"Tell her what else," Mr. Rose coached, rubbing his hands gleefully.

"I'm gonna get us a limo and take you to one of them fancy restaurants in the city, maybe go to a jazz club after, drink some champagne, do some dancin'."

Why? I thought. Why me?

Mr. Williams was bright-eyed, going on about his ideal date, while Mr. Rose urged him on from the sidelines. They looked like squirrels begging nuts, their faces full of expectation.

"Then after we hit Mama's, maybe we keep drivin' on down to Vegas, do some gamblin', find us some fine blow . . ."

I shook my head. "Hold it. First of all, it's against policy to even talk about anything of a personal nature, let alone accept dates. Second, just a few hours ago, you wanted to put out a contract on me, and now you want to take me to dinner? And did you ever think I might be married or have a boyfriend?"

"Policy can be broken for a stud like me," Mr. Williams said, unabashed.

"In six months he won't be a prisoner anymore either, so the policy doesn't hold," threw in Mr. Rose.

"And I was only tryin' to scare you wid that story 'bout havin' somebody cut you up." Mr. Williams laughed.

"And we both know you're single," Mr. Rose said, winking at Mr. Williams.

"Yeah," said Mr. Williams. "Women who got men are fat and easy. You're too skinny and nervous to have a man."

Tuesday
2 A.M.

Too skinny and nervous? Is the nervous part from not having sex? I thought only the skin was supposed to go bad. Oh God, now I'm worried that everybody who sees me is thinking, Poor thing, she isn't getting any. What can I do? Is it my fault that my sex drive—tired of neglect—just up and drove away?

How does the skinny part fit in? Too desperate to eat?

Full moon tomorrow. Thank God I'm off. Pia has some kind of surprise for me and Simon. Hope she hasn't baked another one of her Far East concoctions. The last one worked well as a doorstop, but Simon chipped a tooth before we knew better.

Part of Dr. Meyers's atonement as imposed by Mr. Pope was to make a formal apology to each of the nurses involved. Butter wouldn't have melted in his mouth as he told each of us he was sorry for being such a dick. He was so mortified, he resembled the face on a bottle of poison.

Simon left me a list of fish baits that he wants for Christmas: rattling flatwart, super-dawg crankbait, slo-poke jighead, power slugs, professional crappies, chewee juice leeches, and worm weights. This request comes from some-one who does not fish . . . doesn't even own a rod. I do not understand the adolescent mind, although I myself had one at one time.

I keep thinking about Honey's communist-pinko speech. But, as Beth later said, what do you expect from a woman who is a member of the Los Angeles chapter of the Click Clack Club? Anybody who dedicates an hour a month to perfecting the art (?) of attracting male attention by the racket she makes while walking in high heels, cannot be taken seriously.

When I left, Mr. Pope was sitting in the waiting room holding his head. I stopped to ask if he was okay, and he said he had a bad headache. Thinking I would give my ho-listic pressure-point cure a try, I took his hand and told him that with minimal cooperation on his part, I could make his headache go away.

He got all smarmy and weird like he'd peed himself and said, "Yeah, but I'm married."

Maybe Williams and Mr. Rose aren't pulling my leg. Maybe I really do look as hungry and desperate as those tired, fading secretaries one sees hanging out in fern bars on Friday nights, looking for love and affection.

Oh, please God, let this skinny and nervous little body have some sleep tonight.

When Pia's third negative HIV test came in, I planned a cel-ebration around her favorite edible, the stinking rose. There was baked garlic for appetizers, garlic bread, a cream-of-garlic soup, and pasta primavera in heavy garlic sauce. For dessert, I made garlic ice cream from scratch and served it in prechilled bowls with sprigs of parsley.

The event had been memorable if only for the fact that for several days afterward we dared not come into contact with others who had functioning olfactory glands. I recall that even Mooshie slept under the bathtub for the duration, and would hold his breath when I picked him up to talk.

To show her appreciation, Pia invited me and Simon to din-ner and told us there would be a surprise. With Pia, this could mean anything, from a serving of her onion coin cakes—onion pancakes with foil-covered dimes folded into them: a 1956 *Women's Home Journal* idea that struck her as "cute"—to an evening of tweezing each other's eyebrows.

Simon was skeptical as we headed up the dirt road to her geodesic dome set on the top of a hill in Tiburon. He'd met Pia during our nursing school years and taken to her immediately. But even though he'd known her for twelve years, he still had reservations about her unpredictable, crazy side.

Dinner was just shy of normal—spaghetti and tofu squares in strawberry sauce as a main course, and peanut-butter-and-jelly-stuffed celery stalks for dessert.

When the last string of celery had been coughed up, rechewed, and swallowed, Simon wandered off into the living room and occupied himself by sampling Pia's extensive tape collection on his Walkman. In the kitchen, Pia's and my postmeal-cleanup conversation ran to shoptalk, her constant stream of boyfriends, and my lack of same.

"Your problem, Ec, is that you don't put yourself out there," Pia said, taking a covered bowl from the refrigerator and setting it on the table between us. "You've got to make yourself more available if you want to meet men, Ec. You have this one job where you don't meet any men except sick or injured ones, and your other job forces you to lock yourself away in that haunted room you call an office, with a computer for sixteen hours at a time."

I peeked through the plastic wrap covering the bowl. It was full of oatmeal, cold and gelatinous, the way oatmeal often goes when it's been refrigerated. "Oh hell, Pia. I don't know how to meet men. I've never been one of these modern women who know how to think with their thighs. I'm shy, plus the only instructions I ever got on how to meet a guy was to go slap him on the back and say, 'So! How about them Mets, huh?' I tried it once at the library. The guy, who was in the sports section, kind of looked at me weird and moved to the psychology section without so much as saying, 'Shoo.' "

"Psshhh, he was probably gay or had a jealous girlfriend loitering down in the romance novels," Pia said.

"But that isn't the only problem I have with men," I said. "When I finally did land a date, the guy brought me to his apartment *before* dinner. That worried me, but what really sent me running were the three bags of disposable toothbrushes he kept on a shelf over his bathroom sink."

Pia put a bag of powdered sugar, a bowl of softened butter, two plastic place mats, several Tupperware containers, and two tablespoons next to the bowl. "All I know is, there's a man out there waiting for you and you're standing him up." In a wistful tone, she added, "You're cheating someone wonderful and yourself out of a lot of loving."

"Oh please, Pia," I scoffed. "You're almost as much a melodrama junkie as I am. If I'm supposed to meet someone, I will. My only responsibility is to screen all applicants to make sure they're functional, healthy people."

I watched my fellow nurse spoon out a clump of oatmeal, shape it into a ball, coat it with butter, and roll it in powdered sugar. The result looked much like a golf ball. This masterpiece she placed neatly in the corner of one of the containers and regarded with great satisfaction.

"Well, he's not going to come to your front door and knock, Ec." Pia put the other spoon in my hand and indicated I should follow her example with the oatmeal. In the background, we could hear Simon singing along with whatever song was blasting through the earphones. The random, off-key wailing sounded a bit like Billy Joel's "An Innocent Man," or "Happy Birthday."

"When I'm supposed to meet him, I will." I rolled the porridge as though I'd been doing it for twenty years. "I've already got it fantasized out—it'll be over the cabbages at Safeway. He'll ask if they're the seedless kind and how to tell if one is ripe. . . . Speaking of seedless, what are we making here?"

"It's part of the surprise." Pia got out some raisins and stuck a few into each golf ball. "Tell me again what that psychic guy told you?"

I smiled at Pia's memory for romance-related detail. Several years before, I'd taken care of a patient who was supposedly a renowned psychic. As soon as I walked into his room, he told me I was many centuries old, that I was a writer and had a musically inclined son who kept to himself. Then he asked if I had met David yet.

"He told me that I'd have a wonderful, life-altering relationship with a man named David, and he was right."

Pia paused in her rolling. "You've met someone named David?"

"Yep. He's the romantic interest of the main character in my next book."

"Tsssssssh. Main character, my ass. What about *you*? What are you doing about meeting the real life-changing David?"

I patted her hand, leaving a small peak of oatmeal where I'd touched. "I'm doing exactly what I'm supposed to be doing. I'm making these weird oatmeal balls in your kitchen."

The first Tupperware box filled, we moved on to the second.

"Don't worry, Pia," I said evenly, "I've got it all figured out. I'll end up as a lonely old woman in a rocking chair with a cat on my lap, writing Harlequin Romance novels for the romantically disabled and automatic-weapons handbooks for militant nurse radicals. I'll be fairly content, but in poor health because there won't be a doctor left in the country who will treat me without wanting to kill me."

When we had three full boxes of oatmeal balls, Pia gave Simon and me each a pair of her leather riding gloves. She then had me exchange my skirt for an old pair of her jeans and my stockings for a pair of wool socks. Dividing the load of Tupperware containers and two thermoses of hot cider, we headed out over the Tiburon hills toward the stable where Pia kept her horses.

Our way was brightly lit by the moon, huge in the clear midnight-blue sky. We walked through the cool, surrounding silence, involved in our own thoughts, until Simon stopped dead in his tracks. Running into him, we stacked up, in imitation of the Three Stooges.

"Wha—?"

Simon clapped his hand over my mouth and pointed. No more than twelve feet up the trail stood a bobcat holding a limp jackrabbit in her mouth. Although she stood as still as a stuffed lion in a museum scene, I sensed that she was irritated by the encounter, impatient to get home with her groceries.

Paralyzed by indecision, we engaged in a stare-down for fifteen or thirty seconds while each of us tried to think of what could be done to break the Mexican standoff.

Pia, in a moment of insane bravery, stepped toward the cat and raised her arms. "Scat!" she hissed, continuing to advance on the animal. When she was close enough to have touched the cat's nose just by extending her arm, the animal turned and loped up the hill with her kill.

"A strong spirit has presented herself to us," Pia said solemnly. "The Miwoks would tell us this is an omen."

Simon rolled his eyes.

"Of what?" I asked. "A decrease in the rabbit population?"

Pia did not change her expression. "This is a good omen. The wildcat is a romantic symbol of female strength and sensuality. The rabbit is a symbol of productivity. I think . . ." She narrowed her eyes and looked up at the moon, sniffed the wind, and then let her gaze settle on me. "I think you will marry a true warrior within a year and have one more child."

Simon and I roared with laughter. When I could finally stand up straight, I wiped away my laugh tears and slapped her on the back. "Jesus, Pia, you've been living in that dome too long—some of those cosmic rays are getting at your brain."

"Okay," she said, and resumed walking. "Ye shall see, O ye of little faith."

Pia outdid herself on the surprise, thus putting homemade garlic ice cream so far to shame as to wipe it off the slate. A moonlight horseback ride over the hills to the Bay—can't get much better than that at any price.

We'd been riding at a leisurely pace for the better part of an hour, singing three-part harmony on as many country-and-western songs as we could remember the words to, when the trail ended at the edge of a flat, wide-open field.

I don't think any of us breathed as the magic crept in around our small group. Even the horses, sensing a change, picked up their ears, paying attention. Giddy on fresh air laced with sweet grass and wild thyme, we all felt somehow indestructible.

Simon and Pia glanced at each other, then, without a word or signal, broke into a full gallop across the meadow.

Pia took the lead, then lost it to Simon. Whooping at the top of their lungs, they raced the length of the field and back along the edge, near the trees. Like ghostly riders, they disappeared from view in the long shadows of the scrub oaks, only to reappear a moment later, spectral in the midnight brightness.

By the light of the moon, my son's face was totally alive with the rapture of the moment. His long body crouched forward, flat against the horse's neck. His light, fine hair and the black mane of his horse flew wildly together, then apart as the wind broke and flowed over their bodies.

All images to stay in my mind a lifetime.

The oatmeal balls, believe it or don't, were not all for the horses. Simon and I had to be coaxed, but once we got over the idea of it, and saw how much the horses enjoyed them, we ate our fair share.

In truth, the taste wasn't really half bad.

Wednesday
6 A.M.

I'm punch-drunk on no sleep. Legs feel like rubber bands, my mind is a bowl of Jell-O. If this is written in English, it'll be a miracle.

Got home from Pia's around midnight only to find a weepy message from Beth in the ER saying she'd broken her ankle and gone through a glass door during a code on Mr. Galante.

She was running out of the room to get the pacemaker insertion cart, when she slipped on a glob of defibrillator paste and went headlong through the door. She said the crack of her ankle was so loud, Risen and Chris heard it out at the desk. She lacerated one ear and three inches of scalp.

She's already freaked about making ends meet on disability, but this isn't the main reason for her tears. What I suspect she's really upset about is not being able to dance, for this is the addiction she has used to replace alcohol.

I took her home, and spent a long time calming her down. When she was able to listen, I told her that without the replacement addiction, she was going to need support twenty-four hours a day, and although I loved her, I couldn't be the one to give that to her.

I said what I should have said months ago—that it was time to get on with her recovery and go back into AA, where there were people who understood and could really be of help to her. Don't know if I got through, but I think it is Beth's only chance for survival and happiness. I don't envy her—I think she has some old pain to sort out.

Got to sleep now or I won't be worth a rat's ass at work. I've willed myself to dream of flying horses.

TEN

> "There was never any yet that wholly could
> escape love ..."
>
> LONGUS, *Daphnis and Chloe*

IN THE FINAL MINUTES OF 1988, I watched the festivities from a table littered with paper plates, crumpled napkins, clear plastic cups, and noisemakers, all in various stages of mutilation. I think it was the noisemakers that started the depression. They got me dwelling on the fact that time was marching on. Actually, time danced erratically rather than marched, although sometimes it felt more like it was plodding.

I reflected on the fact that I'd been plodding right alongside of it—alone. Evidence of my solitary state was all around me: the party consisted of 101 people—fifty couples and me. Even the band members had been accompanied by their significant others.

The old sadness began in the center of my chest and crept slowly toward my throat, like a cat slinking onto the kitchen table for the turkey. I fought the melancholy by imagining what Dale Carnegie, the Emily Post of Positive Thinking, might have to say about my plight.

Looking dapper in his New Year's hat and tuxedo, Dale's advice was to recall and dwell on the good things that had happened during the soon-to-be-past year.

Okay. Good things. Let's see. . . . Well, I had my health, and I'd been able to check off five items from my Things I Want to Do Before I Get Too Old or Die List: hang glide, take a hansom cab ride through Central Park, cruise in a glider without throwing up, snorkel, and rock climb. That left only 347 more things to accomplish.

I continued to be pretty busy on the lecture circuit, and although the editing policeman was constantly at my back, my second book was progressing on schedule.

Oh yeah, and none of my close friends or family had died.

Dale Carnegie (he resembled Bill Graham playing Father Time on New Year's Eve) was smiling. "See? You're a lot better off than most. What's a little loneliness compared to all these marvelous things?"

I was about to shrug in reluctant semiagreement, when the mixed and negative events that had transpired during the year demanded equal time by filing through my mind in a slow death march. The positives stood aside to let them pass through.

First of all, life at the hospital was becoming more stressful and intense each day. True, the critical care units were enjoying the advantages of the new wing, but the administration was screaming poverty and tightening the screws on the nurses. As the politics got dirtier, nurses began to lose their patience (no pun intended, although it was a distinct possibility). It was no longer a battle limited to the rabble-rousers, either. All the nurses were fed up.

We were already limping under the strain of the unsafe work loads, when the administration cut the budget yet again. The straw that broke our injured backs, however, was the discovery that several of our benefits had been reduced or discontinued without our knowledge.

My tolerance for the administration's nonsense was at an all-time low. I was outraged at not being able to give my patients the care they needed. After twelve years of the same old story, I was more prone to flying off the handle, then going home and being tortured by nightmares about patients left suffering because of something I did not have time to do.

Then I awoke at two one morning to find a strange man standing over my bed, going through my purse. Never having been burglarized before, I wasn't quite sure what was considered proper behavior under the circumstances. The police were shocked that my first reaction had been to pummel the guy, then jump on his back screaming obscenities that made harsh reference to his mother.

On his way out, the thief made the further mistake of grabbing Simon by the neck and dragging him along. Although the police said he'd done this to get me off his back, so to speak, it prompted me to kick him in a most delicate place. He loosened his grip on Simon and went limping off into the night. It was enough to keep my nightmares fueled and my neck veins distended for a week.

I don't know if the burglar incident had anything to do with his decision to move out, but a few weeks later, Simon discussed with me and his father his need for more male influence in his daily life. "Male bonding" we call it in progressive California, although, helping him move to his dad's, I felt in touch with the primitive; I was giving my son over to the men of the tribe in order that he might go through the necessary rites of manhood.

Cutting the apron strings was all fine and healthy, but the repercussions of Simon's move were to come for months. The most immediate effects were the hollow silences in the cottage (similar to those heard inside a recently vacated shell), and having no one to cook for (a cooking-for-one cookbook was *too* depressing).

About three weeks after he left, I found myself missing Simon and all his wisdom, humor, and good advice, and his weirdness. I yearned to find him in front of a mirror, pulling his face into amazing contortions, or hear him talk in his sleep.

I began waking in the middle of the night, all in a terror over the slightest noise. The cottage, which had always seemed cozy, was now enormously cold and empty. My journal entries grew by pages—not that I had more to say, I just didn't want to face the hours of tossing and turning in insomniac frustration. More than ever, I was plagued by a loneliness that stung constantly, like being out in an endless hailstorm without protective clothing.

Of course, my friends were charitable and forever tolerant of their fifth wheel. Out of the kindness of their hearts, they made a point of inviting me to weekend dinners. It had to be a strain on the host, because the number of chairs never came out even. I can't tell you how many times I ended up eating at a card table tacked onto the end of the paired-off grown-ups' main dining table. It was reminiscent of the Thanksgiving dinners of my childhood, except my cousins weren't there to share the isolation.

The mental image of Dale Carnegie faded positively from my mind. Relatively speaking, I had a good life—I just didn't have a personal life.

Jolted out of my reverie by the blasts from a hundred noisemakers, I found myself awkwardly drifting through a sea of fifty embracing, kissing, dewy-eyed couples.

Before the midnight minute was up, I slipped into my coat and drove home, kissing the back of my hand.

On January 2, I purchased a rocking chair and resolved that I would focus my energies on my inner spiritual journey. I had visions of myself as a wizened, silver-haired old woman serenely rocking in my chair in the desolate desert of New Mexico or Arizona, totally blissed out on inner peace like some eccentric Castaneda character. I was committed to working on being content with the idea of living my life out single. I had already spent the majority of it single—I didn't imagine the loneliness could get any more uncomfortable than it already was.

I was wrong.

No matter how much I meditated or read or wrote, I couldn't squelch the lonely, sad feelings. On my more pathetic days, I even cried over romantic commercials, or movies where the couple ended up together after 108 minutes of conflict and emotional trampolining. It got so bad that in airports I would begin to sob at the sight of parting and reuniting couples.

Now, at this point in my life my personal jury was still out on the subject of divine intervention. A lot of the time, it seemed like there was never anybody home up there, no matter whom I chanted or prayed to.

I was soon to have an experience that would convince me not only that Someone was home, but that Someone was paying close attention.

Some people I know have a real talent when it comes to ESP.

Take my younger sister, Mari, for instance; she'll have one of her "special" dreams about a person she knows, and bingo—one to three days later, they drop dead.

Janey and I have always had a type of ESP direct line between us. If I think about wanting to talk to her, it's a sure thing that within twelve hours she'll call. When I answer the phone, the first words out of her mouth are, "Why are you beckoning me?"

I have been told that on a metaphysical level, I am an open book. At various times, total strangers have approached me with information about myself that no one knows (or would *want* to know) except me.

So I wasn't too surprised when I received a letter at the end of July from an elderly man in Maryland who wrote to say he'd enjoyed my book and wanted to give me something in return. His "gift" was the last two pages of the letter:

I have never written to an author before, but I felt you would not mind, especially since I see that you are now going through a difficult time in your life. When I focus on you, I feel the pain of loneliness which will not let you sleep in peace.

You do not believe you will find that love for your life. You go so far as to surround yourself with the accoutrements (I see a rocking chair?) of an old widow. You alone are the architect of this misery. Now is the time to renovate.

Hear me when I tell you that because of all the lives you have touched, you have a bank account of love stored away that is beyond your wildest dreams.

You've been making deposits for years into this account, but as yet you have not made any withdrawals. Why don't you ask for some of that love back? I must warn you however, be very specific about what you ask for.

Goose bumps went up on my arms, not so much because this man obviously had some psychic connection into me, but because I felt what he'd told me to do was a magic formula of a kind—a modern-day version of the genie in a bottle.

The first day of August holds a fascination for me, I think because I have always thought of August as the most romantic month of the year. With this in mind, I waited out July, planning exactly where to go and what to ask for.

On the morning of August 1, I eagerly marched out to the ocean. The deserted beach was my bank; the waves were my teller. I was there to make a withdrawal of love. Speaking aloud, I gave my first specification: I wanted a normal, nice guy—no more abusive, woman-hating misogynists. No rescuers or victims. No addicts looking for a co. Someone who could say the word "commitment" without clenching his jaw. The rest was standard personal-column fare: happy, healthy, unafraid to love, communicative, gentle, with a strong sense of self, practical, intelligent, reasonable, willing to work at making it work, loyal, trustworthy, offbeat, affectionate, possessed of a good sense of left-field humor, athletic, handsome, and on and on *ad nauseam*.

A week later, the one man in a thousand answering this very description walked up to my front door and knocked.

His name was David.

A sable-brown cat hung over the man's shoulder, playfully licking his ear while marking the side of his face. The man I recognized as a resident of the apartment building that faced my cottage—it was the cat that stumped me. This cat *looked* like the Moosh, but Mooshie was a spoiled-rotten animal who wouldn't allow a stranger closer than twenty feet, let alone permit himself to be held by one with outward displays of feline affection.

I made no move to claim the animal, who was purring—a noise foreign to *my* Mooshie. Now, if he'd been wheezing or growling . . .

"Isn't this your cat?" the man asked, smiling a wonderful smile. "I found him in the middle of the street, getting off on watching oncoming traffic dodge him. I've seen him on your porch and I figured he belonged to you."

I studied the animal more closely. It *was* the Moosh, unless there was another chubby Burmese in the neighborhood wearing a neon-orange collar with neon-green bells.

Disbelieving, I reached for my cat, who refused to be separated from the guy's shirt. From his curled position on the man's shoulder, Mooshie shot me a deadly glance that clearly read: "Get lost. You've had your chance—I'm in love with somebody new."

The only way I could lure Mooshie away from his rescuer and into the house was with a can of tuna, a treat reserved for his birthday and Christmas.

Stepping into the front hall, my neighbor showed an interest in the unusual wicker walls of the cottage, which led to my standard history tour of the place, which led to casual conversation about who we were and what we did for work and why we'd never met before, since I'd lived there for seventeen years, and he'd been there for almost three.

I recounted that I had waved and smiled at him once as I was driving out our common driveway, but he hadn't returned either gesture. At the time, I shrugged it off, figuring that like so many good-looking men in the Bay Area, either he was afraid I was just another lonely single woman desperate for a date, or he was totally self-absorbed.

He remembered the gesture, he said, but was too taken

aback by the sight of a cat draped casually over the top of my head to respond.

At some early point, I asked him how he had avoided the draft during the Vietnam War. He roared with laughter. When he got his breath, he looked at me like I was from another planet and mentioned something about conscription and graduating from kindergarten during Vietnam.

Silently, I calculated that when he was going into the third grade, I was hanging out in People's Park ("You hung out in parking lots?" he asked) and taking part in antiwar demonstrations in Berkeley.

Then he asked me outright how old I was when John Kennedy was shot. (I was a junior in high school. He was a junior in his playpen.) And that was when we first realized there was an age difference of fourteen years—his favor.

I don't recall everything that was said that night, but I *do* remember that we sat at my kitchen table talking until three the following morning, and it was the most comfortable, honest time I'd ever spent with a man in my life.

That was the first night. With the exception of the evenings I worked, it was the same every evening for the next three weeks. David would come over after work; we'd have a light supper, build a fire and talk until three, sometimes five the next morning.

At that rate, it wasn't too long before we realized we knew each other better and had more in common than anyone else in our lives, including best friends with whom we had histories.

In our fourth week of averaging four hours of sleep a night, David was accused of drinking on the job, and my switchboard ladies were so fuddled, they were threatening to strike. Since we were both still operating motor vehicles every day, we decided in the name of safety to call it a night no later than midnight.

Shortly after we'd begun the new eight-hours-of-sleep routine, we were saying goodbye at the front door one evening when I caught a glimpse of him that stopped time and sent shock waves through me. Blame it on the soft laughter, the dimples, or the brown eyes—whatever it was, it took my breath away, leaving me confused and sleepless.

Before that moment, the thought of having a romantic interest in David never entered my mind. After all, this was a "kid" and I was an "adult." True, he was older and wiser than I in a lot of ways, but still, fourteen years' difference . . .

The confusion was turning my mind into a battlefield when I finally took hold of the situation and spent a day talking myself out of the idea of David as a lover. Being anything more than good friends, I decided, was out of the question. Intimacy always had a way of turning my relationships into relationshits. Besides, it was ludicrous to think a man as young and handsome as David would be interested in me as anything other than a friend. Relieved, I put the flowing juices back into cold storage, and the wild urges to rest. David would remain a most precious friend and never know of my silliness.

Everything, I told myself, would be fine.

Two nights later, we were playing cards in front of the fire, discussing America's methods of disposing of our dead. I recall I was going on about my thoughts on cremation versus embalming, when David, looking pale, laid down his cards.

"Echo, what the hell are we doing?" His voice was unsteady, and he was sitting on his hands. Mooshie jumped off his lap, a resting place he did not part with easily.

"We're playing cards and talking about how—"

"I mean you and me. What are we doing?"

A surge of panic instantly crawled up from the knot in my stomach to my throat, spread out into both temples, and rendered me immobile.

"You've got to know that something more is going on here than a couple of friends playing cards," he said.

For a few moments there was silence except for the fire making autumn-sounding crackles. I had just realized that I'd ceased to breathe, when I heard myself say, "What did you have in mind?"

David took a deep breath and reached over to touch my hand. "I think we should . . . be together."

It was the first time we had actually touched. My switchboard ladies went tilt and passed out. In a fuguelike state, I watched myself stand, walk behind his chair, and put my hands on his shoulders. I laid my cheek lightly against his hair and thought, Is this the one who has been chosen for me?

No.

Yes.

No. I need more time to think.

Yes. You've thought it to death already. Nothing more to think about.

I'm scared.

As well you should be after six years of celibacy, but take comfort—it's like riding a bicycle.

I'm too old. Christ, I'm a bifocal candidate already.

Give it a break. You're more of an adolescent than your son. Everybody says so.

David's too young.

He's older than you in every way except on his birth certificate.

What will people think?

Oh, come on. Since when have you ever in your life cared about what people think? Is this the same woman who dances on narrow railings of high bridges and shouts her left-field, harebrained ideas from rooftops at the drop of a hat?

What are we getting ourselves into?

Is this the original Ms. Adventure speaking?

(David reached up and covered my hands with wet and icy palms.)

What if I fall more in love with him than I already am? I don't want to get hurt.

Who is this in here with me? What happened to the old battle cry of: "I'd rather die on the dance floor than be a wallflower on the sidelines"?

Okay. Okay. You win. Lead me into the Colosseum. Onward Christian soldiers.

Taking my own deep breath, I closed my eyes and kissed my gift.

ELEVEN

"Modern nursing in a sentence?—Florence doesn't live here anymore."

ECHO HERON, R.N.

IN THE UNNATURAL ORDER OF THINGS, there are night shifts. Unless you are biorhythmically unique, a vampire, or a raccoon, working nights has about two hundred disadvantages to two advantages.

During my nightmare as a rookie working nights on the isolation ward, I discovered that besides sleep deprivation and the annihilation of one's social life, one of the other 198 big disadvantages is that a normal assignment usually includes nine to twelve moderately heavy patients per nurse. Out on the med–surg floors, that's considered a good night. Then there are the bad nights when one nurse can be assigned up to twenty patients without benefit of float nurse, orderly, or other nursing staff.

Of the two advantages, one is that most management people have gone home, which allows us to do our jobs properly. The other advantage is that most physicians sleep at night.

But if working night shift on the floors or in the units is bad, working emergency room night shift is a horror story. ER nurses know there is an unwritten law stating that after midnight the stranger-than-fiction cases are supposed to crawl out from under the porch steps and make their way to the closest ER.

Zombie shift stretches from seven P.M. to seven A.M., and although there are nurses who actually like working this shift (extras from the cast of *Night of the Living Dead*), Redwoods policy stated that all on-call staff must fulfill their standard night shift obligation of two zombie shifts per month, or else.

The way this most inane of rules worked was that the staffing office would pull a regular ER night nurse off her schedule and put her on a day or an evening shift—usually at an inconvenience to that nurse. This task completed, staffing would pull an on-call ER nurse from her usual day or evening shift—again creating havoc—to fill the empty night shift they had just created. All this was done for the sake of satisfying the policy that on-call nurses were required to work a specified number of night shifts per month.

For want of a plausible excuse, staffing office countered that other than satisfying rules, the switching around served to keep day and swing shift nurses' "night skills" up-to-date. I am here to tell you that treating a gunshot wound or splinting a wrist at three A.M. isn't any different from doing it at three P.M.

Although ER's head nurse himself had documented that I was an unsafe night shift worker, he nevertheless insisted that I fulfill my two obligatory zombie shifts each month. That the doctors complained I began slurring my words and walking into solid objects around four A.M. could not override the importance of the regulations.

In October, my zombie shifts fell on a full moon. I am not a day sleeper, but I knew from experience that I had to be ready for the insanity that was sure to be waiting for me when I arrived at seven P.M.

Sliding into my bed at two in the afternoon, I told myself I would not sleep, but only rest for three or four hours. In punishment for all those weeks I had defied him while on my talkathon with David, the sleep god put me in an immediate state of drool-depth REM unconsciousness.

The full-length feature was a strange one, as midday dreams often are. It began with a repeat of my Mafia/FBI-thugs-chase-Echo-through-dark-old-houses-and-city-streets dream. From there, I found myself in 1920s Paris, in a small apartment built into the upper right corner of the Arc de Triomphe. I was married to Dr. Cramer and hugely pregnant with our first child.

My job was working night shift in the Louvre, restoring paintings of the Dutch masters by candlelight because the Parisian curators felt the colors would be truer to the original. Instead of paints, however, I was attempting to revive the paintings with defibrillator paddles and syringes of lidocaine.

On this particular night, I was working on Dou's *The Woman with Dropsy*, when to my horror, the paint transformed itself into Goya's nightmarish *The Old Woman*. The old crone came alive, crawling toward me, screeching the question asked in the painting—*"Qué tal?"*

When she reached my throat, *The Old Woman* changed into a version of *The Last Supper* where Jesus and the apostles immediately took on the appearance of Snow White and the twelve dwarfs.

I was working desperately to reinstate the original painting, when Snow White turned into a demon wielding a baseball bat. The monster's face was a horror of fangs and yellow eyes as he brought the bat down on the head of Judas-cum-Dopey. Blood spurted out of the painting and ran in streams down my face and arms. In that dreamworld type of frozen panic, my first thought was of Dopey's HIV status and the safety of my baby.

Miss Milks appeared out of the nowhere of dreams with a slip of paper disclosing that the blood, now dripping into my eyes and mouth, was indeed HIV-positive.

It was one of those dreams that evoke mysterious and unidentifiable emotions; the kind that ride on your shoulder, nagging at you long after you wake up.

"Stay with me, Osbert, do you hear?" I felt for the green plastic airway and the ambu bag I had placed between the mattress and the steel frame of the gurney. "Cooperate, Risen, and I'll throw in a twenty."

I didn't expect a laugh, really, but I prayed for at least a smile. But no, Risen lay death-still, looking pretty dusky at that. Other than an occasional grunt, he hadn't been able to communicate with us, and the police as yet hadn't come up with the details. All we knew was there had been a 911 call from Risen's apartment, and when the paramedics got there, they found him on the floor, unconscious, his skull crushed.

I pushed the gurney as fast as I could toward the scanner, sweat drenching my scrubs. Considering Risen's weight, and the fact that I was pushing against the deep-pile carpet in the main hall (one of administration's many demonstrations of how they take nurses into consideration), I was doing all right. That is, until I ran into Mr. Cooney cleaning the carpet in front of the scanner door.

"Gotta get in there stat, Mr. Cooney. Move aside, please."

Mr. Cooney had never forgiven me or Pia for putting ideas of coronary troubles in his head, no matter how many times we tried to convince him that we'd probably saved his life by making him feel sick enough to seek help. Turning a deaf ear, he complained that if he'd never known about his hypertension, he would have been fine and not having to take "goddamn pressure medicine" every day. He refused to listen to our tragic-stroke stories about other people who also never knew they had high blood pressure and were now vegetables, or dead.

"Floor's wet," he muttered, making no move to get out of the way.

"Mr. Cooney," I said, my voice granite, "I've got a nurse here with a crushed skull. If you don't move your ass, I swear I'll pick you *and* that goddamned machine up and throw you down the hall." I glared, daring him to argue the point further.

Mr. Cooney ignored me and looked at Risen closely. Surprise and dismay instantly replaced the dull, smug expression. "Jesus! It's the male nurse from the heart unit. He looks bad. What happened to him?"

"We don't know, Mr. Cooney, but I've got to get him in there stat."

With the grace and speed of a much thinner, younger man, Mr. Cooney heaved the carpet machine out of the way and pushed the gurney into the scanner room. "He took care of me real nice up there," he said, returning to his beloved machine. "He's a different sort, but I hope the young fella is gonna be okay."

A garbled "Thampks" came from the gurney. Risen's eyes rolled around under closed lids.

I almost cried with relief. "Hey sweetie, it's Echo. Are you awake?" I picked up his hand and kissed it. "Tell me your name."

"Sandy. Bastard."

I laughed. "Sandy Bastard. Good name. Who's the president of the United States, Risen?"

"Mr. Cooney."

"You're very close, actually, but not quite. Risen, listen, you're in the hospital. You've got a bad head injury. Can you tell me what happened?"

Sandy Bastard checked out again, and the fear-laced depression settled back into my temples. Taking care of a fellow nurse, especially in a trauma situation, was a different kind of caretaking experience altogether. For me, it was as if I became that nurse, watching and feeling everything done, critiquing my own competence from another consciousness. The other side of it was, of course, that there were no sickbed lies when it came to taking care of a medical professional. You couldn't tell another nurse that everything was going to be okay when it wasn't. You couldn't stall for time in giving out the diagnosis or prognosis.

The hardest part, though, was that this patient was family in the truest sense of the word. Being objective was sometimes impossible.

The X-ray tech and I pulled Risen onto the narrow scanner table and strapped him down securely. I arranged the IV lines and placed the monitor in a spot where I could see it through the observation glass of the control room. With the volume control set to max, I could begin Risen's admission notes and "watch" the monitor with my ears. Risen's rhythm was steady, exactly matching the tempo of my least favorite song in the world, "Mack the Knife."

I took a last set of vitals, kissed my co-worker on the cheek, and sank down into one of the physicians' overstuffed office chairs. Peeling the exam gloves off my sweating hands, I shook out my feet, which felt like footballs filled with hot water.

It was only midnight, but business had been nonstop since seven. When we came on duty, Gus and I hadn't even made it to the end of the pneumatic door runner before Dr. Kin nabbed us both for assistance with a drunken man who had sustained a deep laceration from hip to ankle while trying to negotiate the barbed-wire fence his wife had put up in front of her bedroom door.

After that came the usual full-moon madness of lacerations, stomach upsets, strange and gnarly rashes, overdoses, and sprained joints, the head injury of a woman who was extricated from a vehicle hanging by its bumper from the rungs of a telephone pole, and a nun who had broken her arm and nose in her sleep—or so she said.

Just before nine o'clock, Dr. Mahoney assigned me to the doom room, where a forty-six-year-old commercial airline pilot was in the process of having an MI. He would have been a piece of cake, except he got a death grip on my hand and wouldn't let go for anything. In my twelve years, I had never seen anyone so scared about being in a hospital. I was sympathetic, although I *did* get a perverse pleasure out of watching him grip the side rails and sweat. Some sort of justice had been served for all the turbulent flights I'd taken where the pilot announced with great urgency that everyone *must* return to their seats—only to leave us in this horrible state of terror, strapped in and hyperventilating for the rest of the trip. As far as I was concerned, they might as well have announced that we were all going to die, and to please prepare for death.

While the tech set the dials for the scanner, I found an admission form and began transcribing the progression of Risen's vital signs from the odd scraps of paper towels and the palms of my hands. I was trying to read the blood pressure smudged on the mound under my index finger when the beat of Risen's monitor rhythm changed from "Mack the Knife" to "Silent Night." The adrenaline rush bolted me into the scanner room in time to see his rhythm go from a bradycardia to a simple flatline.

Screaming for a code blue call, I ripped off the Velcro restraints and gave a hard-fisted thump to the center of Risen's bony chest. Instead of the nice normal sinus rhythm I prayed for, the pattern on the monitor changed from asystole to fine ventricular fibrillation. Still a disaster, but better. At least there was some electrical current to work with.

"Damn it, Risen!" I inserted the airway into his mouth and fitted the oxygen mask over the lower half of his face. "Don't do this to us."

As I positioned Risen for a couple of quick breaths, my fingers sank into the mushy area that was the back of his head. It felt very much like picking a cantaloupe out of a basket and finding the underside has rotted away.

I hadn't given one full breath before Dr. Menowitz and the code team crowded through the door with the crash cart. Stepping away to let the respiratory tech take over, I had to raise my voice only a little to give report over the controlled noise level familiar to night shift codes (as opposed to the chaotic, wild noise of day shift codes).

Someone shoved the greased defibrillator paddles into my hands. On automatic pilot, I charged the paddles to 300 joules and placed them in the appropriate places on Risen's chest.

"Clear!"

The respiratory tech and the nurse doing chest compressions jumped back from the scanner table. I made sure no part of my body was in contact with Risen or the table, and clicked the discharge buttons.

The jolt lifted Risen's thin body off the table.

An eternity of two seconds had to pass before the heart's

new rhythm would register on the monitor screen. Everyone's mind raced during this time, catching up, planning what drug to give next, what action to take. Was it time for more epinephrine? Should we defibrillate again? Intubate now, or hold off for a minute or two?

I pulled myself out of the medical brain scramble; there was enough medical talent in the room already to resuscitate an army of codes. Instead, I focused on Risen. The angular, thin face was the whitest shade of pale. Even his freckles were faded to the point of looking like pieces of gray ash settled across his nose and cheeks. I slipped my hand in his and squeezed. It was strange to see another one of us, the healers, in the position of needing healing.

"We're back in business, folks!" someone shouted. Risen's rhythm started with the beat of "Angel Baby," jumped once, and accelerated to an epinephrine-induced "Let's Spend the Night Together." The lab tech laughed and the respiratory tech sighed in relief. The supervisor told a quick joke about Saint Peter and a doctor.

I put myself back in the game by relating what little I knew of Risen's health history, per Dr. Menowitz's request—like the fact that he suffered from asthma, and had contracted hepatitis when he was in nursing school, that he took steroids for bad allergies, and was prone to getting bronchitis, and that he was gay, and—

The sound of me sucking in wind drew Dr. Menowitz's attention. He caught the panicked expression and followed my gaze to my hands—my bare hands, which were covered with blood.

"Not too bright, Echo." The words were harsh, scolding.

I nodded and moved toward the sink. As I scrubbed Risen's blood off my hands and from under my nails, I kicked myself for luring Mooshie into tearing up the two loathsome hand monsters before leaving the house for work.

Wearing a fresh pair of exam gloves, I placed myself close to the head of the gurney.

"Risen?"

The nurse strained to open his eyes. "Ec?"

"Yeah. It's me. You're okay, just hold on."

"Ec?" He seemed to be in a vacant state of disbelief.

"Yeah, Risen?"

His mouth moved ever so slightly, skirting around the edges of whispered words. I put my ear to his mouth.

". . . die?"

The word was so faint.

I rubbed his shoulder until I could get my throat to work. "No, Risen. You're not going to die." I leaned down again, close to his ear. "And if you try it again on my shift, I'll assign Ginger to you, and that will, in your famous words, really put your knickers in a twist."

I held my breath, praying for the right response.

Risen smiled a brief, wan smile.

I invited the policeman to fill out the report on Risen at the table in back of the physicians' station. Armed with his own personalized Dunkin' Donuts mug, and a half dozen jelly doughnuts, Officer Lansing contentedly dunked and chewed while going over his report sheet.

"It must be a drag having to work with a pervert, huh? Christ, I'll bet the patients go crazy when he swishes into their room."

I paused momentarily in my search through the "sacred instruments" cabinet and threw the man a sharp look. "Actually, Risen is a great guy and a really good critical care nurse."

Busy licking a dribble of strawberry jelly off the report sheet, Officer Lansing missed both the look and the warning in my answer.

"Well, he's got lousy judgment in people. His live-in sweetheart has been making the rounds of the Castro Street leather bars and baths for the last two years. Seems that every time your friend went to work, his friend went cruising."

A sadness surrounded my heart as I recalled all the dozen or so quick phone calls Risen had a habit of making during his shifts. I imagined him calling his apartment, never getting any answer, and being left wondering.

". . . so he decided to crack your friend with a baseball bat." The cop was still talking and beginning to chuckle. "When I asked him what a fairy was doing with a piece of sports equipment, the little flit told me they used it for a kind of sport that took more balls than one."

Mid-laugh, the cop inhaled some powder off his doughnut and turned scarlet.

Gripping the long-handled nasopharyngeal clamp, I left the officer choking and delivered the instrument to Dr. Menowitz, who was preparing to remove a rhinestone from the deep recesses of a belly dancer's nasal passage.

When I returned to the back desk, Officer Lansing was still wiping away choke tears.

"Did you check out the name of this guy?" he said. "Sandy Lace. How's that for a perfect queer's name?" The officer put his pen into his shirt pocket behind the oversized brass nameplate bearing his name. "Personally"—the policeman stood and stretched—"AIDS is taking too long. I'd like to see the whole damned lot of fucking perverts drop into the ocean with the next big quake."

I walked behind the cop and pulled the collar of the blue-black uniform shirt away from his neck. "Pretty red there, Officer Lansing," I said.

Uneasy, the cop chuckled.

"Do you know Officer Templeton? Michael Templeton?" I asked.

"Hell yes. Works day shift. Hell of a guy. Nice family. Shit, he almost—"

"I know. He almost died. I was in CCU the night he coded."

Officer Lansing sobered appreciably, bowing his head. "They saved the guy's life."

"*Who* saved his life, Officer Lansing?"

"The docs." He hesitated. "And you nurses helped too. Dr. Ostermann said—"

I held up my hand to stop him, then motioned the man to come closer. Catching the drift of my mood, he defied the small command and did not move.

"Let me tell you a secret, officer. The main person responsible for saving Officer Templeton's life that night was a quick-thinking, fucking pervert flit nurse you would like to see drop off into the ocean with the next big quake."

At two A.M., I got a brief second wind. Unfortunately, so did a lot of people in the community. Gus never blew out of wind to begin with and was moving around at the speed of light, tending to motorcycle chopped meat and crushed bones, overdose madness, and colicky babies.

Melanie, the regular ER night shifter who came on at eleven, took on the arduous, all-night task of restocking the entire department, a job both Gus and I hated. I was assigned to share the patient load with Gus, plus man the paramedic and county radios.

Dr. Menowitz was being particularly "sensitive," or, to be straightforward, he was in an extremely foul mood, as only Dr.

Menowitz could manage. Gus and I tiptoed around him, especially after he went into his Sarah Bernhardt routine and slung an unsheathed syringe against the wall, where it stuck with a twang.

I attempted to humor him out of it by calling him "Robin Hood of the Redwoods," but received such a murderous glare, I didn't try again.

As Dr. Mahoney said, sometimes you just had to let the man be an asshole.

At 2:20, a woman who'd been in a barroom fight was delivered to us with a broken jaw and leg; 2:34 brought a seventeen-year-old who said she drank half a bottle of rat poison. On her heels came a woman who was the driver of the first of five cars to hit a man who, using his Bible as his shield, decided to take a leisurely stroll across the freeway.

"We can't reshoot the X ray until she takes the gun out of her pocket." The voice coming through the receiver was dull and zombielike.

"What gun?" I asked stupidly. It was three-thirty A.M.; I could be stupid if I wanted. I was surprised I wasn't hallucinating yet.

At the mention of a gun, Gus looked up from her pumpkin pie and coffee, alerted to possible fun and excitement. Her dark eyes sparkled in twisted expectation.

It was amazing how differently nights affected our attitudes. Take the alleged rat poison girl, for example. I'm ashamed to say I made a snap judgment of the young lady as a spoiled-rotten, miserable brat. To be perfectly honest, my appraisal didn't have anything to do with the fact that she drove her own Rolls-Royce and lived on Belvedere Island, a place where the lesser mansions went for two and a half mil. Furthermore, the fact that she was openly hostile about "Mummy and Dhaaaaaad" having gone off and left her in the hands of the governess and chauffeur while they went shopping in Monte Carlo didn't play into my personality call. It didn't even have anything to do with the fact that she wore a tire chain over her black leather jacket and had one of those hairdos that defied the laws of gravity. It really had more to do with the way she told me I could lick her shoes and die, when I offered to help her into a patient gown.

There's nothing like a defiant, depressed, spoiled teenage

girl acting out at three in the morning to make you want to drink rat poison too.

But not Gus. Gus was a saint, cooing and coddling in her own codependent version of a southern Mother Teresa. Using her arsenal of verbal syrup, it appeared she had succeeded in sweetening the battery acid that charged the girl's disposition. By the time Gus left the trauma room, the brat had actually agreed to drink a milk-shake-container of ice-cold, frothy, inky black charcoal.

For those who have never experienced medicinal charcoal, it is a concoction most certainly originated in the depths of pharmacy hell. Initially the fine powder comes to the nurse in an unmarked amber bottle. Unless black staining is desirable, nurses experienced in charcoal never open the bottle without donning gloves, mask, gown, head cover, and, if white shoes are involved, shoe covers.

So protected, Gus hummed while she poured out the powder, added glucose, water, and ice, placed the evil mixture in a blender, and whipped. Into the finished product she stuck a large-bore straw and proudly held up the glass.

"Sure would be pretty with a cherry on the top, don't you think?" she drawled.

Squinting, I couldn't decide if it looked more like a Halloween milk shake or liquid tomato blackrot, but nodded, and followed dumbly to witness the impertinent, adolescent witch actually drink the stuff.

And drink she did, but only after ten more minutes of Gus coaxing her heart out. Wrinkling her pretty upturned nose, the girl followed Gus's directions to take big sips only through the straw and avoid licking her lips so as not to get the black anywhere outside her mouth.

She sipped once, twice, three times—without swallowing.

Dr. Mahoney, roused by Dr. Menowitz to help with the flurry of new activity, stood at the end of the gurney, while Gus and I flanked the sides. We all stared, unconsciously holding our breath. The part Gus neglected to tell the precious teen was how disgusting the stuff was once it was actually in the mouth. All the drug books said it was supposed to be tasteless and textureless, but in fact, it was exactly what you'd imagine fireplace leftovers to taste like.

The girl's cheeks bulged, yet she still went on sipping.

"You'd better swallow," I warned. "Remember what happened to the guy in *The Five Chinese Brothers*."

"Come on now, doll," Gus cooed. "Gotta swallow so it absorbs all that nasty old rat poison. You don't want that black staining those pretty white teeth of—"

The girl leaned forward and sucked a huge amount of air in through her nose. Then she simultaneously gave us double-fisted fingers, aimed, and sprayed the ink over the three of us.

Dr. Mahoney and I saw it coming and jumped back a split second before she let loose. Gus never suspected a thing. Our shoes may have been ruined, but Gus looked like a blackfaced Al Jolson getting ready to croon "My Mammy."

In the end, it turned out the spoiled darling hadn't really ingested rat poison. It was all a ploy to punish "Mummy and Dhaaaaaad" for leaving her behind.

Gus, however, didn't let the incident dampen her spirits. She simply wiped off the worst of the charcoal and sat down to finish her pie and coffee.

I slumped like a deflated balloon and replaced the receiver. Somewhere out in the lobby, a man shouted, "Hip hip hooray," and there was a chorus of laughter. How could people be so up and ready in these hours? Was it all drug-related?

"What is it now, my little prairie doggette?" Gus asked, smacking her lips over her coffee, which had been sugared and creamed to a nice tan color.

"The lady that was in the barroom fight has a gun in her pocket and won't give it up. X ray won't do the films as long as it's on her."

Gus raised her dark eyebrows. "Well now, that's just downright rude. Where I come from, a lady leaves her gun at the door."

I grinned and rubbed a hand over my chin. "Wait a minute. I thought you were from Tennessee, the land of sweet thangs and peachy belles?"

"That's right, honey," Gus said, and headed dutybound, toward X ray. "But don't you go underestimating your southern sisters—if we can handle drinking mint juleps, we can carry a piece."

Gus brought back the firearm, expertly unloaded it, and wrapped it in a pillowcase.

"So, who is he?" she asked, sealing the wrapped weapon in a plastic bag marked "Admitting."

"Who?"

Gus clucked her tongue. "*The* man. The one who's got you glowing like a pink neon tube."

I blushed and smiled. "Oh, *that* man. His name is David and he's wonderful."

Gus let out a scream and flew across the room to administer a bear hug that knocked the wind out of me. "Alllll right, Ecker baby! It's about time, honey. I swear after that last jerk, I thought you'd thrown away the cake and shut off the oven."

Gus had a way of phrasing things. I never knew if they were part of a secret southern language, or if she made them up on the spot.

"So, come on, tell me all about him. What does he look like, what does he do, where does he live?"

"Well, he's great-looking—curly black hair, wonderful brown eyes, trim and muscular. He's a mortgage broker, and we pretty much live together either at the cottage or his apartment." I squeezed Gus's hand, building on my own enthusiasm. "I've never had such a solid and healthy relationship, Gus. We talk about everything, and we honestly like each other for who we really are, faults and all. . . . We've got a lot in common—we have a blast together. Basically, we fit like two gears. Even Simon likes him."

"Does David have any children of his own?"

"No."

Gus hesitated, and I could see a tiny cloud of doubt on the sunny horizon. "Oh. Well, has he ever been married?"

"Ah, well, actually no."

Gus poured herself another cup of coffee. The aura of thrill was dimming. The conversation was going in a direction already familiar to me.

"How old is this guy?"

"Twenty-seven." I scanned Gus's face, hoping for something other than the usual reaction, but no, one of her eyebrows shot to her hairline.

She shook her head. "Oh, honey." She said this in a tender, how-could-you-be-such-an-idiot? voice. "You *sure* you want to do that? I mean, taking up with a young pup like that is kinda like grabbing an alligator by the tail and trying to bite off his snout hairs one at a time."

I blinked uncertainly.

"What I mean is, Ec, you're asking for trouble, don't you think? I mean, where's the future in it?"

"It's a good relationship, Gus," I said quietly. "We truly care about each other. We're friends besides being lovers, you know?"

Gus heard the hurt and slipped an arm around me. "Oh, I'm just an ass. Forget what I said. I'm real happy for you. Honest."

There was an awkward silence. Finally I lifted my head and fixed her with one of my looks.

"Snout hairs?"

"Hey Reverb, grab some Demerol and come here." Dr. Mahoney's voice came from the direction of bed 3, the temporary refuge of the lady who'd run over the poor soul on the freeway.

I signed out the syringe and slipped behind the curtain. A woman of about forty was vomiting into an emesis basin held by Dr. Mahoney. She was one of those totally silent vomiters I admired so much.

"It was not your fault," Dr. Mahoney was saying, gently rubbing her patient's back. "The man was crazy. You just had the bad luck of being in the wrong place at the wrong time."

Susan looked over the woman's head. "Give her fifty milligrams IM. She's got a migraine."

Together, we laid the woman down and turned her onto her side. With my finger, I drew an invisible cross on the upper half of one exposed buttock, made a V in the superior lateral quadrant, wiped it with an alcohol swab, and gave the injection inside the point of the V.

"What the hell was that rigamarole?" Dr. Mahoney asked in puzzled wonder.

I looked at her, surprised and slightly hurt. "I map out my injection landmarks and give the injection in the outer quadrant, like I was taught in school."

"You still map them out, at *your* age?"

I shrugged and sniffed. "Well, it works for me. If you want to go jabbing away at any old place, I suppose that's your prerogative. I happen to think this way is—"

Without any warning at all, the patient on the gurney rolled over and vomited on the floor. The green bile mixed with the black charcoal on the toes of our shoes.

Looking very Abraham Lincoln–ish, Dr. Bell nodded a silent greeting to the four of us and poured himself a cup of coffee. It was common practice for the specialty guys to stop by ER on their way out of the hospital, checking to see if they were needed.

Not only were Dr. Bell's services not needed, but we were all idle, due to a welcome momentary lull in the onrush of wounded or demented masses.

In the soft light of the desk (we'd turned down the headache-producing fluorescents), I noticed we were all dressed in shapeless scrub tops and pants. It looked a whole lot like an adult slumber party sans pillows, blankets, and teddy bears.

Dr. Mahoney waved from her mat on the floor without pausing in her sit-ups. "Fifty-six. You're here either very early or very late. What's happening, Al? Fifty-seven."

The surgeon took a minute, thinking carefully about his reply. He was a man of few words. "I got that kid who walked onto the highway with God."

Melanie, who was sitting on Dr. Mahoney's feet, raised her eyebrows in silent question.

"Oh," said Gus, sipping her fourth cup of coffee, "some poor guy thought that if he carried his Bible, he could walk out onto the freeway and Jesus would protect him from being hit."

"Sixty-two. Five cars got him," panted Dr. Mahoney. "The first lady who hit him said he looked like a bouncing rag doll being gored by the cars' hood ornaments. Sixty-three."

"Yuck," I chimed in. Against my wishes, the image was instantly filed for future use in my nightmares.

"Damn near ruptured every organ in his body," added Dr. Bell thoughtfully. "When I opened him up, his insides resembled a fruit salad."

I wished to God I could drink coffee. People who drink coffee can do just about anything they want, any time they want.

Personally, I was near my breaking point. I could barely walk, let alone reason, and yet Dr. Mahoney and Melanie were locked into the minor surgery room, halfway through Jane Fonda's advanced workout tape while discussing Dr. Menowitz's personality in high-tech psychobabble. Dr. Menowitz and Gus were in the pelvic room with a possible ectopic pregnancy, who I'll bet drank coffee too.

Since my legs had buckled out from under me twice, I was allowed to stay at the desk to answer phones and listen for the radio. As soon as I sat down, my head fell onto the clerk's desk, came to rest on an eraser, and I was out for the count.

As for what happened next, I have to rely on Dr. Menowitz's eyewitness account. Apparently the triage buzzer went off twice. In my fog I must have mistaken the buzzer for the paramedic radio signal, because I dutifully stood (leaving, I might add, a large drool spot on the desk blotter), but instead of going for the radio console, I went to the sink, turned on the faucet, leaned close to the spigot, and gave my call letters. The cold water woke me up enough to realize where the noise was coming from and what was required of me.

The buzzer sounded a second time and I wheeled about, moving in the general direction of the lobby. Dr. Menowitz said I tripped over the clerk's chair, bounced off the wall and a corner of bed 6, then off the front of the clerk's desk and toward the black runner. Dr. Menowitz gave me a gentle push to keep the momentum going, and I sailed into the lobby to see what was the matter.

The black almond-shaped eyes stared at me, pleading for help. The woman's typically wide Chinese face, with its high cheekbones, was neither pretty nor plain. It was simply Chinese.

She stood tensely, wearing a shapeless, pilled sweater and baggy faded jeans. Gesturing with her hands and arms, she spoke again in the thin, breathless voice that seemed common among Oriental women.

"You nurse?" she asked, her dark eyes wild and haunted. "Come wi' me now. Mother very sick. Come now to car. Too old. No walk. Come, please."

She took me by the arm, leading me toward the entrance doors. Fully awake, I pulled out of her grasp and grabbed one of the orange wheelchairs parked against the wall. "Okay, kid," I said, smiling. "You lead the way. I'll be right behind you with the rescue chariot."

The woman stopped, looked at me with a puzzled, disapproving expression. "No understand. You come wi' me to sick mother." Her hands were shaking, and I saw they were red and chafed.

I dropped the smile instantly. This was a serious situation; flippancy was grossly rude. Gesturing that she should walk in front of the wheelchair, I spoke with much gravity. "I come with you now," I said, mimicking the choppy Chinese cadence. "Please. Go to the old mother."

With an almost inaudible "Ah, aiiee," she ran in front of me, frequently turning to make sure I was keeping up.

Outside in the fresh air, I looked up into the clear night sky. The woman in the moon winked at me, probably laughing at the very idea of having a cleanup crew for her mischief. I'd probably laugh too, watching mortals run around like wild hens, trying to save people from themselves and each other.

In the middle of the parking lot, parked between a BMW and a Winnebago, sat a black 1978 Pontiac without benefit of bumpers or rear window. The four brand-new whitewalls didn't quite match the rest of the car.

The woman began chattering in Chinese, pointing into the backseat. Peering through the window, I saw only a small bundle of dark and tattered blankets. I set the brake on the wheelchair and opened the door.

The smell of urine and decaying flesh hit me like a brick. Automatically, I put my hand to my mouth and stumbled back, gagging. There was something ominously familiar about the poisonous stench. Only twice before in my life had I smelled something like it; one was Wheelin' Wilma, the other the dead-fish-and-gull collection wagon on Bradenton Beach during red tide.

The woman, still chattering in Chinese, caught my actions and switched to English. "So sorry. Mother very ill. Bad fever. Too sick for bathing. You give medicine now? She well soon. Smell go away."

Relying on intestinal fortitude, I took a long breath of fresh air and tugged on a frayed end of one of the blankets. The whole pile slid easily toward the door. My unnatural curiosity made me flip back the top blanket.

Two feverish black eyes stared at me from a very old Chinese face. Framed by sparse strands of stiff gray hair, the puffy yellow skin of her forehead and cheeks was mottled with raised patches of an ugly rash I guessed to be filth-related.

The crone's dry, arthritic hand snaked out of the blankets and found my wrist. As she pulled herself close to me, her face twisted into a hideous, grinning mask. In the eerie light of the moon, I saw a cavernous mouth filled with blackened stumps that had once been teeth. In some places the stumps looked like they had been broken or filed into points, as if to facilitate the chewing of meat and other tough foods. The tongue, by trick of shadow or light, appeared to be a swollen, black tube. Her laughter rose in pitch and volume until it resembled a

peacock's scream. The piercing sound seared through the stillness of the night, hit the back wall of the building, and rever-
berated all around us.

I tried to pull back, but the insane grin and impenetrable
eyes held me motionless, teetering between rational thought
and terror. Seeing my fear, the daughter spoke to the old
woman sharply. The woman abruptly ceased laughing and let
go of my arm.

I snapped out of my paralysis and cleared my mind enough
to think about the best way to transfer the woman from the car
to the wheelchair. Before I had a chance to act, the daughter
hoisted her mother up, blankets and all, and swung her into the
chair.

The daughter smiled for the first time, explaining, "Old
mother very small. Weigh like baby."

By the time I wheeled my odiferous patient into the space of
bed 5, my olfactory glands had been insulted to the point of
shutting down. The hellacious smell now seemed to be only a
faint unpleasant odor, like a slab of blue cheese sitting out in
a hot, unventilated kitchen.

To save time and trouble, I picked up the bundle of rags and
lifted her effortlessly onto the gurney. The daughter had spoken
the truth; the woman could not have weighed more than seventy pounds, nor stood above four and a half feet tall.

The old woman rested her head against my face, thus
forcing me to notice the large areas of bare scalp covered with
ringworm. Perhaps it wasn't quite as disagreeable as Wheelin'
Wilma's lice-and-cockroach-infested hair, but when things got
this bad in the realm of personal hygiene, one didn't want to
spend much time making definitive distinctions between bad or
worse.

Several of the ratty blankets had fallen away, and in the
place where her feet should have been were two tiny, misshapen, brocade-covered stumps.

In my Chinese-fascination phase of life, which came on
shortly after moving to San Francisco, I had learned about the
long-outlawed practice of binding the feet of girl children.
Among upper-class Chinese families, "lily feet" were not only
a measure of a woman's attractiveness, but were also considered a sign of superiority and breeding. Since binding rendered
the feet useless, these women would never have to work. They
were meant only to be waited on and served, lifted and carried
from place of rest to place of rest.

I pointed at the stumps. "Lily feet?"

The old woman cackled, nodding her head violently. A piece of dried food flew from what was left of her hair.

While I donned a gown and changed my gloves, I explained to the daughter that I needed to undress her mother and get her into a patient gown.

"Old mother will not allow," the daughter said, obviously frightened. "She never take off clothes. Same clothes she wear to honor dead father. It has been many years past. If she take off clothes, old father spirit punish her. He go inside the heart and make more sickness."

"Wait a minute." I bit the inside of my lip. "Are you telling me that your mother hasn't been out of these clothes since your father died?"

She nodded.

"How long ago did your father die?"

The woman counted on her fingers, figuring out loud in Chinese. "Two year, four month, twelve day."

I didn't believe anyone could wear the same clothes for more than a week, let alone two years, although Simon had tried it on occasion. Intrigued as to what would be under the garments, I touched the waistband of the old woman's pants, praying I would not have to look far to find an opening. Having sensed my intention, she plucked my hand away and bit it, scolding me in a sharp screech. The bite wasn't hard enough to break the skin, but it was hard enough to hurt. I don't know why I was shocked. After all, these clothes were worn in honor of her dead husband. Who was I, this brazen American amazon, to tamper with her sacred memorial outfit?

"Explain this must be done," I told her daughter firmly, rubbing my hand. "The doctor cannot tend to her unless she is undressed. She must cooperate or the clothes may be ruined."

Obediently, the daughter translated what I'd said. She sounded much like someone rapidly reading a page of abbreviations. There was a cross fire of angry shrieks between the two women, which stopped abruptly when the old woman slapped her daughter's face. The younger woman did not so much as flinch or give any indication she had been struck.

The old woman shot me an accusing look, but in her eyes I read resignation. She gave a stiff, proud nod and was silent.

I was already feeling uncomfortable with the situation. Now I felt guilty.

Without looking into her face, I untied and removed her

thin, frayed belt and handed it to her daughter. The old woman began to whimper in singsong, "I-yieeee. Ahhhh. I-yieeee." Determined not to let her laments affect me, I went for the safety pins holding the front of her shredded silk overblouse. The fabric was stained to stiffness with grease, dried mucus, and old food. As I fumbled with the catches, the tension rose appreciably.

"I go now," the daughter said, opening the curtain. "No watch. Come back later."

"Wait. You've got to translate. You can't leave your . . ."

I watched the woman fly down the runner and out the doors.

Okay. Perhaps there was some old Chinese law that made it illegal for a daughter to see her mother humiliated by insensitive amazons.

Looking back at the mother, I shrugged apologetically. In silent retaliation, the woman stuck a bent and gnarled finger into her nose.

"How lovely for you," I said, gritting my teeth. My stomach went into a slipknot.

The old mother replied in Chinese with an evil gleam in her eye and left her finger where it was, thank Buddha.

Formalities out of the way, I completed the removal of the overblouse, careful not to fold it for fear it would crack. The black cotton jersey was next. As I pulled it over the woman's head, the sleeves stuck at the upper arms. That was when I noticed the sticky ooze that covered the jersey from elbows to shoulders.

I touched the areas, and had the strangest sensation of sticking my fingers into hot, lumpy mud. The woman howled violently in protest and, I realized now, pain.

"Oh now, you sound like I'm skinning you alive," I said, and gave the shirt a firm tug. It gave way. "It couldn't hurt that mu—" I recoiled against the side cabinet in revulsion, biting my lip for a reality check as I did so.

Hundreds of rubber bands, pieces of string, and old bits of wire were wrapped tightly around the woman's arms from her shoulders to below her elbows. In several open places, the thick purulence undulated, alive with maggots.

The old woman was delighted with my reaction. Grinning, she pointed proudly to her rotting flesh and shrieked something in Chinese. She rocked back and forth in a frenzy, her cackling laughter grating on my nerves like a Whitney Houston record played at high speed. In those crazy eyes, I saw the subtle void that is the calling card of senility.

I was shaking by the time I summoned up the guts to unfasten the six or seven rusty safety pins guarding the opening of her pants. Fearful of what was under the garment, I gently pulled the grossly soiled silk material over her hips. The sharp ammonia smell of old urine burned the insides of my nose, so that I had to fight not to rush.

The pants stuck at midthigh, where two bands of sticky pus had soaked through the material. Above that, her belly and groin were caked with dried stool and dirt.

I found a bottle of irrigation saline in the bottom drawer of the side cabinet and poured most of the bottle over her legs in hopes of loosening the material.

Her whimpering changed to shrill shouts. Striking out in rhythm with her rocking, she clawed at me, managing to lay open the skin of my right arm above my glove. (For two weeks afterward, the deep scratch would stay infected despite a round of antibiotics.)

When the crust had softened enough to relinquish the fabric, I gritted my teeth and pulled her pants all the way off. Both legs had been bound, ankle to midthigh. Thinned out by the saline, pus ran freely from between the pieces of string and whatnot. The maggots, thicker here than on her arms, were falling in clusters onto the clean white sheet that covered the gurney. I swept them into a plastic debris bag and pulled my surgical scissors from its sheath. Beginning with her arms, I cut away as much of the old string and rubber bands as I could.

By the time I began on her legs, I was perspiring. When the outermost layer of debris was cleared away, I put up the side rails and, using a childlike form of sign language, indicated to the woman I wanted her to rest. She grinned that crazy grin, made the okay sign, then laid her head back and closed her eyes tightly.

I covered her with a clean sheet, mostly to hide the hideous sight from view. Grabbing the end of the sheet, she pulled it over her head. From under the linen came loud and exaggerated snoring sounds mixed with small fits of cackling.

I found Dr. Mahoney and Gus at the back table, debating how strong to make the coffee for day shift. Susan wanted it to be triple jolt; Gus thought single strength would be sufficient. Both of them were vibrating.

"You aren't going to believe this one," I announced, and sat down. Looking at my watch for the first time since I'd gone to the lobby, I was surprised to see it was six A.M. "I'm not so sure I believe it myself. If I wasn't so tired, I'd probably be in a corner somewhere begging for someone to wake me up."

"Let me guess," said Dr. Mahoney. "There's a woman over there who gave birth to a litter of field mice and she wants to know if it's safe to breast-feed."

Gus wrinkled her nose. "From the smell, I'd say it was our San Rafael lady who wears those black rubber boots for months at a time without taking them off."

I regarded them both, noting they had dark circles under their eyes despite the coffee. "Not bad, but no cigar. You know about the old custom of binding feet in China?"

They both nodded.

"Well, there's a senile Chinese lady over there who has tried to bind herself out of existence."

The two of them looked at each other, then back at me.

"She's got ten, twenty layers of rubber bands and string tied around her upper arms and legs that have been on there for months, maybe years. She's supporting hundreds of feasting maggots." I sighed. "There's so many of them, I think they're the only thing giving her clothes shape."

Neither of them moved, their expressions doubtful.

"Go look for yourselves if you don't believe me."

Dr. Mahoney wearily got up from her chair and addressed Gus. "Embellishment comes so easily to writers. Did you read how she portrayed me in her book?" Susan headed toward the curtain of bed 5. "She took a perfectly sweet, gorgeous, serious woman and made me look like a sarcastic, ball-busting neurotic. I don't know where she gets that stuff."

She disappeared behind the curtain and within a second had changed into her professional voice. "Hello, I'm Dr. Mahoney. I hear you're not feeling so well. Boy oh boy, something doesn't smell so nice, does it? Ah, now why don't you let me take a look here at . . . Now, now, no hitting or biting. I need to see where the hurt is. I'm going to take a peek under this corner and we'll . . ."

I counted to two.

"Holy Jesus, Mary, and Joseph!" Susan's head popped out from the curtain. "Order a CBC, SMAC, sed rate, and chest X ray for starters. We need some vital signs, and whoever brought this woman in, Reverb, get them in here stat."

* * *

The daughter sat in the farthest corner of the waiting room staring at her hands. When I touched her shoulder, she jumped.

"Doctor wants to talk with you now. You come with me." Expecting the woman to follow, I headed back into the department. When I got to bed 5, however, she was nowhere to be seen.

I went back into the lobby and saw that she had not moved.

"Why don't you come and talk to doctor?"

When she looked at me, I saw that she had been crying.

"Old mother die. She sick long time. I do nothing. Her mind sick. I do nothing to help."

The entrance doors opened, allowing a blast of cold air and Dr. Cramer to enter. I hugged myself against the chill, studying the errant daughter. From the lines in the woman's face, I could see that her life had been neither happy nor easy.

I took her hand in mine. "Look, the doctor has to ask many questions, and she can't do that without you. In this way you can help the old mother now." Mentally I rolled my eyes at myself. I sounded like David Carradine in *Kung Fu.*

She hung her head farther down than I would have thought possible for her neck, then rose from her chair. Sadly, she motioned for me to lead her to her shame.

Monday
10:30 A.M.

Only a few lines. When I drop the pen for a third time, I'll stop. I must remember to fall asleep on my side so there will be no chance of aspiration during the deep unconsciousness that will soon follow.

I worked overtime on zombie shift—a first and, I hope, a last for me. By the time we got Mrs. Lin onto the slide board and to the fifth-floor tubs, it was eight-thirty, although I wouldn't have missed sliding her into the whirlpool for anything. There was something absolutely satisfying about watching the maggots and other debris wash out of her flesh. From there we took her straight to surgical reception, where Dr. Bell was ready for her. If I thought I could have stood without assistance, I would have liked to watch the debridement, but by that time, I was slurring and bouncing around like nobody's business.

Dr. Menowitz walked me to my car and apologized for his

weirdness last night. It's the same old thing, except his rut is getting deeper and his burnout is scorching the edges of his sanity. I think Dr. Neidler's suicide affected him more than he'll admit. They were the same age.

I asked if he would show me some of his latest writing, but he's a stubborn cuss and maintains nothing is ready yet. Checked on Risen before I left. The ICU nurse said Dr. Schupbach thought he'd be fine, although there is some real concern over his HIV status. They drew blood for the test without his knowledge. I believe this is illegal, but I'll admit I have a vested interest in knowing. The idea that his lover has been screwing around indiscriminately makes me go into panic supreme. Sandy Bastard is right.

Risen has played all the nurse's roles: indispensable healer, martyr, saint, superman. But, like most of us, he has neglected to take care of himself, continuing to play rescuer in his personal life, eventually—inevitably—to fall as victim.

Tuesday afternoon I face Miss Milks. Oh joy. My one day off and I get to spend it with the chimney.

When I arrived at the cottage, David had laid out a small meal for me and warmed the house. When he left for work, he kissed me and asked, "Have I told you yet today that I love you?"

I am already used to the neighbors' wounding comments and questions. As an example, the one next door who had her cap set for David had the green-eyed gall to ask how long I planned on baby-sitting. Jim and Liza have both stopped calling. Whenever I talk to Bill, Moira, or Shelly, they don't mention my relationship, and if I bring the subject up, they become deaf mutes.

I can't figure out if my friends are simply having a hard time adjusting to seeing me for once in a healthy relationship with a good person, or if they're all worried that David is going to desert me and they'll have to rush in and pick up the pieces.

As far as I can tell, I don't have one friend who takes my relationship with David seriously. Even Janey sighed and said she had no idea how badly I wanted another child.

How backward this culture is! It is perfectly natural to see a woman of thirty with a man of fifty or older. People don't even notice. But put a younger man with an older woman, and that's something perverse—unnatural.

*The therapists say the older women/younger men combi-
nation frequently works well. I wish*

*Oops. Excuse the drool. Must have gone right out. Don't
remember what I was going to wish for, but I have only two
more hours to sleep before I have to go back to the Stephen
King cavalcade of horrors.*

TWELVE

"The life we have chosen as nurses . . . is not for the fainthearted. It demands uncommon fortitude."

GERALDINE FELTON, R.N.

NORMALLY I AVOID THE MOVABLE BOX like the plague, which leads people to believe I enjoy the exercise of stair climbing. The simple fact of the matter is, I am claustrophobic and acrophobic. That is why, once I am actually trapped in an elevator, I will talk to anyone about anything to keep my mind off the fact that I am far above the ground in a small, closed box, hanging by a couple of relatively thin cables, and I cannot get out until the mechanical doors say I can.

Because there were only ten minutes before I needed to report for zombie shift number two, I succumbed to taking the elevator to ICU to see Risen. In the iron maiden with me were Gus, Dr. Macmillan, the P.M. nursing supervisor, a med–surg nurse, and a Filipino respiratory tech steering a piece of equipment unfamiliar to me.

My nerves were straining at their sheaths. I was *sure* the elevator motor was chugging and groaning more than it should. Even though this same elevator had been running for thirty-two years without incident, I was positive that on this particular night, on this particular ride, the elevator would snap its cables and plunge us all to our bloody and horrible deaths.

Before we made it to the second floor, my palms were wet and I could feel the acro/claustro phobias in me rising for a good old-fashioned hysterical scream. Wildly, I looked for something to distract my thoughts and fixated on the respiratory tech's strange machine.

"Excuse me," I said, wiping the sweat off my upper lip with a trembling hand.

The man smiled.

"What is this machine? I've never seen it before."

"What?" The man's eyes grew round with surprise. "You no see a fuk machine before, lady?"

A sudden heavy silence came over the elevator. Everyone stiffened and stared down at their shoes or at the invisible flies on the floor. Under her breath, Gus twittered. Dr. Macmillan and the supervisor blushed vividly.

I thought maybe the man was mispronouncing the brand name of the machine and looked for the word "Fuchs." It said "General Electric."

Okay, so there had to be some mistake. I'd give the man a chance to correct himself.

"I don't think I heard you correctly." I cupped my ear and leaned toward him. "It's a . . . *what* machine?"

He tapped the top of the clear hood. "Fuk. A fukking machine, you know?"

The nursing supervisor, Dr. Macmillan, and the ICU nurse all moved simultaneously to push the third-floor indicator button. None of them was going to the third floor, but it was clear they desperately wanted to be anywhere but in the elevator.

As soon as the doors opened, everyone evacuated the elevator except Gus and me and the respiratory tech.

The doors closed and we started upward.

"So, how does the fukking machine work?" Gus asked with a smile.

"Oh, very easy," said the respiratory tech, totally oblivious to the fact that he had just forced three people to go places they didn't want to go. "Put in water, plug in wall—make big fuk."

"Big fuk?" repeated Gus. Her voice and eyebrows went up on the word "big." "I see. Well, I sure could use one of those at my house," she said, smiling innocently. "You wouldn't happen to know what gender it is, would you?"

The man smiled uncertainly. "No generator. This electric fuk machine."

Gus took in a deep breath. It squeezed out of her as a soft, wheezy snort.

I thought sober thoughts: Risen. HIV. Maggots.

Mercifully, the door opened onto ICU. The man waved cheerily, wheeled the machine of dubious function out of the elevator ahead of us, and disappeared into the room across from Risen's.

I glanced at Gus out of the corner of my eye. "If you start, I swear I'll—"

Gus let loose with one of her Cousin Ralph laughs.

Running as fast as I could, I got into Risen's room and closed the door behind me before I could so much as guffaw.

There were already ten or so get-well cards taped to Risen's wall. Someone had broken rules and allowed several vases of flowers to be brought in and placed around his bed.

"Risen?"

There was no response except the sound of his respirations under the green nonrebreather mask.

"It's Ec. Are you okay?"

I waited, knowing for certain there wasn't going to be a response. Behind me, the monitor bleeped out an even, reasonable rhythm; "Take Me Out to the Ball Game" fit well.

"I want you to get better, Risen. I want you to take care of yourself. We're going to get our knickers all in a twist if you don't come out of this as soon as you can." I rubbed his feet with lotion, doing range of motion so he wouldn't get foot drop. Risen had one set of long, narrow, utterly strange-looking feet.

"We've already seen you rise once from the dead. We're waiting for the second coming."

Through the front window, I saw the Filipino tech busily moving about the patient's room next door. He had placed the machine directly next to the bed. The hood was extended over the patient's face. From a graduate, he poured the water into the machine and, true to his word, plugged it in.

"I've got to go to ER for zombie shift now, but I'll come up to see you tomorrow and give you all the gossip I can find."

Risen's feet twitched.

"Have a good sleep, but don't overdo it, okay?"

Next door, the machine began to fuk.

I found a somewhat downcast Gus leaning against the counter at the central station, drinking coffee and talking with a group of ICU nurses. As soon as she saw me, she checked her watch. We had two minutes before we were expected to walk the black runner.

Silently, I directed Gus's attention to the room where the

machine was hard at work billowing out steam over the patient's nose and mouth. As the light broke, she started to laugh.

I made a mental note that when Risen awoke, I must be sure to tell him about the infamous fog machine.

"Abandon all hope, ye who enter here," Sarah said, sweeping past us into the utility room. The sounds of turmoil coming from the main room told us she wasn't kidding. We stepped around the corner to scan out the action before actually entering the gates of chaos.

Two children in the minor surgery room were screaming bloody murder; one was having his leg stitched by Dr. Menowitz, the other was being prepared for stitching by Dr. Kin and Melanie. In the main room, Don ran from gurney to gurney administering treatments and comfort.

I peeked through the two-way mirror of the orifice room and was surprised to see four of Rescue 56's crew. Dr. Papaneau, a staff psychiatrist, was speaking to them from his seat on the Pap smear worktable. His tie hung loosely from his shirt, and he had bags under his eyes. Overall, the group looked as though they'd witnessed a massacre.

Without a word to each other, Gus and I stowed our purses away, did the change-of-shift narcotic count, and sought out Sarah.

"Believe it or not, Don and I are left over from days." Sarah leaned wearily against the clerk's desk. "Katy called in sick at the last minute, and staffing said they couldn't find anybody to replace her, which I knew was major bullshit, so I called Melanie myself."

Gus sucked in a breath and made "Uh oh" eyes.

"Oh, screw them," Sarah said, and brushed back the hair from her face. "I look at it from the point of view that I'm saving them the cost of a lawsuit. . . . So, Melanie has been here since five, and Don has offered to stay past eleven if needed. Menowitz and Mahoney called in Dr. Kin to help cover until things settle down, which I don't—"

Ileta interrupted by holding the phone out to Sarah. "Phone call, honey," she said in a soft, apologetic voice. "It's your kids again wanting to know when you're coming home."

Sarah talked to her children, while Gus and I politely eavesdropped on the maternal apologies and excuses that were familiar to us both. Nurses' children do not have an easy time.

They share their parent on holidays and weekends, and rarely see them when they aren't bone tired.

"Drs. Mahoney and Bell are in the trauma room with the surgical team," Sarah continued, before the phone was even back on the receiver. "I think they're pretty close to moving the patient upstairs. The second they're out of there, Echo, I want you to clean and restock the room. Gus, you need to stay out here to help Melanie and Don process the people for Menowitz and Kin. The orifice room is out of bounds until Dr. Papaneau finishes debriefing Rescue fifty-six. When he's done with them, Don, Dr. Mahoney, and I are going in for our debriefing."

"Jeez, what war happened that you all need a debriefing with a shrink?" asked Gus.

Sarah turned to leave, her face assuming a deep color, as though she were either having a hypertensive crisis or fighting back tears. "To be honest, Gus, I really don't feel like talking about it right now. Just go do what I've asked you to do, okay?"

Gus winced, removed a new-patient chart from the foot-high pile, and wandered toward the waiting room. I wondered how long it would take her to realize there wasn't any place to put the patient.

"A debriefing in ER?" I heard her say as she disappeared down the black runner. "Like, wow."

Wow was right. To have a debriefing in a unit such as ER was a remarkable event. It was a service usually provided to the staff of a floor or unit that had experienced a strain sufficient to break down the staff's morale.

I had been a part of one debriefing which involved a CCU nurse who, over the course of several weeks, began showing signs of a mental/emotional breakdown. We all encouraged her to seek help, but she refused to hear us out. Since her nursing care was without fault, our hands were tied, even though we were all witness to the bizarre behavior she sometimes exhibited among her peers in the sanctuary of the nurses' lounge.

Nealy and I had worked with her the evening she went home, killed her three-year-old daughter, and then attempted to kill herself. "In a profession such as yours," we were told by the debriefing psychiatrist two days later, "you handle an inordinate amount of stress, and no matter how many defenses you build, or how many coping mechanisms you use, some days it gets to be too much."

I pushed open the trauma room door and drew back at the sight before me.

Some days, I thought, *it gets to be too much.*

Big man though the patient was, it was hard to believe that so much blood had come from one person. There were places on the floor where puddles of it had formed. A bright red quilt of various sole patterns covered the area, broken only by a random, long smear where someone had slipped.

Walking through the sticky, congealing mess, I headed for the equipment carts, the soles of my shoes making a noise like *kruuupt, kruuupt, kruuupt.* Between the respiratory tech and a surgical nurse, I got a glimpse of the patient, intubated and unconscious, lying naked on the gurney. A unit of blood was being pumped through one of his four IV lines at a fast rate, while volume expanders and a bag of antibiotics ran in the other three.

The focus of attention lay below his waist. I deliberated for a moment, then stood on my toes to get a better view.

The severed section of the man—his inner thighs, penis, testicles, and lower abdomen—was mottled purple. In an almost perfect upside-down U, the cut began just above the pubic bone and ended halfway down each of his thighs. It was exactly as if someone had used a large U-shaped cookie cutter to carve out his groin.

Dr. Bell concentrated on the wound while the plastic surgeon listed for one of the OR nurses the various instrument packs he wanted available in the operating room. Dr. Mahoney was scrubbing at the sink, talking to the supervisor in a low tone.

Dr. Bell covered the wound with several sterile towels. "Okay, everybody," he said, slowly removing his sterile gloves, "let's get him up to surgery."

Like a well-practiced caravan, the surgical team and respiratory tech packed up the gurney with monitor and IVs and was rolling out before the rest of us could say ouch.

As soon as the gurney was out of sight, Dr. Mahoney yelled for Ileta to call housekeeping stat. "Tell them to use a strong cleanser on this floor," she said, wrinkling her nose in disgust. "I want that smell out of here."

With the visual onslaught, I had failed to notice the smell of blood that hung heavily on the air. Breathing through my mouth, I began clearing away the debris of empty supply and equipment boxes, half-full IV bags, towels and gauze—everything soaked with blood.

By the time I finished, I was struggling to rid myself of an escalating depression. With eleven and a half hours left to work, I would need to come up with some inspiration other than coffee in order to get through.

Aching for the safe haven of David's arms, I closed my eyes, searching for some peaceful thought. What came to me was not the thought but rather the sound of peace. The fan in the air control vent squeaked faintly in a regularly irregular pattern, perfectly duplicating the sound of crickets. Instantly I was twelve years old, drifting down the Mohawk River on a hot summer's night, feeling warm and fiercely happy to be alive. . . .

"Wipe the smile off your face, Reverb." Dr. Mahoney stood in the doorway that connected the trauma room with the X-ray department. "It seems somewhat incongruous, considering that you're picking up after some major carnage here."

The summer night faded as Susan sat on the exam stool and rolled into the corner behind the crash cart, far out of the view of the door's porthole window. She crossed her arms and leaned her head against the wall.

"What was this all about?" I asked, making a broad sweep of the room.

"Just some poor guy jogging up the wrong street at the wrong time." She paused and removed her glasses with a careful, restrained gesture. "A garbage truck lost its brakes and impaled him against a concrete wall."

"Is this what the debriefings are all about?"

"Only a small part of it." Dr. Mahoney gave way to a shudder. "There was another truck accident earlier that really unnerved the rescue guys."

My mind could not even imagine what would get to the paramedics. They were often firsthand witnesses of the most gruesome of trauma scenes.

"They had a man-down call from a construction site where a crew of Mexican laborers was pouring a cement foundation. When the paramedics got there, the least hysterical of the crew led them to the cement mixer truck and—"

"Stop," I said decisively. "I don't want to hear the rest of this."

"Is this the writer speaking?" Susan said, annoyed. "Aren't

you the official recorder of human folly and all this god-damned man's-inhumanity-to-man-and-himself stuff?"

She's exhausted, I thought, at the end of her rope. Like those who go through a war, she needs to talk about the atrocities.

Dr. Mahoney settled back against the wall again and list-lessly ran a hand through her hair. Her temper had risen and receded swiftly. "The foreman's kid—I think they said he was seventeen—was doing something to the truck while they were off at the other end of the site, and got his shirt caught in the mechanism. The machine pulled him in a little at a time.

"When our guys got there, they managed to extract his legs right away, but finding the rest of him wasn't so pleasant. When Russ found the kid's skull, he got sick and had to be relieved by one of the other paramedics."

The housekeeper came in the door rolling a suds-filled bucket before her. The portly woman stared at the floor and groaned; it was a combo sound of "Ugh" and "Yuck."

Dr. Mahoney dropped her voice. "We ordered sedation for the father and released him to crisis."

I shook away the vision of the boy's death agony and the worse agony of his father. I could not—would not—accept the images my mind was conjuring up.

Dr. Mahoney rose wearily and stretched. For a minute we watched the housekeeper at her task. The water in her bucket had gone from gray to dull red with only the first few turns of the mop.

"The debriefing for you and Sarah and Don is a separate matter, then?"

Dr. Mahoney's face sagged and I was instantly sorry I'd asked.

"Separate *matters*," she said, emphasis on the plural. "Earlier we had a forty-two-year-old woman with an abdominal aneurysm, and an eight-year-old boy who had been hit by a car and partially decapitated. Both of them came in at the same time, code three. Both of them died. The boy's parents were absolutely . . ." She paused. "I guess I don't need to tell you about that, do I?" Susan abruptly searched the room with her eyes, apparently found what she was looking for, and relaxed.

"It was *such* an ugly day," she said in despair, "I'm losing my sense of humor. I don't think I can keep doing this year after year."

I reached out and clumsily hugged the physician. Dr.

Mahoney was not one who gave or accepted physical affection easily, but she squeezed my arm in acknowledgment of my sympathy.

"The husband of the aneurysm woman went nuts, forced his way into the room during the code. Dr. Bell was almost knocked over. For a minute there, I thought I was back in the trauma center in Oakland.

"No more than twenty minutes after those two were given slab tickets, I saw a thirty-nine-year-old librarian who drove himself here, registered, sat in the waiting room for an hour, and then told us this freak story about aspirating a gold crown at the dentist's office this morning.

"Ignoring the advice of his appropriately panicked dentist to come directly here, he went back to work, where, of course, he had more and more trouble breathing.

"As it turns out, he's the nicest, cutest guy you'd ever want to know. Here he is with a stupid gold crown sitting in his right main bronchus and he's trying to cheer everybody else up. He even got Morose Menowitz to make civilized conversation with him."

Dr. Mahoney cast a side glance my way and shook her head. "He was so charming, the thought crossed my mind that I might ask him to dinner or something."

I raised my eyebrows and asked where he was.

"We brought him up to surgery. He coded and died before they even had him on the table.

"He was only thirty-nine years old," she repeated, facing me. A sort of pleading had slipped around the tones of despair. "He woke up this morning, put on his clothes, and had his coffee just like every other day, and six hours later he's dead."

The physician put her hands over her head and laced her fingers together. "Reverb, why didn't I set up practice in a nice, quiet town in the Midwest and tend to colicky babies and old ladies with arthritis?"

"One reason," I said gently, "is because you chose a long time ago to work in the realm of chaos. Since then you've earned your gold membership card in the Sisterhood of Fools Club—you're a drama junkie.

"Another reason is because at the end of an eight-hour day of seeing sore throats and giving fussy babies vaccinations, you'd be bored silly, wondering why the hell you didn't take work in a big city hospital ER."

Sarah tapped on the port window and crooked her finger at

me and Susan. "Dr. Papaneau is ready for us, Susan. Echo, we need you out here to cover while the three of us are gone."

"Oh God," Dr. Mahoney sighed. "It's shrink time for the Death Day survivors."

"I don't care how much they complain and object." Dr. Menowitz addressed me and Gus while he wrote discharge instructions on two charts. "From now on, when I'm here, I don't want any visitors coming back here with the patients unless they're blind deaf-mutes or need someone to translate for them."

"That's going to be tough, Morton," Gus said in a sulky voice.

"I don't care, Augustine. I wasted an hour of my time last night with that woman with the ectopic pregnancy. Would you like to know why?" Dr. Menowitz leaned close to our faces with a forced, full-toothed smile/glare.

Gus and I shook our heads, but we knew he was going to tell us anyway.

"All because her damned sister was in the room. She almost had me convinced her belly pain was due to the pork she ate for dinner. It's a good thing I know an ectopic pregnancy when I see one, because if I'd sent her home with a bottle of Mylanta, she'd be in serious trouble or dead—and so would my career."

He handed the broken ankle's chart to me and the lacerated chin's to Gus. "People can't be a hundred percent honest with us when their family or friends are hanging around, ladies. This woman, for whatever reason, didn't want her sister to know she'd been having sexual relations. As soon as I sent the sister out, she told me the truth."

"So this means when your wife comes in, we can kick you out?" Gus asked. Her face was serious, but her eyes were sparkling.

"Of course," the physician answered stiffly. "I would not infringe on my family's right to privacy."

"Great," I said, addressing Gus. "Then we can pump her for all *sorts* of information."

"Yeah," Gus chimed in enthusiastically, "like if it's true that he really wears Roy Rogers PJs."

Dr. Menowitz half smiled, half bristled. "I doubt you could even get Roy Rogers PJs any—"

"And if he *really* plays the trombone in the closet at three in the morning with nothing on," I said.

"That's absurd. Who said I—"

"Hey, we could ask about how he sings along to Frank Sinatra records in the bathroom when he—"

"I *hate* Frank Sinatra." Dr. Menowitz's face was red. "Who told you this garbage? It's a bunch of—"

"I wouldn't make too much of a fuss about lies if I were you, Morton," Gus said slyly. "We have reliable sources. Remember the time your mother came in when she broke her wrist?"

"*Mom* told you this nonsense?" Dr. Menowitz was taken aback.

Gus and I nodded.

"Yeah," I said. "You remember, Mort. The time she had to ask that you be thrown out of the exam room."

I recognized the woman right off. As a matter of fact, the dressings I'd put on her ankle and arm two weeks before were still neatly wrapped and relatively clean, except for the polka dots of fresh blood.

Through the mess, I could see Mrs. Turner had recently washed and set her thin silver hair. I recalled from her first visit to the ER that she was proud of still being able to take care of her own hair. Considering that she was seventy-nine and people her age frequently lacked the physical ability to reach over their heads and scrub for any length of time, let alone make pin curls, it was an accomplishment. Then again, she had the advantage of having more upper-body strength than most elderly people, since she'd spent the majority of her adult life in a wheelchair due to a run-in with polio, pre–Dr. Salk.

The paramedics had radioed in at 9:02 code three to say they had an apparent single gunshot wound to the head, entry site behind the left ear. As soon as they said they were at the Greenwood Seniors Center, I knew they were bringing in Mrs. Turner.

When the paramedics picked her up two weeks before, Mrs. Turner had told them that her "little mishap" was all a mistake. The story, as she calmly related it, was that she had proceeded to the cliff behind the seniors' apartment building, opened the fence, and, wheeling full steam ahead, flew off the edge. She landed, still chairbound, some forty feet below. The wheelchair, including the silicone-gel seat cushion her husband had given her on their golden wedding anniversary, was totaled.

Mrs. Turner had been disappointed that she miraculously survived the fall with cuts, bruises, and a mild concussion.

This time she was not so lucky (though I am sure Mrs. Turner would have disagreed), for it was clear the moment they wheeled her into the trauma room that she would not survive. The code activities were halfhearted at best. When Dr. Menowitz began ordering the last-minute, cover-your-ass drugs, I slipped out to the waiting room to find Mr. Turner and bring him to the Quiet Room where he could receive the news in private.

Instead of Mr. Turner, I found two policemen waiting for news of Mrs. Turner's condition.

"The husband shot her, called nine-one-one, then left a note saying he was going shopping," said the shorter of the two policemen.

The tall policeman, whose badge was level with my forehead, said, "The neighbors say the old lady has been begging him to do her in for a year or more—ever since she found out she had cancer."

"Well," I said finally, "it looks like she got her wish."

The bag man shuffled behind me, humming "Amazing Grace." In the old days, I would have called him a bum or a hobo, but in these times of obsession with polite new labels, Mr. Breton Birdy was a member of the Ever Increasing Homeless Populace.

Mr. Birdy was also the illegal owner of a shopping cart which he drove about with great pride. This possession placed him in the higher echelons of homelessness, until one of the younger and tougher Homeless Persons decided *he* needed the cart more than the old man. It was this clash over proprietorship that brought the tragic figure to us—although more than likely, it was his need for a kind word and a smoothing of ruffled feathers rather than his minor scrapes, major bruises, and fat lip that made him seek us out.

I helped him off with his bulky corduroy coat, marveling at eighteen outside pockets and ten inner pockets, each one filled with the necessary paraphernalia for street living: toothbrush and paste, gloves, socks, soap, various shoes, watch cap, plastic bags, eating utensils, string, army knife, newspaper, collapsible cup, toilet paper, and a plastic Jesus on a suction cup pedestal. ("I stick him on my forehead when I lay down to sleep. Don't nobody mess with a man wearin' Jesus on his forehead.")

After washing out his wounds, I was making note of his vital signs, when the space on the chart designated "Occupation" caught my attention. In a shaky, old-fashioned hand was printed: "DREAM COLLECTOR."

The lines of his face, deep as cracks in dry mud, snaked about as he explained. "I go out to the streets every day and pick up what them other folks throws away. Folks, you know, they throw away good things—things that got plenty of value still left in them."

He paused to see if I understood. As a lifelong devotee of rummage sales, I most certainly did.

"I get me lots of aluminum cans and bottles and sell them to the recycling place. Then, see, they give me the money and I save it till I get enough to buy me a bottle. Nothing fancy, mind you—don't need fancy whiskey to give me the good dreams. Just the regular stuff gives me dreams that makes me a rich man."

A few minutes after eleven, Dr. DeMarco, the ortho doc on call, brought in his golden retriever puppy for the application of a cast to her left foreleg. As the first canine patient in the history of the hospital, Femur received more loving attention than any patient to date.

By the time she was discharged, Femur had been seen by every doctor still in the hospital, including a urologist, Dr. Bell, both Menowitz and Mahoney, an anesthesiologist, and Dr. Schupbach.

In order to avoid detection by the supervisor nurse, Dr. DeMarco wrapped the pup in a bath blanket with only her muzzle exposed and carried her like a sick child out of the department.

Pete, one of our repeater alcoholics, took a bleary gander at the passing bundle, complete with wagging tail escaped out the end of the blanket. The grizzly old fossil shook his head in befuddled wonder. "Man, I sure hope that guy has good insurance, 'cause that kid is gonna need a lot more medical attention."

Ileta was getting ready to leave for the night when the registration office called to say there was a Mr. Turner in the waiting room, inquiring about the whereabouts of his wife.

I found the distinguished-looking gentleman sitting in a chair against the far wall, wearing a pale yellow cardigan, gray wool slacks, and a plaid tam-o'-shanter. On the bench beside him were several bakery boxes, neatly stacked.

"Mr. Turner?"

The man stood, removed his cap, and offered his hand. "Yes ma'am, that's me."

There was an awkward pause, and we both sat down. Mr. Turner cleared his throat. "How is Agnes?"

This wasn't the question I expected; I was thinking more in terms of his wanting to know what had been done with her body or if the police were waiting for him.

"She died shortly after she arrived."

"Did she suffer?"

"No. I don't think she ever regained consciousness."

Mr. Turner accepted the news with a nod, then solemnly bowed his head. "Thank God. She wanted to be put to rest for a long time, you know. She had a bad cancer in her belly—didn't want to go on with the pain anymore. She'd had it with being sick." The man turned to look at me. "She wanted me to be the last person she saw and touched, not some stranger."

I stayed silent, watching his face. In the careworn eyes there was sorrow over the loss of his companion, but also relief that she had escaped the pain.

He kept pulling the cap through his hand, around and around. "She had me running every which way trying to finish everything on her darned honey-do list. I told her I wanted to sit by her until they came for her, but she said the list was more important." Mr. Turner leaned toward me. "Agnes belonged to the Episcopalian faith," he said. "She wanted the ladies at church to know as soon as possible. It's on the list."

Carefully, as if he had low back pain, Mr. Turner got to his feet. "These two on top are for the doctors and nurses," he said, indicating the bakery boxes. "Agnes had them on the list. A rhubarb and an apple for the medical people, and a pumpkin for the policemen."

The elderly man removed an envelope from his shirt pocket and handed it to me. "That's the name of the funeral home, and inside are the release papers all signed and dated. Agnes made the arrangements herself. If you'd give the mortuary a call for me I'd appreciate it, young lady. I'm going to head on over to the police station now. Thank you very much for—"

"Mr. Turner?"

"Uhn?"

"Why did you agree to . . . help her?"

The old man looked surprised and slightly offended by my question. "Because I loved her, that's why. I loved that woman every day we were . . ." His voice broke and he turned away from me. With a slight wave of his hand, he disappeared through the doors.

The handsome face was familiar, but the switchboard ladies absolutely could not come up with a file from the memory banks. The name, Charles R. Henley, Jr., rang no bells, and his diagnosis—a sore hand—didn't provide me with any clues either. That bothersome, vague brainache that happens when I can't remember someone's name or where I know them from, crept under the switchboard ladies and over my optic nerves and settled in around the sinus cavities. The funny thing about it was that I had a distinct feeling I'd been on almost intimate terms with this guy.

"Why do I know you?" I asked. (Unwritten rule 71: When working ER, it pays to be direct. Subtlety wastes time.)

The patient adjusted the ice pack on his swollen hand and pointed a finger at me. "Yeah, you look familiar too. Do you buy your meat and fish at Cordova's Grocery Market? I'm the managing butcher there."

I shook my head. I couldn't afford to shop at Cordova's. It was one of those California "gourmet" grocery stores that carried lots of expensive and exotic imported foodstuffs, such as jellied livers of South African banana flies and the like. It was so exclusive, in fact, that I wouldn't have been at all surprised to find that the customers were charged admission and hourly rental on the carts.

"No, I'm a vegetarian," I said with an apologetic shrug.

"Do you belong to the Belfast Gym?" he asked hopefully. Apparently he suffered the same memory loss brainache I did. "I work out there every day."

"No, that's not it. Are you a runner? Would I have seen you on some of the trails around the lakes?"

"I'm strictly an indoor-workout person."

My brainache was growing unbearable, warning me to give it a rest. I could fret about where I knew the man from just before I tried to fall asleep the following morning.

"What did you do to that hand?" I asked, in order to divert

our attention. Like hiccups, brainache could sometimes be cured by ignoring it.

"Oh"—he laughed—"my partner slammed the freezer door on it."

I pushed up the sleeve of the man's shirt and took a close look at his hand and arm. Faint scars from long-ago needle tracks lined his inner arm. My memory loss brainache disappeared.

"I've got it!"

"Huh?"

"A long time ago you came into CCU with endocarditis."

"*That's* where I know you from!" He slapped his knee. "You were the nurse who gave me a shower. You got soaked."

"Right."

"I remember all the nurses up there got together and gave me the food from their dinners. I was so . . . Jesus." His smile suddenly slid upside down, and his shoulders slumped. "I was so goddamned sick and wasted, I was pitiful."

"Yeah, but look at you now. You look and sound like you're doing great."

He shrugged in a gesture of agreement. "Well, I said I'd never go back to that life. It's been a long haul, but I got out of it."

Relieved that I wouldn't have to spend any more time being tortured by the *where*-do-I-know-that-guy-from? ache, I congratulated him again, put the ice pack back over his hand, and began taking his vital signs.

"Hey, do you remember that male nurse who came in and fed me?"

I finished counting his pulse. "You mean Risen?"

"Yeah, that was his name. You know, he told me that night that the reason you were all so kind to me was because you had faith in the living. I repeated that to myself about a thousand times a day all through my rehab. It made a difference. . . . Is he still at this hospital?"

"Yep," I answered truthfully. "He's up in ICU." *Because he had too much faith in the living.*

"Next time you see him, will you thank him for me and tell him how much what he said helped?"

"Will do." I said. *As soon as he pulls his knickers out of the twist they're in and rejoins the living.*

* * *

Holding on to her swollen belly, Doris Klanger got up from the chair and walked bent at the waist, wincing with each step. Clinging to her skirt was a scrawny girl of about six.

Having just received orders from Dr. Menowitz about no visitors, I opened my mouth to say the child couldn't come back with her mother, when the man accompanying them slapped the seat of the chair the girl had been sitting in. The explosive violence of the gesture made the three of us jump.

"Get yer goddamned ass back in this chair or I'll beat the living shit outta you," he said through clenched teeth.

The child whimpered into her mother's leg.

"Oh Billy, now don't go yelling at the girl in front of everybody." Even as Doris Klanger spoke, she began pushing her daughter toward him, her eyes hooded with nervous fear.

"Please, Mama." The girl looked to her mother. Her pleading carried a distinct note of desperation. "Please, Mama, nooooooo."

"Get yer"—the man violently slammed his hand against the back of the chair. The small gold loop in his left ear jiggled with the force—"fucking ass"—the slap went harder against the seat—"back over"—the chair rocked with his punch—"here!"

Uneasiness roiled in my chest at the potential of physical violence. I spoke quickly, directing my gaze just over the top of his greased-back hair. I wanted to avoid looking directly into his eyes. "No, really, it's fine if she comes in. We've got a place for kids who want to color health posters—we need more to hang in the lobby.

"Do you like to color, sweets?"

The child gave the man a quick, frightened glance and nodded.

"Okay then, it's settled." I slipped an arm around the girl's thin shoulders and led her away from the deep-socketed, fierce eyes.

"Okay, like I know this sounds totally weird, but me and my friend had to take advantage of this excellent full moon and these excellent waves to exercise our boards. It was so radical, man. I mean, it was superior surf."

"You mean until the excellent shark came along and tweaked your little butt with his superior sharp teeth?" I cut away what was left of the surfer's shredded wet suit and poured antibacterial solution over the uneven gash on his hip and buttock.

The adolescent sucked in a quick, yelping breath and bit his pillow. His friend, interrupted in his task of working over a pimple on his neck, gawked. "Oh, gag me. That is like *to*tally gnarly, dude."

Dr. Mahoney took off the gloves, which were now smeared with a variety of Doris Klanger's bodily secretions, and threw them away.

She donned a new pair and leaned toward the woman. "Okay, Doris, we're going to let this culture grow for a few days, but I'm fairly certain you have gonorrhea and you definitely have a severe case of venereal warts. The nurse will give you a shot of penicillin before you leave, but I want you to continue taking the penicillin pills for two weeks. Your partner will have to be treated too."

Looking drawn and pasty, Mrs. Klanger stared silently at the ceiling, her jaw muscles clenched.

"I'm going to swab some medicine on these warts now," Susan said. There was a warning lilt to her voice. "You shouldn't have intercourse for at least two weeks."

"Doc, did you say that the only way I could get these diseases is . . ." Doris groped, then set her jaw. ". . . from sleeping with Billy?"

"Well, if it's true that you've never had venereal warts or gonorrhea before now, and you haven't engaged in sex with anyone else for over two years, I'd say it was pretty certain you got it from him."

"You mean, I couldn'ta got it from my underwear being dirty?"

"Nope," Susan said. "It's a sexually transmitted disease."

The woman frowned as she let this sink in. A second later, she pulled herself up on her elbows, anger and disgust lacing her voice. "Doc, after you finish with me, can you take a look at my little girl?"

Dr. Mahoney asked the question with her expression.

"I don't know, doc, but I think she's got the same as me."

"When you see a guy who looks like Harpo Marx come into the room, you'll have to leave, dude." I dropped the sterile towel over the suture set and removed my gloves.

The teenager cocked his head. "Who's Harpo Marx?"

I rolled my eyes. "Okay, when you see a guy who looks like Pee-wee Herman, only with curly red hair, you've got to hightail it."

The young man lying facedown on the gurney groaned. "Oh man, can't the dude stay? He's like my best friend. He's cool. He won't sneeze on the cut or nothin'. I *need* moral support, man. This thing hurts like a mother."

"Well," I said doubtfully, "you can try to talk Dr. Menowitz into letting him stay, but I'm going to warn you right now, he's a very uptight, temperamental kind of dude—like whoever your worst nightmare of a teacher is."

"Wow!" They laughed in unison, their eyes gleaming. "Mr. Owens!"

"Yeah," I said dryly. "Like Mr. Owens, only with a twist of Beetlejuice mentality."

"He's not my uncle!" the child screamed at her mother. She looked fragile in the patient gown, which hung on her like a tent.

"All right now, Cory. I want you to tell the doc here what Unc—what Billy did."

Dr. Mahoney put her hands on the girl's shoulders and turned her so they were face-to-face. "Honey, did Billy touch you down there where I just looked?"

The girl nodded, her eyes red-rimmed and wide. The mother moaned and sank in at the middle, looking as fragile as her child.

"Has he touched you there with his . . . ?" Susan looked to the mother for the girl's word for penis.

"Peepee house," Doris said.

"Did he put his peepee house down there?"

"Yes," Cory answered in a whisper. She pulled at a loose thread in her gown and was silent.

"Did he hurt you?"

Tears gathered in the child's eyes and spilled over. "Yes," she said, hiding her face against Susan's chest.

Doris began to cry. "Cory baby, why didn't you tell Mommy?

Cory looked out from Susan's arms. "He . . . He said if I told, he would kill you and I'd have to live with him forever."

Mother and daughter cried for a few minutes, until Dr. Mahoney gently laid a hand on the mother's arm. "Doris, by law I'm obligated to call Child Protective Services," she said softly. "I can't allow Cory to go back into a situation where there's been—"

In blind panic, Mrs. Klanger stood. "But I . . . I gotta have her with me. You don't understand. If I walk out of here without her, Billy will kill me. He'll know she told. He'll beat me to death."

"Would you be willing to go to a women's shelter and stay there?" Susan asked.

Doris hung her head, her eyes darting about the floor while she thought. I clenched my jaw. It seemed inconceivable she would hesitate for even a nanosecond.

"*Please*, Mama!" Cory begged, crying harder. "Please, please, please. Don't let's see him anymore. He's always hurting us. He's a bad man, Mama."

"Okay," Doris said with finality. "I don't know how they'll keep him away from us, but I don't want him around me or my kid no more. He's going to try his best to kill—"

Outside, we heard loud shouts and then a sound like someone falling against the wall. Susan and I rushed for the door, only to have it jerked open from the other side.

"What the fuck's going on in here?" Billy stood in the doorway, his fists clenched. He flicked a half-finished cigarette to the ground and roughly grabbed a paralyzed Doris by the arm and thrust her into the main room. "Goddamned cunt. Git the hell back in the truck right now!"

Cory cowered, but before either Dr. Mahoney or I could pull her out of the man's way, he'd seized her by the hair and yanked her off her feet. The little girl began to scream wild, high screams. He backhanded her and tossed her after her mother. She landed on the floor near where Doris had fallen.

"I'm gonna thrash the shit outta both of you," he yelled after them. They scrambled to get up off the floor. "You ain't gonna walk for a month."

He whirled around and held a warning finger to me and Susan. "And if you two cunts make any trouble over the lies them bitches told you, I'll carve yer fuckin' faces apart."

Dr. Mahoney was trembling. Had I not known her, I might have mistaken it for fear instead of anger. She slapped his wrist out of the way as if it were a fly. "You will not abuse that child again! I'll personally see to it that you—"

Snarling, the man put his hand over Susan's face and shoved. Dr. Mahoney toppled backward into the wall.

Torn between running away from and running at the man to

slug him, I yelled for help. I decided to at least try to slow the guy down and was raising my arms to knock him off balance, when I saw Dr. Menowitz and an armed security guard headed toward the room.

Thinking along the lines of Kevin McCarthy in the original version of *Invasion of the Body Snatchers*, I imagined Dr. Menowitz to be secreting a syringe full of Thorazine behind his back that he would jab into the maniac's rear end. If it worked for Hollywood, it would work on this stage.

Billy turned to follow my gaze.

It wasn't until then that I noticed Gus and the surfer dudes, eyes big as saucers, peering out from behind Dr. Menowitz.

"Did you see that old lady's face when that dirtbag dude jumped over her bed?" The two teenagers laughed with that cracking, halfway-to-men laughter that always put me in mind of young animals undergoing hormonal experiments or donkeys braying at each other.

"And when the sheriff yelled, 'Halt or I'll shoot your fucking head off'? God, that was *so* radically cool, man."

Another peal of guffaws.

"Stop moving or you'll get a suture where you don't want one," said Dr. Menowitz, smiling in spite of himself.

He had reason to feel good. Even though the man escaped, Dr. Menowitz *had* managed to get him into a half nelson almost long enough for him to be apprehended, but not quite.

"Sure, Mr. Owens." The patient giggled. "We're cool."

"Cory and her mother get into the shelter okay?" Gus asked.

I nodded, mouth full of my beloved graham crackers. It was coming up on three A.M., and the masses either had been treated or were temporarily resting, thinking about being treated.

Dr. Menowitz had gone to the doctors' room to sleep, while Dr. Mahoney continued to fill out her police report. Every so often she would stop to rub the back of her head and say, "That bastard!" Melanie was doing some sloppy sipping of her coffee and filling in the restocking list as she picked at the last of Mr. Turner's rhubarb pie. Gus sat sullen, uncharacteristically at rest.

I looked at her for a time while I chewed. She'd been too long without a smile.

"Okay, what's the problem, Gus?"

"No problem," she said, and drank off the rest of her coffee.

"Give me a break."

"I haven't got any extra to give you." She smiled a little.

"Stop it and tell me why you're so quiet. Are you drinking decaf or something?"

"I got some shitty news to tell you, Ec."

I swallowed and bit into another grahamie. "Not another fecal disimpaction? At three in the morning? Give the patient some Feen-a-mint and tell them they can come back any time after seven-thirty."

"Your friend Osbert is HIV-positive. All the information points to the probability he's been positive for a long while."

The graham cracker turned to sawdust in my mouth, and the switchboard ladies went numb at their posts.

"It's what started the fight between your friend and his lover," Gus said, avoiding my eyes. "Osbert found out the results of his test yesterday morning and confronted the guy. They'd both been HIV-negative when they started living together four years ago. Osbert didn't have a clue that his significant other had been screwing around for the last three of those."

Suddenly very much awake, I stood and walked toward the black runner. "I'm going for a walk," I said.

Melanie grabbed my hand. "Hey, sorry about that. Anything we can do?"

"No. Just cover me while I take a break."

"If you're worried about yourself, Reverb, don't," added Dr. Mahoney. "I know about the gloves. It takes more than that."

Gus was putting on her sweater. "I'm going with Ec," she said to Melanie. "I won't stay but a minute."

I started to protest, but shrugged and let her follow me out to the ER parking lot. We sat on the edge of a large planter pot, hugging ourselves to keep warm.

"*Are* you worried about being infected?" Gus asked finally.

I shook my head. "Nope. That's not the way I'm scheduled to die."

I stared at the moon, letting myself be hypnotized by the delicate light, and thought about the rest of Risen's life. He would regain consciousness in a day or two, maybe with a physical residual from the injury, maybe not. When his mind cleared, he'd remember the fight and his AIDS test. Of course, he'd be fired before he even left the hospital, and then he'd get

some kind of disability and live like a leper, taking his AZT
every four hours until he died. One year? Two?

Then his name would be sewn into a quilt with thousands of
others. Under his name, someone might take the time to add
"Our sweet nurse." And Risen, the bighearted, talented artist,
our funny, gossipy brother, would be gone from our lives.

Gus put her arm through mine and hugged closer. "Life can
be so shitty sometimes. It's not fair."

"Yup, and there's nothing we can do but go on."

We sat in silence until a very loud IV pump alarm echoed
from somewhere on the fourth floor and down across the parking lot.

"So how do you think you're going to die?" Gus asked,
wearing an amused, tongue-in-cheek expression.

I pursed my lips, looked down into my lap, and smiled.
"Oh, well, my sister Mari had one of her special dreams recently and saw me being abducted by sadistic editors, put into
a room made to resemble the Schenectady library, and given
nothing but Danielle Steel novels to read."

Gus's closed mouth hid a ball of laughter. "You know how
I want to die?" she asked.

I shook my head, already laughing. "How?"

"Very quickly."

9:30 A.M.—no clue as to what day it is

*By the time we left, the "dirtbag dude" had not yet been
picked up. How do people get so screwed up—so far away
from life? Couldn't they repair their lives? What does it all
boil down to? Education? Money? Fate?*

*I don't have the words for how it felt to come home and
crawl into a warm bed next to David. Let the maniacs roam
free, they cannot hurt this peace ... even if David's snores
are enough to wake the dead.*

*My last patient of the morning was a genuine limited-
heartbeat-theory patient. For years I've heard of these people who believe in the idea that we are all given so many
heartbeats per lifetime, and if we exercise, we will die
sooner than if we remain sedentary.*

*It was no wonder the guy weighed 279 pounds. He was a
character, although he wasn't a Wildroot cream man who
put good grooming first: when he rolled in, he had a roach
egg stuck to the front of his shirt. Oh, shades of Wilma.*

Gus's last patient took the prize: He was a thirty-two-year-old San Quentin prisoner who came in—talking and answering questions appropriately—with a new No. 2 pencil stuck into the corner of his right eye, and through the length of his brain. It was very odd to be talking to a guy who was blinking around an eraser.

Seems the white supremacist gang didn't appreciate his lack of racist ideology, and decided to hold him down while the leader hammered in the lead.

David listened to the events of my shift and said that no one in their right mind would do what nurses do to make a living. It's good that he's figured this much out in the early stages of the relationship.

Just realized it's Tuesday and I have an appointment with Miss Milks. Must sleep before I see her. Seeing Miss Milks on no sleep would be like going to a Young Republicans party on LSD.

"What's the problem, Heron? Are you looking for a medical discharge from service, or are you suicidal?"

"No, Miss Milks. I made a mistake is all. It won't happen again, sir."

The wizened old lady blew a stream of smoke toward the immense poster that hung over her desk: a red, white, and blue replica of the "Uncle Sam Wants *You*" placards from the Second World War. The addition of the line ". . . to Quit Smoking!" gave it a contemporary touch.

"I thought you weren't supposed to smoke in your new office, Miss Milks."

"I'm not," she said, staring at me steadily, one eye half closed against the smoke.

I crossed and uncrossed my legs. The old lady sat watching me without saying anything for quite some time. I figured she'd had a small stroke and had forgotten who I was and why I was there. The ash on her cigarette was growing longer, the glowing part coming closer to her fingers. It was making me very nervous.

"Nice poster you got there, Miss Milks."

"It bites the big one," she said absently, and took a deep drag.

At once, she spat out the cigarette and threw it into her ashtray.

"Rats!" she said, spitting into her hand. "I *hate* it when that happens!"

"Miss Milks?"

The disgruntled old bird gave me an evil eye. "Aw, those goddamned filters. I hate those things! It's like sucking cement through a banana. Then you end up smoking that damned crap at the end: plastic and old men's whiskers, is what it tastes like. Ought to be some law passed against it. Filters are the ruination of a good smoke in this country."

"Had many chances to taste old men's whiskers, have you, Miss Milks?"

An arthritic digit pressed the tip of my nose. "Watch it, Heron. I might look like an old fart, but I haven't even *begun* to pass wind. Now, roll up that sleeve and pump up those pitiful strings or I'll report you to the brass for insubordination."

I saluted and did as I was told.

The stairwells of Redwoods Memorial have provided the stage for many a scene and the speaking place for many a gossip. If inclined to eavesdrop in those stairwells, one could overhear all the inside details of who was sleeping with whom, how often and where; who was angry and why; who was happy and why; and if you were lucky enough, top secret administrative information. To get an earful of a lusty tryst was rare, but known to happen on nights.

Being small and enclosed, stairwells invite these sorts of happenings and loosening of the tongue by giving a false sense of security and privacy—much in the same way the cabin of an automobile fools people into believing they can freely talk to themselves and pick their noses behind the wheel and not be observed.

Because I know this about the stairwells, I was uncomfortable when Gene, ER's head nurse, pulled me aside on the landing between the third and fourth floors.

"Heron, I need to talk with you."

I had to physically check the urge to run away. Gene came to Redwoods straight from the administrative offices of a private, tightly run East Coast hospital. Unfortunately, he'd never been able to adjust to California's laid-back way of life and remained an excessively rigid, regimented individual, especially when it came to managing the nurses in his department. I had a sneaking suspicion he wanted us to salute and stand at attention whenever he entered a room. Gus, Sarah, and I were the only ones who refused to cower under his authority, and he openly resented it.

In his usual manner, he stood at a slouched sort of attention: an odd combination of preppy Ivy Leaguer and reform school psycho-rebel.

"Effective today, there's been a change in policy for the on-call staff," he said, and rested a hand on his hip.

I stiffened and waited silently. The man brought out a wariness in me that was more instinct than personal taste. His thinly disguised hostility toward the female nurses was, to my mind, something to be heeded; a hair trigger waiting for a tiny bump.

"In order to retain your on-call position in ER, you must now work at least one full weekend a month. We're also going to require three night shifts per month instead of two, and during the holiday season, we've increased the required number of legal holidays worked from one to two."

My heart bounced off my stomach, which had turned into a hard block of cement. "But I'm already working two weekends a month in CCU and two of the five holidays. I might be able to swing the extra night, but if I work a weekend down in ER, that leaves me with only one weekend to myself. I'm not crazy about the Christmas season, Gene, but having only one holiday off isn't fair—especially for the nurses who have kids at home."

"That is your problem." He shrugged and clucked his tongue. "If you can't fill the requirements, you'll be stricken from the on-call list."

The old anger that always came with management's tyrannical manipulations settled in my throat like a burr. "May I ask who made these decisions, and were any of the on-call people consulted about this ahead of time?"

Gene did a hasty bit of mustache grooming. I thought I saw him smile briefly. "The director of ER and myself made the policies. We didn't feel under any obligation to consult with the nurses, since all we'd get would be a bunch of hysterical flak."

"Can you tell me what the reasoning was behind your and Dr. Manville's decision?"

The man laughed and began walking away. "Forget it, Heron. It's done. Either come down and sign your agreement to meet the new obligations, or present your resignation. I don't have time for political sermons."

"Wait a minute, Gene."

He stopped and turned, his face set in a moue of contempt.

"What if none of the on-callers are willing to go along with this? Most all of us work elsewhere as part-time staff. People like Gus have families to consider. They aren't going to give up a third weekend a month."

The man shrugged me off with peevish impatience. "Like I said, Heron, either agree to it or quit. There's plenty of people who're begging to work ER."

"Yeah, but who are they, Gene? Are they trained? Are they certified mobile intensive care nurses? Have they been there for years and know all the doctors' individual quirks? How can you arbitrarily make a decision of this magnitude and force it on us? Do you really think that no one will go to the union with this? What are your—"

Gene held up a hand and started down the stairs in the true tradition of administrative tactics—hit and run. "You can do whatever you want. Go to your union. Start a riot. You're wasting your time. Sign the contract or quit ER."

I felt like I'd been slapped. I loved working in ER with all its crazy excitement and drama. But at the same time, didn't I need to take care of myself? I wanted more time, not less, to spend with Simon, David, and my friends. I needed to have more than one weekend off a month to at least pretend I was among the normal.

The old rage bit my throat. I was sick and tired of playing defense. I leaned over the railing, noticing that there were three other people on various floors doing the same thing. "Hey Gene?"

"Heron?" He was on the landing below mine, but did not stop descending.

"You and Manville can take your new rules and shove them far, far up."

From somewhere on one of the landings above me, somebody applauded.

Tuesday, October 17, 1989
11:00 P.M.

A day to remember for a lifetime.

I went home after seeing Miss Milks and Risen to treat myself to an afternoon of cooking. So lost was I in the culinary art that I did not hear the front door open.

I did, however, hear the footsteps in the hall. I looked at the clock. Five was too early for David, and it was not likely to be Simon. I don't know why exactly, but for a moment while I waited with my spoon, instead of terror I felt such a hope.

And there was David, home early, Mooshie hanging over his shoulder, both man and beast purring and smiling. In that second I loved the man so much, I'm surprised the force of it didn't knock him over.

I burst into tears and could not stop crying long enough to assure a confused David that I hadn't hurt myself and no one had died. His cure for whatever ailed me was to put me to bed with promises of Chinese soup and hot tea.

On the bed, I was trying to explain that the tears were because I had never been so happy in my life, when Mooshie's ears suddenly lay back. Puffed up to twice his size, he let out with a mournful yowl and flew under the bed.

Astonished by the cat's sudden, strange behavior, David and I laughed, until I heard the customary low rumble that precedes the shifting of the earth.

The top of the four-poster began to sway gracefully, and when I looked into the hallway, I saw that my eighty-pound gilt-framed mirror was swinging like a straw in the wind. When the desk in my office slid out into the hall, I told David we needed to stand in the doorway.

A true Connecticut Yankee boy, he laughed and said, "Oh, it's just a small one, don't worry." I relaxed for a second or two, but then thought, What? Are you nuts? This is it, and what the hell does an East Coaster know about earthquakes anyway?

Giddy with the excitement that this was the big one I'd been waiting twenty-two years for, I looked into the hallway to get my bearings and saw the house rocking literally from side to side on its foundation.

When I heard the bookcases topple over and crash, I grabbed my now unsmiling David by the collar and pulled him to the door and out of the house with the intention of standing in the middle of the parking lot.

I was stopped cold at the sight of the blacktop undulating, as if it had a life of its own. Figuring it was still safer than this rickety old cottage, I kept one eye on the power lines overhead and one on the ground for cracks.

I turned to yell at David to watch for power lines and re-

alized he was not behind me, or anywhere to be seen. I ran back to the moving house, imagining him knocked unconscious by the huge mirror. Instead, I found him on hands and knees trying to coax Mooshie out from under the bed.

When I asked him what he was doing, he replied, "I couldn't leave the Moosh. The poor little guy might have been crushed."

Who is this man? From what heaven did he drop?

As soon as I could get an open line, I called to make sure Simon was safe. He was in a car and didn't feel a thing. His father, however, is missing. He was coming home from Oakland.

We are without gas, but are lucky in that we have electricity and partial phone service. Still, the neighbors have all gathered to share meals and comfort. I called hospitals around the Bay to offer my services, but they have more people than they can use.

2:30 A.M.

Thank God. All my sheep are safe. Patrick just sent word to me and Simon that he was one of the last cars off Interstate 880 before it collapsed. With the bridges closed, he has been helping the rescue teams take the bodies off the ramp.

Mooshie is curled up on David's chest and is licking his nose. I have to put this away and pull Moosh off him, before the poor man passes out from a lethal dose of cat breath.

THIRTEEN

> *"Of all the professionals, nurses perform the most intensely personal services for all people in extraordinarily vulnerable positions. Occasionally we hold a person's life in our hands; almost always his dignity."*
>
> LEAH L. CURTIN, R.N.

THE DOG DAYS OF SUMMER were on us before anyone had a chance to stock up on long johns and wool socks. The San Francisco Bay Area was in its fifth year of drought and colder than most people from other parts of the country would believe—that is, unless they could afford to be tourists on the Golden Coast, paying premium dollar to freeze their buns off in August. ("But this is *California*, Marge—how could it *possibly* be colder than Muskegon?")

We were coming up on the first anniversary of the big quake, even though the residents of the Bay Area had been constantly assured by seismologists that the *reeeeally big* one was going to happen any day. No dignified, laid-back Californian took them seriously after the first week, and the expert predictors were soon looked on as minor cranks—Criswells of the cracks.

Redwoods Memorial had been the first hospital on the block to go millions into debt by building a new wing. CCU moved into its new digs, twice its original capacity, without a hitch and was running like a top. With a few modifications, we adjusted to the design problems that someone would have done well to consult about with a nurse *before* the building was built.

The best feature of the new wing was the abundance of windows overlooking the estuary and the surrounding marshes.

Every room on both the acute and intermediate units was flooded with natural light and birdsong, creating an ambience of peaceful comfort for the patients.

Our job descriptions were yet again expanded when the open heart surgical program was established. Besides being trained in the techniques and procedures used to care for these patients, we were also required to develop and institute effective educational and rehab programs for the patient as he went through the preop and postop phases.

New staff nurses were hired at a faster rate than the old-timers were quitting. The unit had progressed as a whole, but the feeling of family had been entirely lost among the staff.

The newer generation of nurses, fresh out of school, seemed unwilling to "bond" either with the tenured staff or with each other.

I mentioned this to Annie, who told me that an every-man-for-himself attitude was being encouraged so that each nurse would become an independent working unit. "Too much tight knitting," Annie told me, "made for petty jealousies and cliques." When I reminded her that a family atmosphere made for a strong working team and provided staff members with much-needed emotional support, Annie countered that this created personal loyalties rather than loyalty to the hospital.

With Annie clearly gone promanagement, the unit became an impersonal, cold shell. Pia, Beth, Nealy, and I were the only ones left of the original CCU family. Feeling displaced, the four of us watched in disgust as the administration went unchecked, committing political atrocities left and right. (I likened it to Reagan and Bush appointing one Republican to the Supreme Court after another.)

Either the new grads didn't know any better, didn't care, or had been so intimidated by management, they kept their dissatisfaction to themselves.

There was one hot issue, however, that was causing even the new grads to bleat.

We knew something was fishy when CCU management bypassed budget restrictions and began hiring per diem nurses at an astounding rate. When we had accumulated the largest nursing population of all the units in the hospital, management started to grossly overstaff the shifts. As a result, the "overflow" of CCU nurses was floated out to other units or the medical floors on a daily basis.

Nan finally confided to Pia that the reason CCU nurses were

getting the float shaft was that an under-the-table deal had been struck between CCU management and administration which entailed the intentional overstaffing of CCU for the express purpose of using those extra nurses to fill in the "staffing holes" in the rest of the hospital. This scheme cut the need for Redwoods to hire, at a higher hourly rate, outside agency nurses to fill in the gaps. In a word, CCU nurses were being farmed out for general use without their consent.

The worst side of it for the nurses, besides the obvious lack of say as to where one worked, was that such a large proportion of CCU staff was floated out each shift that CCU itself was frequently left understaffed. This made for larger patient loads for the nurses remaining on the unit.

Civilized mutiny came in the form of decentralization, a widely used practice in which a unit agreed to be its own staffing and scheduling agent, independent of the hospital. While it meant a lot of sacrifice and pulling together, it also meant that no nurse had to float anywhere if she didn't want to. True to form, Redwoods Memorial was one of a small percentage of Bay Area hospitals that had not decentralized their critical care units.

Falling back into old patterns of sticking my neck close to the swinging ax, I borrowed Mercy Hospital's written protocol on decentralization, tailored it to CCU's needs, and presented it at a staff meeting. The idea was eagerly accepted by float-weary staff. Thus it was agreed that they would have three months to read the information, think over the pros and cons, write down suggestions, and check off their names if they were interested in having it brought to a vote. The four CCU management people, it was understood, would not take part in the poll.

The overall enthusiasm was impressive. Easy, I thought. No one except the management's yes puppets would vote against the system from which we would all eventually benefit.

One might think from this display of fancy, and rightly so, that I will never learn.

"You're a vegetarian, right?" Chris asked with a nervous smile. Behind me, manning the monitors and phones, Phoebe giggled. Chris rolled her chair closer to mine, and opened a chart bearing the name DeGraff.

Chris was one of my favorite day shift nurses to follow, mainly because she gave succinct reports and managed to maintain a sense of humor throughout the worst. I was, however, suspicious of the smile.

"Yeah—why? Is my patient a steer or something?"

"Well, not exactly," said Chris. "But he *is* more vegetable than a plate of brussels sprouts."

I put my head down on the desk and groaned.

"You'll recognize him. He's the man who arrested the first time about two years ago at the—"

"Nursing home in San Rafael?" I finished for her, my memory having served me again. "He's the man who's married to that . . ." I searched for the right word. It was difficult to come up with an accurate description for Mrs. DeGraff.

"Cruel and unusual viper who walks like a woman?" suggested Chris.

I nodded. The dreary particulars of Mr. DeGraff's life, which had left him as the contractured, aphasic homunculus in bed 22, stemmed mostly from the fertile ground of alcoholism and an unhappy marriage to a scornful woman.

Granted, as the long-suffering wife of an austere and emotionally absent man, Mrs. DeGraff may have had good reason to want revenge. It was the degree to which she had taken her vengeance that was diabolic. The worst part about the sad affair was that she used the medical system and its servants to do the torturing.

I pulled the covers off the odd-shaped lump in bed 22 and took in the pitiful sight of Elmer DeGraff. The shrunken body was held in a tightly curled fetal position (knees actually touching chin) by permanently contracted muscles. The only thing animated about the man was the left side of his face and his wiry white eyebrows.

After the first stroke, which left him without speech, Mrs. DeGraff put her husband in a nursing home widely known for its low rates and poor care. Left unattended and marinating in his own urine, he developed bedsores first, then infections and general wasting away because no one bothered to feed him. Contractures—the shortening and fixing of muscles in one position due to improper positioning and/or lack of motion—left his limbs frozen into a grotesque pretzel-like configuration.

When the county closed that nursing care facility, Mrs. DeGraff begrudgingly put her husband in another, better-managed nursing home, where it was soon discovered he had prostate cancer.

Mrs. DeGraff stubbornly disregarded the advice of her husband's physicians, refused to examine the quality of his life, and insisted he be subjected to the full course of surgery and chemotherapy.

Soon after these insults had been carried out against his body, Mr. DeGraff, in silent protest, had a cardiac arrest. At the time, Mrs. DeGraff would not allow a death-with-dignity order to be written, her only concern being that everything possible was done to keep the man alive.

Now, six months later, Mr. DeGraff had again tried to defy his wife by having another cardiac arrest. Even as CPR was initiated, the charge nurse had called Mrs. DeGraff in desperate hopes of obtaining authorization to stop.

Is he suffering? Mrs. DeGraff had asked.

Yes, he's in horrible pain, the nurse assured her.

Good. Keep him going.

The lump in the bed glared at me with piercing, cold blue eyes. Mr. DeGraff was irritated by my presence; he wanted to be left alone to die—not turned and tended to.

"Sorry, Mr. D., but I've got to turn you and take your vital signs." I took hold of the pull sheet and pulled the lump of a body toward me.

He was small—or maybe he only looked small because he was all curled up—but he sure didn't weigh small. It was like trying to pull over a grand piano. Incredulous, I looked for the bricks hidden inside his gown, and finding none, tried again.

I'd pulled him almost all the way over, when the corner of the sheet slipped out of my hands and he fell back to his original position. From the deep tangling of his eyebrows and his breathless grunts, I guessed Mr. DeGraff was cursing me in aphasic.

"Do you need a hand?" The voice, of the slippery, yodeling variety, belonged to a tall man who looked like Mr. Peepers on drugs. He entered the room and turned Mr. DeGraff easily with one hand.

I sighed a disappointed, feministic sigh; male muscle mass had once again scored a point. "Thanks. Who're you?"

The thirty-something guy held out an amazingly long-fingered hand. "Dr. Voorhees. I'm the new, independent guy around here. Call me Eric."

I took the hand timidly, only because his fingers reached past my wrist. It was a weird feeling. "I'm Echo Heron, the old, codependent hag. Call me Ec."

"I know who you are," he said. "You're the anarchist. I heard you speak at a nurse solidarity rally about two years ago."

"So, I guess I need to ask if you hold grudges."

"No." He laughed and unwound his fingers from my arm. "I thought you were a little hard on the docs, but nothing most of them didn't deserve."

I slipped the disposable rectal probe onto the thermometer and lubricated the tip. "Yeah, well, it's a different view when you're looking up from under someone's heel instead of down at the tip of the shoe, you know."

Dr. Voorhees nodded as if he did know, and warmed up the head of his stethoscope by placing it under his arm.

As I proceeded to insert the thermometer, I discovered the small, odiferous pool of liquid stool that had collected under Mr. DeGraff. Automatically, I folded the soiled blue plastic pad over on itself and began gathering towels and washcloths. While I drew a basin of soapy water, Dr. Voorhees listened to the patient's lungs and heart, did a good head-to-toe assessment, then took his blood pressure, pulse, and respiratory rate. He wrote down his findings on the back of a paper towel and stuck it in my pocket.

"How are you doing, Mr. DeGraff?" he asked, pushing back a shock of the man's wild gray hair.

Mr. DeGraff turned on him a hostile yet pleading look.

"I'm really sorry, Elmer." Eric Voorhees shook his head. "I'm working on your wife, but she's tough. She doesn't want to give up the fight."

Spreading out towels and fresh soil pads, I glanced at the physician and wondered if he knew the double meaning of what he'd said. Dr. Voorhees returned my gaze in a way that told me he knew perfectly well what the score was between the man and his wife.

"I'm trying to get Mrs. DeGraff to give us permission not to resuscitate," he explained. "I've told her unless I get it, I'm signing off the case. Mr. DeGraff here has made it clear he doesn't want to prolong his life." He leaned over to face Mr. DeGraff again. "Do you still feel that way, Elmer?"

Mr. DeGraff purposely closed his eyes and opened them again:

Yes. Please.

"Elmer had some pretty good foresight," said the physician. "A couple of months before all this happened, he made out a living will stating that in case of his physical and/or mental debilitation, he wanted to be allowed to die without any heroic measures. He had his family doctor look it over and sign as a witness, but unfortunately, never gave him a copy." Dr. Voorhees took two exam gloves from the box on the bedside table and slipped them, with some stretching, over his extraordinary fingers. "Mrs. DeGraff said she couldn't remember there ever being any such document. Right, Elmer?"

Mr. DeGraff blinked twice.

Dr. Voorhees indicated I should change places with him. Thinking he wanted to listen to Mr. DeGraff's lungs again, I did as he asked—except instead of checking his patient's lungs, he began washing down his backside.

"You get a couple more clean washcloths and wash his face and hands," he said. "I'll clean up the mess."

I was dumbfounded. "Wow. Since when do doctors clean up messes?"

He smiled as he put the soiled washcloths in the hamper and found two more. "I was trained well by the nurses over at Pacific Beach, plus my last girlfriend was a nurse." Eric changed the water and added more soap. When he had a good suds, he began to wash the patient's shoulders and pitifully misshapen spine. Elmer let out a moan of pleasure, and a lot of the frown lines in his face eased out.

"Are you just trying to make a good impression, or are you like this all the time?" I asked, washing the grime out from under each of Mr. DeGraff's yellowed and broken fingernails.

"When I've got the time," he said, "I don't mind getting to know my patients from the nurses' shoes. It's good for me." The young physician patted the man dry and dusted him down with cornstarch powder.

"Yeah, but aren't you afraid one of the other doctors is going to see you doing this and you'll get called a sissy for playing with the girls?"

"I'm used to it," Dr. Voorhees said, and slipped a fresh pad under Elmer's hips. "When I was an intern, my best friend used to kid me all the time by saying, 'Uh oh. Eric's going to lose his deity card—he forgot to wear his arrogance again today.' "

"What did they tell you about me?" Miss Racklyn asked in a voice that had not yet decided which gender it belonged to. I couldn't tell from her tone or her perpetually sour expression whether she wanted me to know about her or not. I decided to divulge only the bare bones of what I'd been told, since most of what Chris had said was extremely unflattering and could be easily construed as defamation of character. To say, for instance, "They said you were a manipulative, certifiable crock," would not have been to anyone's advantage.

"Well, I know you're here because you suddenly started having atypical seizures five days ago and the docs can't find any neurological reason for them, so they want to rule out cardiac arrhythmias as possible cause."

I also knew that the forty-one-year-old had been claiming to be "mentally disabled" since she was twenty-one, and was having her "seizures" on command—approximately one every fifteen minutes while awake and only when someone was present. There was an obvious absence of the usual warning aura and the postictal state.

The precipitating factor of the initial seizure was the receipt of a letter from some government office or other stating in so much bureauspeak that her disability case had been reviewed after having fallen through the cracks fifteen years ago. The department felt it had been diddled long enough, and had redetermined that she was mentally fit enough to seek gainful employment, and thus, her disability payments were hereupon discontinued, and don't let the door hit you in the ass on the way out of the system, thank you very much. Signed, Mr. So-and-So, Director.

Dr. Hunt—Miss Racklyn's internist—and Dr. Schupbach could find no reasons for the atypical seizures, but since Miss Racklyn had already filed a suit against several government agencies, they thought it best to cover all bases and bring her into CCU for twenty-four-hour monitoring.

Fanny Racklyn bristled at my apparent lack of information.

"You should have also been informed that I can have a seizure over the slightest thing. My door has to be closed at all times, since there mustn't be any noise, or unnecessary light, except from the TV. The only things I can hold down are Mars bars, pizza, and diet Coke, so don't bring in any other food or I could seize just from the smell of it. I'll let you know about an hour before I want to eat, so you can run and pick up the pizza. It's gotta be steamy hot or you'll have to reheat it for me. I won't eat a cold pizza." Fanny stopped, took a deep breath, and forged ahead. "I need my sedation exactly when I tell you, and I need to be moved in the bed. You have to—"

In my haste to stop her, I accidentally bit my tongue and winced. "Wait, wait, wait," I said, without using my traumatized tongue. "What do you mean, you need to be moved in the bed?"

Fanny seemed irritated by the obviously stupid question. "You'll need to turn me and rearrange my limbs. I'm afraid if I move too much, I'll dislodge something in my brain." She studied me to see if I'd buy this somewhat flawed invention, but I was preoccupied with making sure I hadn't amputated my tongue. While the limping, bleeding creature was checking itself over as only tongues can do, the burly woman reached down and got herself a Mars bar from the bottom drawer of her bedside cabinet—a feat not many nonathletes could do from a lying position.

"And you've gotta whisper because if you—" She stopped and began to sniff like a bloodhound after the scent. "Holy mackerel, are you wearing perfume?"

"No perfume, Miss Racklyn. Just good old stick deodorant. Lime, I believe."

"Go wash it off." She shooed me away. "I'm not supposed to smell anything that has chemicals in—"

Miss Racklyn's right arm went straight up into the air and began to tremble; then her left leg shot out from under the covers to execute several interesting tai chi kicks Chuck Norris could have used. Thrashing from side to side, the woman stuck out her tongue and began to flick it around like a snake possessed. I noticed, too, that she never let go of her Mars bar, and was careful not to squeeze it too hard. When she began rolling her eyes Eddie Cantor style, I stopped watching.

I have seen seizures, and I have seen seizures. Whatever Miss Racklyn was having, it was not a seizure and it was not Saint Vitus's dance—it might have been Clarabelle-itis's Antics, though.

Through the artifact jiggling its way across the monitor, I deciphered a fairly normal sinus rhythm. When I turned back, I caught Miss Racklyn watching me with a steady gaze. The instant our eyes met, she began the Eddie Cantor routine and, with purpose, pulled off her lead wires, one at a time. She had to search for the V6 lead, which Chris had placed too far to the side.

Phoebe came to the glass window and pointed at the monitor with a what's-going-on-in-there? expression. She did a double take on Miss Racklyn's contortions, cocked her head in wonder, and returned to the monitor banks.

As I watched the fantastic dance of distortions, I became more and more disgusted that someone would go to such lengths to avoid taking responsibility for her own life. Maybe it was a deeply repressed streak of Republican surfacing, but as a taxpayer, I resented Miss Racklyn's lifelong free ride. If she was clever enough to have fooled the system, she was clever enough to hold a job. And anyone who could perform these gymnastics was certainly able-bodied enough to work, including as a longshoreman.

"When you're done, Fanny, would you put on your call light? I'll need to rehook your leads and do your assessment."

Immediately the woman jerked her arms and legs in one, two, three final twitches, like a cartoon character in its death throes, and went completely limp. With a soft puckery sound, she dropped her jaw and let a gob of saliva, tainted with Mars bar, spill out onto the pillow.

"When you regain consciousness, Fanny, let me know."

I turned. The call bell went on.

When I turned back, Miss Racklyn was still playing dead. I reached over and turned off the call signal. "You rang, Miss Racklyn?"

Miss Racklyn's round, lashless eyes fluttered open. "What happened? Did I have another seizure?"

"I don't think it was a seizure, Miss Racklyn. I'm not sure what that was. Pretty aerobic stuff, though."

Fanny commenced to have a tug-of-war with the corners of her mouth. The child within her, I am sure, wanted to giggle at her own pranks. To stop the oncoming glee, she frowned and raised her voice, continuing with her list of demands. "I also need to be massaged every couple of hours, and I'll need you to brush my teeth for me at bedtime and first thing when I wake up. Plus, I need to be flossed after every—"

The "need to be flossed" part was the straw that landed on my tilt button. "Miss Racklyn?"

She took a generous bite—like two thirds—out of the Mars bar and gave me her innocent attention.

"Fanny, listen. I have three other patients besides yourself to care for tonight. If you want to hire a private nurse or a personal secretary while you're here, you're going to have to arrange to have one brought in at your own expense. As for the pizza and Coke, if Dr. Hunt wrote you an order for it, well, it's your cholesterol and triglycerides, but remember, this is a critical care unit, not a Chuck E. Cheese pizza parlor. I'll do a lot of things, Fanny—I might even be talked into doing my Marlo Thomas imitation of 'That Girl'—but I don't do pizza deliveries and I don't floss other people."

I turned to go, and remembered something else. "Oh, and I think you're perfectly capable of rearranging your own limbs. You're too young to be suffering from FMPS."

"FMPS?"

"Fluff My Pillow syndrome, Fanny. A bad habit to get into. It might go over big in Beverly Hills hospitals, but not here." I paused. "And if I were to dispense with my deodorant, Miss Racklyn, you really would have a seizure."

"What's with Linda Blair?" asked Beth, indicating Fanny. "I went in to answer her light and she performed the jumping-bed scene from *The Exorcist*, then asked me to arrange her limbs and do her mid-evening flossing."

I gave Beth an amused glance. "Yeah, and what did you tell her?"

"I asked her why she felt she couldn't do her own flossing and rearranging, and she said it was because she was a very special person." Beth snatched the pen out from behind Phoebe's ear and searched for a blank patient info card among the paper rubble that was the clerk's desk. "When I asked her why she thought she was so special, she said because when she was in school, the counselors put her into all the special classes."

After Beth and I set up the rooms for her two new admissions—a postop four-vessel bypass graft and a fulminating pulmonary edema—we turned Mr. DeGraff and "rearranged" Fanny's limbs. Having an audience of two was more good fortune than Fanny could bear, for we had no sooner finished than she had a seizure to beat the band. Beth and I had to physically restrain her from flinging herself off the bed.

Well trained by Alcoholics Anonymous (or, as she referred to it, the Big Double A Club), Beth dealt with Fanny's attempts at manipulation by being bluntly to the point. This did not go over well, however, as evidenced by Fanny's ordering Beth out of her room and throwing a half-eaten Mars bar at her retreating back.

"So, have you heard the latest episode of *As Redwoods Rotates*?" Beth asked when we'd returned to the nurses' station.

I shook my head. Since Risen's departure, gossip was not as easy to come by, and hanging out in the stairwells seemed too desperate.

"What's your friend's name? The Southern gal who works ER?"

I set down my pen, heart pounding. "You mean Gus?"

She nodded. "Last Wednesday swing shift, the supervisor told her she had to stay to cover a sick call on nights because they couldn't find anybody else to come in. Your friend had already worked day shift, then covered a sick call on evening shift, which meant if she did the night shift, she would have worked twenty-four consecutive hours—so she refused to stay. The head nurse had to be called to take the shift."

I whistled under my breath and made the face Lucy Ricardo always made after Ricky bellowed, "Lucy? I think you got some 'splainin' to do." Gene's reaction to being called at midnight with the news he had to work a night shift because his staff had all refused to cover must have been something to hear. I would love to have seen the hole in his ceiling where he'd gone through the roof.

"She came back to work two days later," continued Beth, "and immediately got into a heated argument with the head nurse. He threatened to suspend her for abandonment of her patients, so when Gus told him he couldn't do that, the confrontation escalated and the guy went ballistic. She's filed harassment charges against him."

I forced myself to take a deep breath and let go of the initial anger. I even managed a smile. Ever since Gus filed a grievance against the hospital over Gene's changes for on-call work obligations, she'd been on the warpath with the man. Only the holiday issue had been won on that round, but it was enough to get Gus labeled as a rabble-rouser. Gene wanted her skin and he wouldn't rest until he got it.

I sighed and shook my head. "Yeah. Well, I wish her luck."

"Wow." Beth pulled back, regarding me with a certain amount of disbelief. "That's pretty tame coming from you. I figured I was going to have to physically restrain you from tearing down to ER and hanging the guy by his nuts."

"Not anymore," I said softly. "I'm cooked on politics."

"Hold it." Beth rolled over to my chair until she was knee to knee. "I don't believe this is Echo Heron speaking—champion of nurses' rights and the disturber of shit."

"Believe it," I insisted. "I'm tired. All that hassling and defending for the good cause, and inevitably always losing out to the greedy guys with all the power?" I looked at my co-worker and set my jaw. "It gets old, Beth, especially when you can't win and you know it'll never stop.

"Take this latest incident: Gus will go through the stress wringer—she'll lose sleep and income, she'll be publicly humiliated and have her emotions turned into mincemeat. In the end—provided she doesn't get a judge who has his fingers in the hospital corporate pie—she'll be reinstated to a job where she'll always be subject to abuse. And *then* what? Gene or somebody else will persist in making her life miserable. They'll single her out and fault her for the smallest thing, possibly even try to take her to court again. They'll wear her down until she quits." Fiercely, I pulled Fanny's perfectly normal lab reports off the printer.

"And in her place, they'll put a new grad who won't receive half the pay or benefits Gus gets and won't rock the boat besides. It's fruitless, kid." I stopped, sorry I had let myself get worked up. The beast of frustration residing in the space next to my ulcer was beginning to snort fire.

"I suppose this means you're giving up on the decentralization policy?" Beth's expression was one of annoyance. "You've got to know that nobody is going to pick up that ball if you drop it, and we desperately need to get this unit decentralized."

"I'll finish what I've started, Beth, but I'm not going to prolong the misery after that."

"What about your lectures?"

"Different can of beans altogether. As long as I'm out of the direct line of fire, I can boost nurses' morale and teach them how to fight the power and control mongers until I drop. It's easier to fight other people's battles when you're in the foxhole wearing a business suit and a bulletproof shield. If you . . ."

Beth's attention shifted to something over my left shoulder. From her expression, I assumed either Death or Gene himself was standing behind me.

"Call me a taxi, right now."

I turned to face the voice and saw a fuming Fanny Racklyn holding two hospital blankets rolled up under one arm, a pillow and her purple canvas duffel bag under the other. She looked strange standing there in her street clothes. Instead of the helpless, bedridden patient, she was now a four-foot-eleven-inch gnome in garb of oversized yellow sweats with a red handknit Santa Claus cap to top off the image.

Neither Beth nor I spoke right away, probably out of sheer wonder at the bizarre though endearing sight before us.

"I said, call me a taxi." Fanny stamped her foot for emphasis.

"Okay," said Beth in that deadpan tone of hers. "You're a taxi."

I shot Beth a chastising scowl and went to Fanny. "What's the trouble, Miss Racklyn?"

"I don't want to stay here and be ignored." Fanny pouted. "You haven't been in to see me for twenty minutes, so I'm going to Mercy Hospital—they have nicer nurses."

"What," I asked, "would make me a nicer nurse, Fanny?"

This seemed to tip the delicate balance of Fanny's reasoning power, for her eyes began to frantically canvass the nurses' station as if for snipers. After a bit of shuffling, she rallied. "I want a back rub and a story about a beautiful princess."

The childish innocence of her request melted me. I put my arm around her broad and muscular shoulders, meaning to guide her back to her room, and found it was like trying to move the Rock of Gibraltar. "Okay, okay," I said, giving in. "I'll give you a back rub and a fairy tale about a princess, but you've got to promise you won't do your seizure thing until I'm done."

Fanny thought about this for a long time. While she thought, I tried to take the blankets out from under her arm and inadvertently got into a silent tug-of-war which I clearly lost.

Finally she nodded. "I promise."

"Good. Now let's get you back into bed and arrange your limbs."

Mrs. DeGraff came into the unit led by Dr. Voorhees. If you could ignore the surfeit of diamonds decorating her person and the fact she was slightly drunk, she could have passed for someone's proper, white-haired old grandmother.

Dr. Voorhees guided the elderly woman to the chair next to mine and held her arm while she unsteadily lowered herself into it. Both Phoebe and I stopped what we were doing to gawk at the dazzle of her gem collection: two sets of earrings (clip-on *and* pierced), a diamond necklace, and a diamond-and-ruby bracelet gaudy enough to make a bat blink. On each finger blazed lots of gold and carats. Rings being my passion, I forced myself not to gape.

"Echo is Elmer's nurse tonight, Mrs. DeGraff. She's going to listen to our conversation and maybe she can help clarify some things for you, okay?"

Mrs. DeGraff nodded impassively in my direction before her attention wandered to bed 17, where Beth was trying to keep her patient from going into respiratory arrest.

"Mrs. DeGraff?" Dr. Voorhees leaned forward to catch the woman's eye. "Mrs. DeGraff, your husband is debilitated beyond our capabilities to help him." Dr. Voorhees opened the chart and took out a packet of lab reports, which he set before her. Mrs. DeGraff glanced at them without much interest, then back at the doctor.

"His prognosis isn't very good. He's sustained enough damage to his heart this time that I expect it may stop again." The young physician took Mrs. DeGraff's hand. "Elmer is in pain, he *wants* to die, Bernice. You need to let him die with some dignity."

"I'll think about it," Mrs. DeGraff replied, smiling. It was strange to see so much coldness coming from such a sweet face.

"I'd like you to let me know before you leave," Dr. Voorhees said. His jaw muscle was jumping from being clenched so hard.

Mrs. DeGraff's smile did not falter. That seemed impressive in a fiendish way, and I decided right then and there this woman needed to run for public office.

"Well, doctor, I might be able to let you know in the morning, but until then, I want everything done to keep him alive." Mrs. DeGraff paused, almost coquettishly dabbing at dry eyes. "You have no idea how difficult this is for me, doctor. I depend on you to make things easier."

I bit the inside of my cheek to keep from groaning. Blanche DuBois was alive and kicking in San Francisco.

Dr. Voorhees watched her without changing his expression. At last he stood with a sigh. "Okay, Mrs. DeGraff, you win. You're the one that has to live with this on your conscience."

"Did you want to see your husband, Mrs. DeGraff?" I asked.

She looked doubtful. "No, I don't think so. Not today."

"I think you should, Mrs. DeGraff," I said as firmly as possible. "He needs to see you."

The woman stood unsteadily and looked around. She might have been looking for her husband's room, but I think it more likely she was looking for the way out.

Taking advantage of her hesitation, I pulled her into her husband's room.

"Elmer?" I touched the man's back, noticing that his shoulder blades, thick, bony protuberances, looked like the naked stumps of wings. Mr. DeGraff opened his eyes. "Elmer, your wife is here."

Bernice DeGraff sat in the chair next to his bed, rested her chin on the side rail, and grinned drunkenly down at him. At the sight of his wife, his eyes widened, then narrowed with cold, intense hatred. "Do you like my new earrings, Elm?" Mrs. DeGraff turned slightly and fingered the lower of the two sets. "I bought them with what I got for that old boat of yours."

Mr. DeGraff's right arm jerked away from his body about two inches. His trembling fist tightened. With each violent jab, albeit short jab, the fist moved closer to his wife's face. Bubbles formed at the side of his mouth as he used the grunting noises coming from his throat to make a specific sound: "Gaaaaa . . . itch . . . itch . . . Ga ga itch."

I had to restrain myself from coaching him on how to make the "b" sound.

Mrs. DeGraff moved back from his pistoning fist. "Your fishing equipment went with the boat, of course. And, oh, I almost forgot—I gave your gun collection to Thelma's boy. I figured you weren't going to use them anymore. You don't mind do you, Elm? I know you don't like Randy, but at least he'll use them instead of letting them sit around gathering dust."

Mr. DeGraff's coloring turned purple. His IV bottles clanked on their poles with the strength of his shaking. Behind me, the alarms on his monitor were going crazy. I didn't need to look at the screen to know the regularly irregular bleeps weren't harmless interference. It was all the warning sign I needed to know the man was going to code.

Quickly, I drew the woman away from the bed. "That's enough. We need to let him rest now."

In a brief, awkward scuffle, Mrs. DeGraff pulled her arm out of my grip and leaned over her husband to whisper in his ear. The violence of his reaction at whatever she had said set him off choking. I half shoved, half guided her to the door and motioned to Phoebe to get her out of the unit. Pulling the oxygen bag from the wall, I fitted the mask over the man's face and gave him a couple of breaths, before the anguish in his eyes made me stop.

Please let me die. Please let me die. It couldn't have been any clearer if he had shouted it over the public address system.

I looked away and found the compassionate eyes of Dr. Voorhees. A world of understanding passed between us in that brief glance. We were guardians of life, but we were also there to provide an untroubled transition into death. In the bible of the caregiver, dignity and comfort in death were as important as healing in life. We'd both held the dying in our arms and been witness to their needs. The manner in which their eyes sought ours and held us until their souls were gone had convinced me years before that we were not meant to die alone, in pain, or without peace.

The monitor alarm went off, loudly alerting us to the ventricular fibrillation presently dividing the screen. Mr. DeGraff's eyes rolled back in his head.

I lowered the side rails with the intent of delivering a precordial thump, except my fist, now hovering uncertainly above Mr. DeGraff, had nowhere to go. His frozen legs and arms had created an almost impenetrable fortress around the center of his chest.

Finally wedging an arm between his knees, I pulled back to execute a sort of horizontal punch, when Dr. Voorhees grabbed my arm. "Don't do it," he said. "We aren't going to put this man through more hell."

"Hey guys, you got V fib in here," Phoebe whispered from the door. "Do you want me to call a code or what?"

Eric hesitated, then shook his head. "We're going to do a slow code—just between us."

At once, Phoebe drew the curtain around the bed while I silenced the alarm. "Okay," Phoebe said, staring at the dying man with an expression of both compassion and anxiety. At the door she glanced back over her shoulder. "Mrs. DeGraff is waiting outside."

Eric walked—slowly—to fetch the crash cart.

I didn't turn around to watch the monitor. Instead, I carefully wiped the sweat off Elmer DeGraff's face with a corner of the bedsheet. His hand somehow slipped into mine. For a block of interminable seconds, I massaged his fingers, and when his body's involuntary struggle began, I inserted an oral airway into his slack mouth and pumped in air. Despite the forced oxygen, his skin steadily grew purplish gray.

Mr. DeGraff's pupils, already dilated and fixed, were turned, unseeing, toward the ceiling. He'd vacated the premises so rapidly, it appeared as though he'd jumped at the small leeway of time we gave him to escape safely beyond our reach.

I closed his eyes and wished his spirit peace. There was no question in my heart that to allow the man to die without interference was morally right. Still, I felt uneasy. Certainly, this was not the first off-the-record, walk-don't-run code I had ever been a part of, but Mrs. DeGraff disturbed me. Who knew how deep her frustration ran, or what she would do once her whipping post was gone?

The front end of the red crash cart came through the curtains.

Eric opened one of the drawers more carefully than was necessary, and removed the intubation tray.

"Is he gone?" he asked.

I nodded and withdrew the defibrillator paddles, spreading the conduction paste over their surfaces. Mr. DeGraff's heart defied the first two electrical shocks, and returned to ventricular fibrillation. With the third defibrillation, his rhythm deteriorated from V fib to the wide, agonal pattern denoting cardiac death.

Eric spoke quietly to his patient while he made a half-hearted attempt at intubation. The steady, soothing stream of words brought up memories of the rare nights my father would sit at my bedside and tell me stories until he fell asleep.

As soon as I sensed that certain change in the atmosphere, which, to my way of thinking, is the final and irrevocable departure of the soul, I checked the man's pupils again. In my charting I would note that they were fixed and dilated. In actuality, it was just one more verification for the chart reviewers that Elmer DeGraff no longer existed.

Blood pressure and pulses weren't obtainable, although his lungs still worked at taking a silent breath now and again. The breaths were reflexive, and could go on for a time after a person was dead, in much the same way the heart could have sporadic electrical activity. I knew the clinical reasons for this, yet I still found it unnerving. Wrapping a body for the morgue in which the heart continues to beat from time to time is an eerie experience.

"Get out the medications," Dr. Voorhees said. "We'll push a few in . . . for the records."

I nodded in understanding. We would do all that was medically required in order to satisfy legal dictates, though it seemed ludicrous to be pushing medications into a dead man.

Taking a soapy washcloth, I washed down Mr. DeGraff's body, wondering how many Normal People would be shocked at what we had done. From the startled reactions I got from my interviews alone, I knew that most Americans didn't realize to what extent euthanasia was practiced in healthcare institutions throughout the country. What experienced nurse hadn't given that dose of morphine to the suffering terminal patient knowing it would ease them into death? And what seasoned physician hadn't run a slow code, or ordered that the patient be kept comfortable at the end—at any cost?

Once, on a call-in show in Texas, I'd been asked accusingly why I didn't consider myself a murderess for having assisted in the ending of other people's lives.

My initial response was to tell the caller that she had to have been there to understand. But lest I be accused of flippancy, I invited her to imagine her dearest loved one as terminally ill. I told her to envision that person during the final days of his illness—not rested, peaceful, and well groomed, as the movies would paint the portrait, but rather, debilitated and crying out with pain that refuses to subside even when the maximum dosage of pain medication has been given.

Perhaps that spouse or child or parent is drowning in his own fluids, having to work at every breath, never able to relax for one minute or else he will suffocate. Picture the skin to be pasty white, gray, or mustard yellow and hanging from his bones because most of the muscle has wasted away. Or maybe this person is bloated from the fluids his heart doesn't have the strength to pump and his kidneys cannot filter. Yellowish fluid seeps from his paperlike skin, which tears apart at the slightest stress. Large pressure sores have developed on his shoulders, heels, and coccyx, but he can't be moved because the chance of breaking fragile bones is great. Infection is constantly present, opportunistic bacteria easily invading the body that has little or no immune system left.

Imagine this person you love suffering day after day, where a minute for him feels like an eternity in hell, then think about the fact that you are responsible for continuing that pain.

I ended my explanation to the caller by saying that I did not feel anything like a murderess, but more like a merciful human being.

". . . and so, the beautiful princess got a job as a stock girl at the local grocery store, started eating healthy foods, got plenty of exercise, lost weight, and made lots of new friends. Then she lived modestly but happily ever after."

Without taking my eyes off Fanny, I tiptoed to the door humming the Winnie-the-Pooh lullaby. The deep, regular breaths that bordered on snores, blew in and out of the gaping cavern of her well-flossed mouth. As I switched off the light, one eye opened and caught me ready to leave. At once she began staging another seizure.

"Fanny, you promised."

One leg fell to the bed, though her arms still trembled, hovering a few inches in the air. I knew unless I threw in extra incentive, she'd break her word.

"No seizure, and I'll make sure the night nurse lets you sleep in instead of waking you up at five to weigh you."

Fanny's whole body relaxed. "Can you tell me another story?" she asked, unashamed.

I started to laugh, until I saw Mrs. DeGraff enter the unit and weave her way toward Dr. Voorhees, whose back was to her. My eyes searched the new widow for a weapon.

"Fanny, I've got to take care of something right now, but if I get some time before you're asleep, I'll come back and tell you the story about the Sunshine Girl and the Frankenstein rabbit."

In answer, Fanny switched on the TV, knit her brows together in a frown, and pulled another Mars bar out from under her pillow.

"What have you done with him?" Mrs. DeGraff asked. Tears rolled from her red-rimmed eyes and down the lapels of her royal-blue wool coat.

"He's in his room. I'll take you to him." Dr. Voorhees placed a hand under her elbow, but Mrs. DeGraff slapped him away.

"You idiot. I mean, what did you do to my husband? You let him die. I told you not to let him die."

Before the physician could respond, Mrs. DeGraff sank to her knees, beating the carpet with her fists. "Elm, Elm, what have they done? What am I going to do without you?"

I was trying to get her off her knees, when Dr. Voorhees reached down and pulled her to her feet. Throwing her arms around me, she buried her head in my neck. Her wiry, white hair felt like coarse steel wool against my cheek.

"He's all I had," she sobbed close to my ear. "He was my life."

I disentangled myself and let her lean against the wall. The combined smell of alcohol/garlic breath, stale lipstick, and Chanel No. 5 was revolting. "Mrs. DeGraff, he's at peace. He wanted desperately to be allowed to die."

"Oh, of course." The woman narrowed her eyes and bared her dentures. "The only thing the dirty bum was desperate about was getting away from me. He was trying to divorce me when he had his stroke. If he'd had his way, he would have ditched me forty years ago."

She looked to each of us for understanding, genuine grief in her eyes. Pressing my hand fervently, she told me in one long whimpery sob how she'd been trying to make him fall in love with her since the day they were married. "I couldn't let him go or I would have been alone. That's what he wanted, you know. He knew how much I hated being by myself."

In the space of a second, her grief turned again to fury. She balled her fists and pressed them against her eyes. "The god-damned louse can rot in hell!" she cried, clapping her hands to her ears, her body bent over as if in pain. "What am I going to do now? He was my life."

I conducted the confused widow to her husband's body, wondering if we were dealing with some kind of complex schizophrenia or a simple case of love-hate addiction/power-control disorientation. It must have been contagious, for I played right into her mental jumble by experiencing both justification and guilt over having helped Mr. DeGraff die peacefully.

At the bedside, she threw herself on him, wailing like a grief-stricken elephant who has just lost its mahout. From the way Dr. Voorhees was nervously shaving the top of his thumbnail with his front teeth, I assumed the detailed horrors of a malpractice investigation were marching steadily through his imagination.

I mentally reviewed the code we'd documented, and then studied Mrs. DeGraff, whose hysterics were part dramatics, part alcohol, and part real grief. I doubted she would ask for an autopsy, nor would she question further what had happened.

What would be the purpose? Elmer had finally escaped her clutches, and her role as jailer/tormentor was over.

"What a case for living wills and health proxies, huh?" Phoebe cut another EKG strip from Mr. DeGraff's "code" and pasted it in his chart.

"Tell me about it," I said, signing off the code blue sheet.

"Hey guys, guess who just rolled into ICU?" Beth moved gracefully around the desk and put her canvas dinner sack, now empty, into the duffel bag she used as a carryall purse. Inside, I briefly glimpsed a pair of scuffed black dance slippers, a doggie chew toy, a half-darned man's sock, and a Huggie diaper—items that perfectly illustrated her present life.

Renewed sobriety and therapy had worked magic for her, engendering a happy marriage, a new son, and a second career as a member of a San Francisco dance troupe. Dobbie, who continued to live with her adoptive mistress, was enjoying her new family status as oldest child.

"Hopefully," said Phoebe, a zealous Democrat, "it's Dan Quayle and Dr. Kevorkian."

"Yeah," I chimed in, "either that or Dan's come to see if they can reverse the zoograft he had done on his brain at birth."

Beth did not smile. "Risen's been admitted to the step-down unit. I think he's on his way out."

Phoebe put a hand to her mouth and sat down. Gooseflesh spread out over my arms and scalp, although I wasn't surprised. I had visited Risen two weeks before and seen reflected in his sunken eyes the impatient specter of death. For over a year he had fought the unbeatable foe. Gravely ill and weak though he was, Risen had managed to hold on, not giving up an iota of his old fighting spirit.

With his bones propped up by no fewer than twenty pillows, Risen conducted daily salons from a brass daybed that was placed directly in front of the large bay windows of his apartment.

Visitors from the gay community and the hospital provided him with a constant supply of the most intimate and confidential gossip. People did not hold back secrets—even other people's secrets—from the dying. We all found ourselves disclosing confidences that we had sworn never to reveal to another living soul. But all one had to do was look in those death-bright eyes to know Risen would not have long to betray our small trusts.

Always the storyteller, Risen charmed us with his hilarious accounts of how straight, middle-class society's knickers got all into a twist when forced to deal with AIDS victims. He made the atrocious, mindless injustices committed against him—experiences that would have driven most to assault or at least to verbal abuse—sound like a stand-up comedy routine. His stories of mothers pulling their children out of his way, or old men attacking him with canes, frequently had us rolling on the floor or running for the water closet.

As he talked, his hands worked constantly, making pen-and-ink sketches of those who had come to say goodbye, or of scenes from the street below, until there were stacks of drawings lying scattered about the floor or on the bed.

The pictures themselves were extraordinary, not only because of Risen's obvious artistic talent, but because they were a visual revelation. Reflected in the faces of his portraits were every reaction, judgment, and emotion a human being might have when sitting leisurely across the table from death itself. The sketches displayed a mother's anguish, a friend's love, a nurse's compassion, an ex-lover's fear, a physician's suppressed anger. Common to all the portraits were the shadings of despair and resignation.

His street scenes depicted everyday life in the gay quarter—men looking for love, men working and playing together, men dressed like women, men loving each other, men dying of AIDS.

"Why couldn't they let him die at home?" I whined. "Risen doesn't want to die in this place."

"Oh Ec," sighed Phoebe. "You know how people taking care of terminal patients sometimes get panicked at the end and run for cover. My brother and I did the same thing when my mother died. See, you guys deal with death once or twice a week—laypeople deal with it only once or twice a *lifetime*. The idea of talking to someone and then finding him dead ten minutes later when you come back from the kitchen with his lunch is too much for most people to handle."

"Yeah, but Risen had nurse friends taking care of him."

"Not every day," said Beth. "On even days, his 'normal' friends took over. Today's an even day."

* * *

At ten-thirty I ran to ICU and found Risen had been transferred to five north, the unofficial AIDS ward of Redwoods Memorial. Since heroic measures for those in the final stages of the virus were rarely requested anymore, the AIDS patients went to five north mostly for last-hour comfort measures. I didn't stop at the desk, but went directly to Risen's room.

Inside, there were two beds: one was stripped down to its green plastic mattress, the other occupied by a young, fair-haired man coughing himself blue. His prominent rib cage worked furiously as the skeletal body fought to keep the breath of life going.

I gave him a few neighborly slaps on the back and poured a glass of ice water. When he'd stopped, I slipped my arm around a bony set of shoulders and held the water to his lips. Before he drank, he smiled at me and gently patted the side of my face.

"Are you okay now?"

"Other than dying of AIDS, I'm fine, thank you."

I giggled and after a second he joined in, although it was difficult for him to breathe around the laughter.

"I thought I'd met all the nurses on five north. Are you new?"

I shook my head. "No, actually I'm looking for my friend, Osbert. The computer had him in that bed." I nodded to the stripped bed. "I think they made a mistake. He's probably next door."

"No mistake," he said, quickly lowering his eyes.

My stomach felt like it had been drop-kicked. I hooked one of my fingers around one of his. It was my way of bracing myself to hear the words.

"He died a few minutes after he was admitted." The boy put his arm around my waist and hugged. "I'm sorry."

We stayed like that until the swelling in my throat subsided and I could speak. "Me too," I said, and stood. "We've lost a very special man."

Tuesday
12:14 A.M.

After work, Beth, Nealy, Phoebe, and I cornered Mr. Cooney and asked him for the key to the morgue. Needless to say, he was reticent, though as soon as we explained, he readily handed it over and asked if he could join us.

Surrounding Risen's slab, we each related a story from his days in CCU. Beth started by telling us about the evening she found him crying after one of his long-term patients had died. Mr. Cooney said he was a fine young man and a good nurse because he never nagged him about losing weight. Phoebe said she had really liked working with Risen because he always took the time to make her laugh at least once a shift with one of his crazy stories. I explained as best I could about what his paintings made me feel. Nealy went last with a story about the night he stowed away in an empty tray cart and had free run of the kitchen. He came back to the unit in the dumbwaiter with two cartons of milk, a gallon of ice cream, and a three-layer chocolate cake.

When I got home, Simon and David were comparing the music of some new rock band—the name of which I can't spell, let alone pronounce—to Cream and Procol Harum. I waited until they were done and told them about Mr. DeGraff and our impromptu memorial service for Risen.

I guess I had expected something more than blank stares—even a hug would have been nice. I retired to the bedroom to nurse my hurt feelings, and of course, have worked myself into my own little self-sorry hole. But it is true that Simon didn't even say hello tonight, and it's the first time I've seen him in weeks. David was also distant, and I guess that he is still disturbed by the conversation we had about our getting a place and officially living together.

He is decidedly reluctant to take that step, and it is rapidly becoming an "issue" in our relationship. Janey insisted that for once in my life, I see the handwriting on the wall and end things gracefully now and on my terms.

It stung so much, I refused to even consider that she might be right. But I keep thinking about the way David's friends look at me when we're out, as if I'm a museum piece or an alien from another generation. And every goddamned time someone has the bad taste to make an age joke, I still cringe inside. I'm getting so tired of forcing the smile and laugh to show what a good sport I am.

I woke up yesterday morning to find David pulling out my gray hairs one by one.

I don't want to think about any of this. As Risen would have said, I have enough on my plate to worry about right now.

I'm tired. My body hates the constant stress at work. I'll write a secret here that I haven't said aloud even to myself: the fulfillment isn't there for me anymore. I don't get excited when someone comes through; I give the credit to fate. Even the idea of working ER doesn't get my blood going half as much as it used to.

On the lighter side: Sean and Cathleen were on the acute side discussing titles for codependent books along the lines of I'm O.K., You're O.K. Cathleen, a maximum-strength codependent, came up with If You're OK, I'm OK, and Sean, the typical avoidance addict, decided her book would be titled, If I'm OK, You Don't Matter. We howled.

I can hear David and Moosh playing their I'll-bite-your-ankle-you-pull-my-tail bedtime game. David's laughter is such a warm and comforting sound; I will enjoy it while it is still mine to hear.

FOURTEEN

"There is no sphere of healthcare that can operate without nurses."

JUDY COLLINS, R.N.

SET SIX INCHES BEHIND A SET OF BARS, the gray metal door boasted four institutional locks and a red "Caution—Do Not Enter—Ring for Assistance" sign. I found a doorbell and pressed. In the distance came the shrill ring of an electric bell. While I waited, I surveyed my surroundings.

Painted that depressing shade of salmon one often finds in funky motels, the cinder-block walls were covered with smudges and bits of graffiti. Penciled on one concrete square was the astute observation "You got to be crazy to come in here!" Next to it, in red lipstick was "Fight hunger—eat the rich," and "All men are dykes." Over the door was a surveillance camera with a Dixie cup jammed over the lens.

Accustomed as I was to the country club posh of Redwoods, the only way I could tell I was in a real hospital and not someplace in Times Square was the PA system paging a Dr. Manly for ER stat, and the distinctive hospital smell of Lysol and dirty socks.

No country club here. This was the heart of the infamous Mercy Hospital, a healthcare institution that was about as frontline as it got. The 302-bed teaching facility, known far and wide for the huge number of patients it could take in and process, could not, by law, turn away anyone seeking help. Mercy was situated in San Francisco's roughest neighborhood, and a large portion of its patients were street people: junkies, gang members, prostitutes, and the destitute gays—human train wrecks often in desperate need of serious medical attention.

Its reputation as one of the most dangerous places to work

was not an exaggeration. Even though a small force of San Francisco police were stationed in and around the hospital, muggings and rapes of staff members occasionally took place.

In 1988, I was allowed for one evening to sit in as an observer at the Mercy emergency triage desk. I will never forget that at the end of the shift, my host, a nurse I'd met at an earthquake trauma workshop, apologized because it had been a slow night.

What he considered a *lack* of chaos consisted of four shootings, three stabbings, four auto-versus-pedestrian survivors, three coding ODs, a near strangulation by hanging, four suicide attempts, and three badly beaten children under five years of age.

There were also five rape cases that came in that night. The victims were two adolescent males, one eight-year-old girl, and a fifty-six-year-old prostitute. The last rape casualty was a twenty-year-old girl who bled to death in one of the trauma rooms. According to the story the police gave, the woman's four attackers raped her repeatedly for over an hour while a group of onlookers cheered them on. When they tired of their sport, they forced an empty wine bottle into her vagina and jumped on her pelvis and buttocks until the bottle smashed inside her.

Footsteps and the jangling of keys opening locks brought me back to the present. The metal door swung open, and a nicely dressed older woman asked to see a photo ID. While I searched for my license, she recited a long, monotone warning about any weapons on my person being confiscated, and having to surrender anything that could be used as a weapon, such as belts, matches, or high heels.

I handed her my driver's license through the bars. She studied it thoroughly, comparing the photo with the human standing in front of her, and when she was finally satisfied we were one and the same (I don't know how it happens, but my driver's license photos always come out looking like someone who has intestinal flu and is in immediate need of a rest room), she unlocked the bars, allowing me to step in as far as the yellow line on the floor. Above the line was the red and white warning "Wait Here Until Search and ID Check Completed."

The door closed with a heavy sound of finality which gave birth to a strong urge to run screaming for the exit. Instead, I smiled and held my arms over my head while the woman ran a metal detector over me and asked if I had any weapons concealed on or in my person. Once I convinced her I was clean of all daggers and firearms, I was given a green stick-on spot to wear on my lapel (rather like the "ripe" stickers on avocados and pears) and told to proceed to the next yellow line.

While I waited, I reconsidered my choice of continuing-education hours. I could have spent twenty or so hours in an oxygen-poor classroom sleeping through dull lectures on eating disorders or menopause as a way to earn the thirty units I needed to renew my R.N. license, but since I had to do this only once every two years, I'd thought I might as well choose something stimulating.

The course I'd chosen, "Management of the Mentally Disturbed Patient: A Practical Experience," sounded like something I would like. I looked around at the prisonlike walls and sighed; next time I'd be more careful and read the course description.

The gatekeeper joined me after several minutes of paper shuffling. "Sorry," she said, "but we have to take every precaution in this unit. It's mostly for your protection. It can get pretty hairy around here—we've had two takedowns just in the last hour."

I nodded, unsure of what a takedown was, but my imagination was having a ball. Oh well, it was too late to be turning back now. And as Gus would have said, I'd already stepped in it, so I might as well continue on and make an effort to enjoy the stink.

It was this thought that stuck in my mind as I passed through the final barred door, which read, "Ward Twelve—Psychiatry."

"I began working here right after I graduated from nursing school," said the eyebrowless but otherwise nondescript woman who was to be my mentor for the day. She picked up the report sheet from the counter, and as she did so, cast me a sidelong glance.

Valerie was a refrigerator person—cold and loaded down with hundreds of containers of moldy, leftover problems from an unfulfilled life. She was the type of middle-aged woman who wore no makeup, but always had her hair sensibly cut earlobe length, who lived alone in a small apartment that smelled of frying butter, wore turtlenecks with large, wooden bead necklaces to divert attention away from her double chin, and owned a short-haired, neurotic, yappy dog, upon which she doted.

When Valerie called the night before to remind me for the fifth time not to wear a uniform or nursing shoes, I'd gotten the impression she either had a bad memory, or was one of those humorless nurses who paid an inordinate amount of attention to detail and always thought logically—Nurse Spock types.

"A show of medical authority might set some patients off," she'd said. "This is a plainclothes kind of nursing—we're undercover helpers, dressed to blend in with the crowd."

I had a good guffaw over that one; when I was doing my psych rotation during nursing school, the thing I found most disturbing was never being able to distinguish the staff from the patients. It was a notion that was confirmed by one of the team leaders when she told me, "Basically, the staff are patients with keys."

"The first thing I learned was how to set limits," Valerie said, plucking at one plump, age-spotted hand. "No dancing, no sex, no hitting, and no stripping. The second thing I learned was to be on my toes and to always be aware of the space allowance between the patient and myself."

"Jeez," I said, smiling, wanting to break her deadly serious tone. "If I'd known this was tantamount to suicide, I would have increased my life insurance. I've got to be at work by three. Should I call in dead or gamble on getting out of here alive?"

"Oh, well, I suppose it's not that bad," she said, laughing weakly—a task she managed to execute without smiling. "But make sure you stay right with me.

"The general routine is to get report on everybody and divide the patients up. Then we go check the charts for orders and interact with the patients, making sure everybody is medicated and under control. We also take care of any medical necessities like taking vital signs if needed, dressing changes, treatments, whatever. After lunch we have a mandatory community meeting for patients and staff."

"When you say you interact with the patients, what do you mean?"

"I mean"—Valerie clucked her tongue impatiently—"we give out meds, and provide them with an opportunity to talk to us. If we have to redirect their energies—"

"Redirect their energies?"

The nurse seemed irritated by the question. "We have to limit their input," she said tersely. "It's difficult for some patients to handle a lot of stimuli either from us or the other patients, so we keep it simple and tell them what to do—give them strict limits so they won't act out their hostility or their delusions. If we let the patients do what they wanted, this place would be bedlam's battleground inside of an hour. These patients have very little impulse control. Basically, they're here so we can protect them from harming themselves or anybody else."

Valerie looked down into her lap as if there were a script there. "Oh, by the way, if you hear someone yell 'Staff'? It means someone is getting hurt. Either a patient is endangering his own or someone else's physical well-being. The word 'staff' has the same effect here as 'code blue' does in the cardiac unit, only instead of a crash cart, we respond with a show of force to get the patient restrained and to the ground."

"That's a takedown?"

"Uh huh, and I'm sure with the way things are going so far, you'll see at least one." Valerie sighed. "The manics have been keeping each other going the last few days, and we've got several patients suffering from delusions who are really crazy—one of them jumped out of the window yesterday."

"Oh my God. Did the person die?"

"No, but he did end up with two broken wrists and a fractured ankle."

"Was he trying to kill himself, or what?"

"Oh no, no, no. This guy isn't suicidal, he's delusional. He jumped because 'They' activated the big magnet hidden under the street and it pulled him out the window."

"Who're They?"

Valerie smiled wanly. Her teeth were the color of an old porcelain sink. "Miss Heron, They take many forms. Usually they're the voices who live inside the patient's mind and tell him what to do."

My own smile faded into a nervous, worried tic. Did my switchboard ladies qualify as Theys?

"Anyway, there are twenty-one patients and six of us to control them. If you hear 'Staff' yelled, run—do not walk—to this room and don't come out until you don't hear any more screams."

"What do I do if somebody tries to talk to me? I mean, should I make believe I'm mute, or . . ."

"Be natural, and don't play into any of the patients' games. You can say you're a visitor, but try not to engage anyone and do not allow anyone to touch you." Valerie fingered a loose thread on the sleeve of her argyle sweater. "Things escalate very quickly with our patients. It's important that you stay right by me."

"I promise I'll be stepping on your heels."

"Good. Just make sure nobody is stepping on yours."

The dayroom was a large, bleak place. The presence of twelve or so yellow plastic chairs, two blue Naugahyde couches, plus the concave security mirrors set high on the hospital-green walls, gave it a flavor of state-funded institution, circa 1955. The room was deserted except for an older woman with dull reddish hair sitting on the couch. She had on her winter coat.

"Good morning, Shirley."

The woman smiled pleasantly at Valerie. For a minute I thought she must be a staff nurse, since this person was a far cry from the shrieking wild beasts for which Valerie had prepared me. "I see that you're going home today. You must be very happy."

The woman giggled. "Yes. Yes. Yes. Yes. Yes. Oh yes. Yes. Home today home today home today yes yes yes home today home today yes yes ye—"

"Stop repeating yourself, Shirley," Valerie commanded calmly. "Is your husband coming to pick you up?"

The woman's hands and fingers suddenly went into hyperspeed action, flittering up and down in front of her—like a saxophonist playing a busy piece of jazz, but without the sax.

Valerie imitated her. "What's this?"

Indignant at Valerie's lack of skill, the faded redhead pushed the nurse's hands down. "Not like *that*," she said, resuming the bizarre hand movements with more vigor. "Like *this*!"

"And what does this"—Valerie adjusted the erratic movements—"do?"

"It keeps the radiation particles away," Shirley said. "They told me it's my protective shield."

"*Who* told you it's your protective shield?" I asked.

Shirley frowned. "I've already told Valerie about Them."

"Would you tell me, because I don't know about Them?"

The woman looked to Valerie for permission. Valerie nodded.

"They put a transmitter in my brain on December seventeenth, 1978. Their voices come through and talk to me."

I nodded. "Uhn huh. And where do the voices come from?"

"Out there," Shirley said, pointing to the windows.

I said something vague, like "Oh," and Valerie captured the woman's flying hands. "Shirley, would you like some medication before your husband gets here to pick you up?"

Shirley shook her head violently. "Not now. They don't like me to take medicine—it gums up their machines."

I caught my laughter before it became audible, and turned away as though searching for something, like either the invisible saxophone or Them.

"Well, I hope everything goes well at home for you, Shirley." Valerie shook the woman's hand.

Shirley knocked at the side of her head a few times. "Oh thank you, thank you thank you thank you thank you thank . . ."

"Transmitters planted in the brain is a very common delusion," Valerie said as we headed down the women's corridor. "I swear, the basic story is so consistent that I almost wonder sometimes if it isn't true."

"How can she be sent home like that?" I asked, recalling as I spoke how a neighbor of mine had recently knocked at my door at six A.M. to tell me there were snakes in the trees between our cottages. "They," she said, wanted her to catch and varnish the reptiles so she could sell them as canes to old men.

"She manages with the help of her husband," Valerie said. "He brings her in when she gets too crazy for him to handle. Then about six weeks pass and he starts missing her and wants her back. By that time, we've readjusted her medications so she's not so wild.

"The husband sat in on our community meeting a couple of days ago and one of the patients asked him how he could stand dealing with her. His answer was, 'Well, I know she's a little peculiar, but I love her and she's mine.'

"I wish they all had somebody like that. People like this next patient we're going to see are completely without support from . . ."

Valerie paused to watch a pile of crumpled laundry tottering toward us. Beneath the sheets and blankets were two slippered feet and the lower portion of a set of spindly legs knobby with blue varicose veins.

The tune "I've Been Working on the Railroad" came from the center of the moving hill, only with different lyrics and in a Spanish accent.

"Oh, I be workin' on de laundry, clean all de filth away. I be workin' on de laundry, gonna bleach out all de gray ..."

"Gabriela?" Valerie stopped the moving hill by taking an armful of sheets off the top. The short Mexican woman stopped singing and peered curiously over the sheets.

"Gabriela, what are you doing?"

"I clean de ladies' rooms. I clean de bathrooms. I clean de beds now," she said innocently.

Valerie cocked her head, evaluating the situation. "Oh. Well, that's nice of you, but you can't disturb China and you can't go into the seclusion room. Do you understand that?"

"I no talk to little China." Gabriela made a quick adjustment of her hairnet. "I stay away from isolation. Dat's de devil in dere."

"And you can't go into the men's corridor."

"Oh no. De men, dey are more filthy. I wait. When dey go home, then I clean."

"No, Gabriela, even if they go, you can't clean in the men's corridor. You can clean only the dayroom today."

Gabriela nodded, taking back her sheets.

"Out-of-control obsessive-compulsive with some probable psychosis going on," Valerie explained when Gabriela had shuffled out of earshot. "She cleans."

"Like what?"

"When she first got here, it was mostly herself. She used to take six or seven showers a day and could go through a sixty-four-ounce bottle of shampoo in two. We put her on water-use restrictions. Now she cleans everything else. Last week I caught her in the garbage bins. She had sorted out the garbage by category: wrappers were neatly stacked, papers were un-crumpled and in piles, the Styrofoam cups were washed and dried. I got to her as she was starting in on the wet garbage, polishing old banana peels."

"Do you think I could take her to my house for a day or two?" I asked.

"She'd be more trouble than you think," said Valerie. "You'd find her washing the neighbors' dogs, or taking down laundry from clotheslines all over town and bringing it home to wash."

"So what do you do with her?"

"Adjust her drug levels until she's manageable, then send her back to her normal life."

"Which is?"

"She's been a housekeeper at the Holiday Inn for the last twenty years."

We'd come to the women's corridor and were standing in the doorway of a room that contained four beds (three of which were stripped, compliments of Gabriela).

The fourth bed was occupied by an extraordinary-looking young Chinese girl. A Chinese Rapunzel, her thick hair hung down over the side of the bed and cascaded onto the floor. It was so long, and she was so petite, that had she been standing, I believe it would have trailed behind her, like the train of a long, black veil. Wrapped waist to toe in thick gauze, she lay on her side rocking, her thin arms clapped over her ears.

Valerie pulled me back into the hall. "Her name is China," she said in a low whisper. "She's twenty-one and is—was a student at S.F. State. Seven weeks ago, she was raped by a street gang. After they finished with her, they shut her hair in a car door and dragged her for about two miles. By the time they let her go, more than half of the skin and muscle had been burned away from her buttocks, legs and heels.

"Her family is traditional Chinese. In their eyes, this daughter has brought shame upon the family. Her boyfriend doesn't want to deal with it, and she didn't have many friends to begin with. One girl from her art classes at State came by to see her once, and never came back."

Valerie went on but I stopped listening, as I am in the bad habit of doing now and then. My mind boggled for the millionth time at the kind of mentality it must take to do these things to other people. Beyond that, what mother and father cast off a daughter whose life had been shattered, and what sort of friend was it who failed those in desperate need?

". . . suicide precautions," Valerie was saying. I noticed she had that beleaguered look about her nurses often have when talking about a patient who doesn't have much hope of recovery. "She won't cooperate with physical therapy and she really doesn't talk much. Mainly, all she tells us is that the spirits made this happen because they didn't like her.

"The first week she was here, she wouldn't take water or

food and certainly not meds, so we got a court order which gave us permission to do whatever we had to to keep her alive and comfortable." Valerie searched around her pockets.

"She's at the point now where she'll take her meds and fluids and some foods on her own, but there's still no real communication going on. Last week she tried to drown herself by holding her head in the toilet. Before that, she tried to strangle herself with her hair." The nurse found what she was looking for deep in her skirt pocket. She pulled out a roll of exotic-looking peppermints and offered me one. "So now she has to be observed twenty-four hours a day."

"How long will you keep her here?" I crunched up the pungent sweet immediately. Valerie would savor the wafer until it dissolved.

She pushed a shock of graying hair behind her ear and shrugged. "Until we're reasonably sure she won't harm herself."

The "reasonably" caused me a moment of doubt. "Then where will she go?"

"We'll try to find relatives or someone in the community to take her, and if that doesn't pan out, we'll wait until a space in a halfway house opens up. As long as she's clothed and fed and takes her meds, she can stay out in the community."

As we entered the room, Valerie nodded to an older man sitting in a red Naugahyde chair in the corner. Ignoring us, China continued to rock, her delicate, pale face turned toward the wall. The gentleman put down the book he'd been reading and stretched before introducing himself to me as Graham, a mental health volunteer who sat with China in the mornings.

"China ate a sweet roll and drank two cups of tea for breakfast," he said, and left quickly, presumably for his break. Later, I realized his hasty departure probably had more to do with his being one of those Normal People who didn't like to see the tragedy under the bandages.

"That's wonderful, China," Valerie said, spreading out a large sauna towel on the unoccupied side of the girl's bed. "You need lots of fluids to heal." She opened the bedside cabinet, which was loaded with boxes of dressings and jars of Silvadine cream. "Now, do you think you can roll onto your stomach over here for your dressing change?"

The girl kept on rocking. I wondered if she could hear anything that was said, or if she was so far down the black hole, she was impervious even to sound.

"I need you to lie on your stomach so I can change your dressings, China." Valerie waited a few seconds, then, in one smooth movement, turned China onto her stomach.

During the dressing change, China never indicated that she felt anything. I cannot fathom what kind of control that must have taken, for when the last layer of gauze was removed and I saw what was left of her legs and buttocks, the skin on the backs of my legs came alive with an ache of its own.

With a sterile tongue blade, Valerie spread the creamy white Silvadine over the holes, filling them in. The scene, if one had the imagination of, say, Clive Barker, invited the image of a nibbled gingerbread person being refrosted.

Valerie talked to her patient from unwrap to rewrap, trying to elicit responses but meeting only with deep silence. When she had taped the last bit of gauze securely around China's toes, Valerie left me alone with her while she went to pour the girl's medications.

I tentatively sat on the bed. It was an unconscious gesture on my part to pick up her hair and stroke it. "You have such beautiful hair, China. I'd give anything to have hair like yours."

For one moment the girl stopped rocking and arranged her body with a sinuous movement. She raised her eyes to my face, allowing herself to glimpse mine. "No," she whispered, hoarsely. "It's bad hair. It's ugly. The spirits hate it."

I had not expected her to respond and was momentarily panic-stricken over what would be the best thing to say. I made an effort to smile. "I think, then, that the spirits are blind. In my eyes, you have beautiful hair."

Her eyes stayed on mine for one more second before she threw up the cloak again and recommenced rocking.

I reported the incident to Valerie when we were headed back to the dayroom for the midmorning snack event, but couldn't judge from the noncommittal tilt of her jaw what she thought about it.

In the dining room, we passed Gabriela, who was once again loaded down with a mountain of laundry. Some sudden suspicion caused Valerie to frown and look back over her shoulder at the squat figure waddling quickly toward the laundry room.

Fresh fruit, granola, and toast were laid out on one dining room table. Pitchers of cold milk and Styforoam cups had been placed on the one next to it. Around this meager display of nutrition was an assembly of folk who made up a virtual smorgasbord of psychological aberrancies.

My eye was drawn to the tallest fellow in the gathering, an emaciated man whose arms and face were all bones and veins. He was attempting to wash his face with a piece of toast. Satisfied with his ablutions, he went through the apples and carefully selected one from the bottom of the bowl. "I'll get it!" he yelled. "It's for me." He put the apple to his ear and began having a conversation about joining an Arthur Murray dance studio. The conversation was quite animated, though he seemed to have trouble modulating his voice. From a normal tone, he would slide up and down octaves and decibels, so that it became a workout for the ears.

I noticed that no one else was paying much attention to him, but rather to the fight that had broken out between a girl with a shaved head and an anorexic-looking woman. They were held back from each other by several members of the staff.

"She touched me with her banana!" screamed the shaved woman. "She's trying to inject me!"

"I did not!" The thin woman waved her banana in the other woman's face. "I didn't want to. She made me."

The thin woman pulled out of the staff's grip and punched the bald-headed woman in the stomach. The bald woman doubled over and collapsed.

Valerie shoved me behind her. With vertiginous swiftness, three staff members had the woman with the banana on the ground. As she went down, her banana went flying, landing on one of the yellow plastic chairs. A man sitting in the next chair over picked it up, put it in his shirt pocket, and resumed talking to the security mirror on the wall.

"Martine and Ellen set each other off constantly," said Valerie when she returned. "We try not to let them near each other, but sometimes it's unavoidable."

"What are they in for?" I asked, in mind of a B movie I'd seen called *Women's Prison*.

Valerie pointed to the previous owner of the assaultive banana as she was being led away from the group. "Martine was found walking naked down Market Street with a pigeon on a leash. She was headed for the top floor of the Bechtel Building, because the pigeon told her he was going to teach her how to fly. . . . Ellen is delusional and manic-depressive."

"Why the shaved head?" I asked.

"She got ahold of the men's razors one morning, shaved off all her hair, and put it in a pillowcase. When we asked her why she did that, she said the hair didn't belong to her and she had to give it back."

"To whom?"

Valerie gave me a you-know-the-answer-to-*that*-one look.

"To Them?"

"Who else?"

Luncheon was served buffet style in the dining room. I found this a curious way to go about a meal in a psych ward, seeing as how these patients seemed to need structure, not freedom of choice.

The line moved at a snail's pace as we waited for each patient to act out to some degree with the foodstuffs. A man who wore a bicycle helmet and a pair of adult diapers (outside his trousers) was having a difficult time choosing a dinner roll because he was afraid it might hatch on his plate, and another who saved his bowel movements and presented them to staff as presents had to wait for orders from his voices before he could decide between the cauliflower and the peas. The person who delayed the process the longest was Ellen. She held her fellow therapized sojourners entranced when, after loading her plate with a pound of mashed potatoes, she sculpted the powdered spuds into a large phallus.

Valerie and I chose a table with two patients. Martine, the delusional pigeon lady, sat to my left, and across from me was a paranoid schizophrenic named Peggy who moved her dinner roll around the table as if it were a Ouija board.

"Steve, the man you saw talking into the apple earlier? He was a former cardiovascular surgeon at Mercy," Valerie said, giving my plate of peas and mushy cauliflower the disapproving fisheye. Vegetarians, even in California, are frequently an object of ridicule at the table. (To try this at home, tell a gathering of carnivores that you don't eat anything that once had eyes, and watch them react.)

"He nicked himself on the wrong patient and came up HIV-positive two years ago. He's been here about two months with AIDS dementia, and he'll probably be here until he dies."

Out of the corner of my eye, I watched Martine watching my peas. Her eyes shone with covetous joy.

"Worst part of it is that he's aware of what's happening to him." With difficulty, Valerie speared her chicken breast and sawed through the soggy, fatty skin with a plastic knife. "Once in a while he becomes rational and talks about it, mainly about what a waste it is, but lately he's been getting worse. The other day I found him trying to brush his teeth with his shoe."

I felt a wet tickle near my wrist and glanced over. Martine was painstakingly placing four of my peas in a neat row on my arm. My mother would have been gratified to see this; she, or her programmed tape, had reminded me during every meal of my childhood that I had not been brought up in a barn, and to get my arms off the table.

"Is AIDS dementia like Alzheimer's?" I asked, aware of a rising nausea related to watching Valerie relish a hefty piece of chicken fat. I turned my head away, only to discover that the line of peas was to my elbow, and that Martine had branched out into cauliflower, using the watery white pulp to decorate my watch.

"Um, kind of, except the AIDS dementia patients are a little more aware, plus they come in and out. Alzheimer patients lose it quicker and stay gone."

Valerie suddenly rose from her seat, straining to see something in the concave security mirror. Wiping her mouth, she set her napkin down and pushed back her chair. "There are two blind spots in these mirrors," she said, "and the repeaters know exactly where to go to be in them."

Unable to get the view she wanted, Valerie finally got up and went around the column to a corner yellow chair. I followed, scattering peas and cauliflower as I went.

In the chair was the same young man who had put the banana in his pocket, busily engaged in a bit of after-lunch masturbation.

"Jonathan, you can't do that here," Valerie said matter-of-factly. Actually, she sounded disappointed she hadn't caught him doing something more destructive. "You need to do it in your room or in the shower."

Jonathan stopped and pulled up his zipper, looking like he'd lost a good friend.

"If you need to, you can finish that in the shower."

The man shook his head. "Can't leave the chair."

Valerie softened. "Of course you can leave this chair if you want to, Jon."

Jonathan shook his head again. "Third yellow chair from the pillar. If I get up, They'll shoot me in the nuts."

"Do you remember what we said yesterday when we talked about this?"

Jonathan nodded.

"Do you remember that you said if you really wanted to, you could stop listening to those voices? You said you—"

In the next split second, Valerie's hand whipped around and grabbed me by the collar. At the time, I was in mid-sit, my rear end just two inches from the blue Naugahyde couch. The action so startled me that I yipped, lost my balance, and toppled over onto Jonathan. Without letting go, she yanked me off his lap and set me on my feet.

The chilling look she gave me—a bug-eyed what-the-hell-do-you-think-you're-doing stare—sent terror through my heart. It was the same look my grade school violin teacher used to give me. I managed to say, "What the hell?" before she whisked me back to the dining room by my sleeve.

"My fault," she said, tugging at the skin of her neck. There were splotches of red all over it. It was the most excited I'd seen her all morning. "I'm sorry, I should have told you. *Never* sit on those blue couches."

I raised my eyebrows until I could feel my eyeliner stretch out and crack.

"Patients use their body fluids to act out. Those couches are shit on, peed on, vomited on, ejaculated on, bled on, or spit on at least once a day." Valerie flushed. "Euew. It makes me sick to my stomach to even think of the bacteria that are collected on those things. Nobody from staff ever sits on them."

"Why don't you sic Gabriela on them with some Clorox and a scrub brush?"

"Gabriela won't go near them," Valerie said. "That should give you a clue as to how dirty they are."

An ancient old man appeared at the other end of the room, carrying a pillow crushed tightly to his chest. In truth, I'd been watching him appear for the better part of fifteen minutes, for he was moving across the room as slow and steady as hands on an electric clock. When I first spotted him, I thought he might have been in some sort of catatonic state, but after a while, I could see a progression toward the nurses' station.

"What's with the old man with the pillow?" I asked. "Looks like he's in need of thyroid medication."

"Mr. Lever? We call him Slow Mo. He's pretty speedy today—usually he's just finished drinking his breakfast juice by the time lunch is over."

Slow Mo slid his left foot about three inches in front of his right and paused.

"His brain transmitter has been giving him the same messages for three years," Valerie said. "They warn him that if he moves too fast, he'll cause the earth to rock and we'll all fall off. He carries the pillow to protect himself from crash landings."

"Doesn't he freak with everybody else rushing past him?"

"He never looks up from his feet." She watched him with what I interpreted as fondness. "And talk about delusions of grandeur." Valerie let go of a tiny smile. "Slow Mo thinks he was responsible for the last big quake because he sneezed by mistake and it threw him off balance."

It was time for Wednesday's community meeting, and everyone was assembled in the dayroom. Extra chairs had been dragged over from the dining room and were now interspersed with the yellow ones.

Martine and Ellen sat on one of the blue couches, billing and cooing like best friends. China was placed to one side of the group, where she sat rocking in her wheelchair. Her long hair was piled behind her shoulders, so that it doubled as a pillow. Looking lost without a pile of laundry or a cleaning rag, Gabriela sat surreptitiously polishing the arm of her chair with the sleeve of her sweater.

Trevor, the staff team leader, made the introductory comments, which were directed mainly at the new patients. This preamble resembled the rules board at the entrance of a reform school: no sexual conduct, no foul language, no hitting, no hurting, no spitting, no smoking, and clean up after yourself.

After the rules came a moment of coughs and seat rustlings. Trevor crossed his legs. "So, who would like to start?"

The standard minute of beginning-meeting silence prevailed wherein everyone feels that panicky pressure of needing to come forth and break the ice but hopes that, by some miracle, no one will say a word, and the meeting will be over.

Martine dashed everyone's hopes by raising her hand. "I'd like to say something." Ellen started to cackle, which made Martine angry, though she giggled in spite of herself. "I want to say that I . . . Quit it, Ellen!"

Ellen was pulling on Martine's sweatshirt, trying to tickle her under the arms.

"Ellen, you need to take a ten-minute time-out in your room, please," Valerie said firmly.

"But she made me—"

"Ellen! A ten-minute time-out. Now!"

The bald woman scratched the top of her scalp with a long, thin finger, then spun around abruptly to punch the arm of the couch. "I won't! Martine made me laugh. She's trying to suck out my brains!"

Trevor stood and pointed in the direction of the women's corridor. There was something so extremely threatening about the gesture that I cringed.

Ellen, however, made a noise like a sumo wrestler expelling an awesome amount of flatus, stuck out her tongue at Trevor, and huffed out—walking backward.

With a relative quiet restored, Martine continued. "I want everyone to stop trying to control my brain," she said.

"No one is trying to control your mind, Martine," said a nurse with a bad case of eczema on her hands and face.

From his seat on the floor, Jonathan innocently raised his hand and said, "I am."

This response must have been irresistible to those short on impulse control, because immediately a chorus of "Me toos" rose up . . . and up, until the whole place was in an uproar, with cries of "*I'm* controlling her brain," and "No you're not. *My* voices are telling Martine what to do."

A squall of slap fights broke out among several female patients, and instantly people were hollering nonsensical things and getting out of their seats. The jumble of sights and sounds was—well, anyone could imagine it, especially anyone who'd ever seen *The Snake Pit*.

Half the staff members sprang for the slapping patients and herded them off toward seclusion. Two patients had to be coaxed out from under their chairs.

I noticed that China's wheelchair, left unlocked, had been shoved off to the side. The girl sat doubled over, clutching her hair in an attitude of self-protection.

Chucking my role as invisible and inactive observer, I wheeled her back to her room and waited for the afternoon sitter to find us.

"Boy, that was something I don't get to experience every day." I laughed, helping the thin girl onto her bed. "Did you see the guy who was making believe he was conducting an orchestra? And the other lady who was dancing over by the—"

"J.J. and Rachel."

I glanced around at the doorway, thinking the voice had come from that direction, but found no one there.

"They're funny," said China.

I knew it was China who spoke because I was staring at her, watching her mouth move. "Who is the old guy who asks everybody to sign his autograph book?" I asked.

"Billy Ball."

"And the guy in the helmet and diapers?"

"Duffy."

I smiled and took her hands in mine. I was ecstatic that she did not pull them back. "Do you know everybody's name?"

She nodded.

"You must have a wonderful memory. I can't remember my own name sometimes."

She looked at me with some concern. "What *is* your name?"

"Echo."

China smiled. "That's pretty."

I almost jumped up with glee. "Thank you. China is a very unique and lovely name too."

She started to say something, looked off into space, and then, as quickly as she had opened, closed her inner door and began to rock.

"Was that a normal community meeting?"

Valerie was sulking, prune-faced and uncommunicative.

"No, of course not." She sniffed. "The patients are usually too sedated to all go off at once like that."

"So what happened?"

"Things escalated faster than we could control. If we hadn't taken command of the situation as fast as we did, someone would have hit the panic button."

"Is the panic button a figurative term or is it a real but—"

"It is the ultimate in takedowns," Valerie said. "Even They have to respect the panic button."

Valerie's keys made a coming-home sound as she nervously jiggled them in her pocket. "This is called a seclusion room." She pointed to the metal door with the one-way mirror. "The patient in here is extremely psychotic and paranoid—probably one of the craziest patients I've ever taken care of."

For a moment the nurse hesitated. I sensed she was wavering between suppression and confession. "Several of the staff honestly believe she's possessed," she said finally.

"Oh, come on."

"I kid you not. I'm an atheist myself, so I don't put much stock in those things, but I will say the lady behind this door is pretty ungodly."

Shading my eyes, I looked through the mirrored window in the door and drew back. The instant, overall impression of what I'd seen was akin to the back room of a carnival freak show.

As we passed into the cell-like room, a coarse, fetid animal smell, warm and heavy, rolled over us. On the bed lay a grossly obese woman of about forty whose thick wrists and ankles were tightly bound to the corners of the bed by heavy leather straps with a steel lock on each one. The cotton patient gown had pulled up over the dark brown flesh of her belly, exposing rolls of fat and a strip of black hair that grew upward from her pubic mound to her navel. The gown itself was wet with urine.

Only after my senses became accustomed to the smell and sounds of that room did I begin to notice finer details, like the chafed skin under her restraints and the open mouth which contained no teeth.

Set deep into that face was a set of strange eyes. I saw a wildness in them that went far beyond the borders of insanity and into a realm that belonged to something very dark.

She seemed to be listening intently to something only she could hear. Several times she nodded or mumbled, "I hear you," as if someone were giving her instructions or relating an interesting story.

She watched mistrustfully as I inched closer to the bed, moving as fast as Slow Mo. When I got within six feet of her, she growled, then let out a high-pitched stream of words, some of which I recognized as Italian and French swear words with Latin phrases from the Catholic High Mass mixed in.

"Her name is Inez." Valerie spoke close to my ear. I was aware of her firm grip on my arm, pulling me back from the bed. I sensed the nurse's fear and momentarily doubted the safety of the leather restraints—it was a slight variation on Fay Wray in New York City on King Kong's opening night.

"The police brought her in after the voice of Satan told her to break into a home in Oakland and kill the occupants. She stabbed a pregnant woman and the woman's twenty-six-year-old brother seventy-nine times, then ate parts of the bodies."

My stomach rolled over. I wished I had not watched Valerie eat that chicken; now all I could picture were strips of skin and yellowed layers of fat.

"The first thing she did before we could even get her to seclusion was try and strangle one of our nurses, so we medicated her big-time for a few days, then let her out of seclusion. She was manageable until the voice began commanding her to take out the wire embedded in her throat."

At the mention of the wire, Inez directed her terrible gaze to Valerie, who averted her eyes. "The whore bitch will burn in hell!" the woman shrieked. "Her blood shall mingle with Satan's and Lot's wife! Suck cock. Suck cock."

Valerie spoke over the cacophony of the wailing. "She was so out of control that she clawed one of her tonsils out with her fingernails and swallowed it. She was working on excising the other one when Gabriela heard her choking and came and got us."

I was trying hard not to gag. "You mean she did an autotonsillectomy with her fingernails?"

Valerie shrugged. "I guess that's what you'd call it. We took her to surgery and had her fixed up. By the time she got back to us, she was raving mad."

The tormented woman at that moment lifted off the bed with a roll of her eyes and a howl that made the hair on the back of my neck stand on end. Valerie jumped back. I took a step closer, unsure of what I had just witnessed, for I thought I saw her lift completely off the bed—as in levitation.

From her pocket Valerie pulled out two prefilled syringes. She uncapped both and waited for her chance, not taking her eyes off her patient. "In the last two days, we've given her so much droperidol, I cannot believe she's still breathing. I don't know why we bother, because nothing affects her—Clonopin, Ativan . . . Nothing."

I took yet another step closer, tensing myself for the violence of the woman's response, though her shrill screams dwindled down into a deep-throated warning growl.

"I'm going to give both of these in her left thigh," Valerie whispered. "If you would stand by"—she took a baby step closer—"to make sure . . . she doesn't try something when I'm not looking . . ." Valerie waited until Inez's attention wandered, then plunged in the first syringe up to the hub of the needle.

Inez snarled. Raising her large, dark head, she bared her gums and howled like a wolf. Had she been in possession of teeth, she could have been Cujo's twin.

The sting of the second syringe sent the woman into a foaming-at-the-mouth frenzy. Her eyes rolled back into her head and again her entire body lifted off the bed, then fell back as though she'd been dropped.

Her head rose from the pillow, swaying eerily, like a snake. She strained forward, I thought perhaps to bite (gum?) Valerie's arm, but instead, she flicked her tongue in and out between her lips, making a sound like a cat hissing.

I leaned forward and waited. And when she twisted around to bellow, I had the better part of a second to see if there were pupils or slits.

It was postluncheon quiet time, when the patients were allowed to watch TV in the community room or smoke on the outdoor patio. Valerie was assigned to the nurses' station, which gave her a chance to recall some of the more illustrious patients the unit had housed. She was relating the particulars about D., a famous poetess who had been in and out of mental institutions since the age of fifteen.

"She'll slice herself open at any opportunity because it's her only source of comfort," Valerie said, munching a piece of melba toast. "The warmth of the blood makes her feel nurtured and loved. . . . Have you ever read anything of hers?"

I nodded, vaguely remembering that her poetry was mostly about death and nonexistence. It was the type of thing people read if they wanted to feel positive about committing suicide or homicide.

"As a patient, she's a drain because she needs constant pampering and reassurance. The minute she doesn't get attention, she's cutting herself up with whatever she can get her hands on. The last time she was here, she hacked open her arm with a piece from a broken dinner plate."

Valerie stopped to answer the phone.

"Linens?" she exclaimed after a minute of listening to the caller. "How many carts did she empty?" Valerie bit her lip. "What did this cleaning lady look like? Uh huh. Yeah. Okay, I'll take care of it. Sorry."

Valerie put the receiver back in the cradle, frowning. "I knew something was going on. Gabriela has emptied the linen carts of clean laundry. We're going to have to put her on a linen restriction."

"Jesus. Linen restriction?"

"Oh yes." Valerie sighed. "We have restrictions on this unit that really challenge the imagination—water restrictions, food restrictions, hair restrictions, clothes restrictions. We even had a vacuum restriction once with this guy who was in love with our vacuum. He insisted his dead mother talked to him through it. He kept sneaking it into bed with him until—"

A young woman wearing an oversized, worn army jacket approached the desk.

"Donna, go stand behind the yellow line, please," Valerie said. I could tell by the way Valerie tensed her jaw, Donna was a difficult patient.

"Open the door. I want to go out." The girl pulled on a frizzy strand of blond-streaked hair. Her hair, sticking out at all angles from her head, appeared to be the casualty of a bad permanent.

"Move away from the desk right now, please. Go stand behind the yellow line."

Considering the determination in the patient's voice, I wasn't surprised when she did not comply with the command. I pressed myself deep into my chair, sensing the arrival of disaster.

The patient stepped out of the light. In the shadows, her deep-set eyes were nearly invisible. "If you don't open the door, I'll cut my throat."

"You need to move back from the desk and take time out, Donna."

"If you don't open the door, I'll cut my throat."

Valerie slid her finger closer to a red button on the desk that had "PANIC" written above it. "Let me get you an Ativan, and then let's go to the dayroom and talk about what's bugging you about being here."

From where I was sitting, I saw Donna's hand slip into one of the jacket pockets. She wasn't having any of Valerie's therapy. "Open the door, or I'm going to cut my throat."

Valerie pushed the red button and rapidly rounded the corner of the desk at the same time the girl's hand went to her throat.

At the sight of the shard of bloodied glass, I leapt out of my chair and lunged for the patient's arm. As I went down under the charging wall of staff members, I heard Valerie curse.

In the crowded scuffle that followed, I was hurled bodily off the patient and into the side of the desk, much like a rejected part from a large machine.

From my observation point on the floor, I counted no fewer than five bodies piled on top of the patient. I watched the melee of arms and legs, feet and shouting heads, until I saw one hand wiggle out, still holding the broken piece of glass. This I carefully removed from the hand's grasp and placed safely in the pocket of my sweater.

Around the heap of bodies was a circle of patients, some rocking, some shouting. Over by the blue couches, which were supposedly pungent with invisible life, the manic cleaner herself was down on her knees sponging off Slow Mo's sneakers.

Then the three doors to the unit slammed open and a barrage of some ten people—nurses and policemen mostly—raced in. This new group of players spread out, "redirecting the energies" of any patients who were standing near the scuffle. I crawled to the desk as inconspicuously as possible and pulled myself up onto a chair.

My initial decision not to choose psych nursing as a career was reaffirmed. Looking on, I couldn't help but think that the only people who'd voluntarily work in a place like this were crazy.

I picked off a large piece of cauliflower residue encrusted on my watch and saw it was two-fifteen. I had to be on duty at Redwoods by three; that gave me forty-five minutes to make an hour's drive and change into my scrubs. Considering the pandemonium, I would be lucky if I got out by four. I admit to being a Type A personality when it comes to being on time; as soon as I suspect that I might be late, my switchboard ladies begin pressing the apprehension buttons, which causes my stomach to produce quarts of hydrochloric acid.

Jonathan, our masturbating banana man, must have read my mind, because he indicated he would escort me to the outer door. For a moment I was dubious, but then I caught sight of Valerie under the bloody but now subdued patient. I pointed to my watch and waved goodbye.

She frowned, her cheeks flaming red.

I mouthed, "Thank you," and she frowned deeper. I handed the shard of glass to a passing staff nurse, and told Jon to show me the way.

He held the last barred door open, and as I passed into the corridor, he closed it quickly behind me. "*That's* the place for crazies," he said, pointing to my side of the bars. "They can get to you out there."

I nodded. "You certainly have a point there, my friend."

He blew me a kiss and closed the inside metal door with a minimum of racket.

I rushed through the double doors and into the almost deserted acute unit—all but bed 20 were empty. Glancing briefly into the room, I saw leather straps hanging from each corner of the bed. I didn't even need to look at the assignment board to know that bed 20 was going to be my assignment for the night—they (as opposed to They) always gave me the four-point leather restraint people. But hey, I'd had a whole morning of crazies. What was one more?

"Five people are getting floated out on your shift, so consider this assignment an even break." Cordelia covered her face, peeked through her fingers, and laughed one of those disgusted, tired laughs that, translated, mean, the joke's on you.

"Ah, Jesus Christ," she sighed, and launched into the familiar, chanting rhythm of the introductory report. "Big Tom Grennan in bed twenty is a fifty-one-year-old patient of Dr. Cramer's, three days out from an inferior wall MI. He's six feet five, weighs two hundred and eighty pounds, and is an unemployed chef and ex–restaurant owner. He's a member of Active Alcoholics and has been dry, against his will, for four days."

I groaned. Cordelia patted my shoulder without a lapse between words. "We first noticed he was going into DTs this morning when he tried to strangle his wife, whom he believed to be cheating on him with the IV pole. It took six people to pull him off her and get him back into the bed."

Cordelia stopped. "Want more?"

"Okay. As long as it doesn't have anything to do with animals or chickens."

"No problem." She looked back at the patient's information card and continued. "His infarction was small, so he's off lidocaine and hasn't had any ectopy and angina for two days. He's being controlled with oral Pronestyl, and we've been giving him Librium around the clock. He's coherent on and off, but when he's out there, he gets like waaaaaay out there."

I considered the gist of the report and felt pretty good; taking care of only one three-day-old MI in DTs was actually a very cushy assignment. I said a silent prayer of thanks, feeling like the girl in the catbird seat. "You know, Cord, this really isn't that bad. I could have been floated to four west and had ten patients."

"Well, yeah, but there's something else."

Cordelia liked surprises and practical jokes.

Expectancy filled the short silence.

"You're going to transfer Big Tom by ambulance at seven P.M. to St. Joseph's CCU."

My smugness waned and I started to say something; my mouth opened, but my tongue couldn't deliver the words. As a result, there was more silence except for the sound of my teeth bouncing off my tooth guard.

"However," Cordelia said, enjoying herself, "Cramer did say he would come in before the transfer and order a big dose of something to keep him sedated until you get to St. Joseph's."

I drew myself up. "Hold on. St. Joseph's is an hour and twenty minutes away and I'm going to be in the back of an ambulance with a two-hundred-and-eighty-pound fresh MI who is going in and out of DTs?"

Cordelia nodded happily. "Yes, you are and may the Force be with you."

"Where are the unsafe-assignment forms?"

Cordelia grinned. "That's what I said this morning too. But then again, I say that every morning." She closed the chart and snapped her fingers. "Oh yeah, one more bad part."

I sank in at the chest. A howl came out of bed 20 that put me in mind of the seclusion room at Mercy.

"The ambulance company won't transfer him unless they get the money up front in cash. Five hundred and fifty bucks."

I let a low whistle drift from my mouth. "Expensive ride. What about insurance?"

"The guy doesn't have any." Cordelia's chair creaked as she stood for her getaway. "That's why he's being transferred to St. Joseph's."

"So what am I supposed to do? I've got about ten dollars on me."

"The original plan was that Mrs. Grennan was going to bring in the money, but she stormed out of here this morning talking divorce, so I think that's out. Mr. Grennan says he can borrow it from his brother-in-law who owns a pizza joint in San Rafael."

"Great."

"Well . . . kind of," corrected Cord. Her eyes flickered, almost imperceptibly.

"I'm going to strangle you, Cordelia."

"The guy can't leave his restaurant, so you have to pick it up," she said, coming over to stand near me—a risky thing to do, considering.

"Do the ambulance people know they're going to have to make a pit stop?"

"Not exactly," Cordelia said lamely.

"Christ, Cordelia! How could you set me up like this?"

Her giggle as she put on her coat added insult to injury. "Oh, Ec, it'll be *fun*."

There came another howl from bed 20, and the sound of the steel locks of the restraint being whacked against the side rails. A man's deep voice boomed, "Heeeeere's Big Tom! Serve 'em up. This round's on Big Tom the bomb. Maria? C'mon baby, get your sweet ass over here and sit on my face."

I glowered at Cordelia from under my frown. "Oh yeah. Some kinda fun we're gonna have here tonight."

Les and Del Proctor, identical twins, rolled the Proctors' Ambulance Service's only stretcher into the unit as I was checking the pretransfer medication order for Mr. Grennan.

"Is the patient ready?" one of them asked.

"No," I answered vaguely, momentarily bewildered by their identical uniforms: jeans, and red satin jackets with gold trim. Over the pockets were embroidered gold dragon emblems and the wearers' first names. The twin with the facial tic was Les. "I've just now gotten the order to medicate him for the ride."

Del, the more aggressive and cheerless of the duo brought out a dingy, stiff handkerchief and blew his nose. "We expected you to be ready when we got here," he said. "The transfer was set for seven P.M. and it's now ten after. I want to be rolling out that door in five minutes. We've got a business to run here."

My temper went up like a flare. Here was yet another man who, once in the hospital world, thought he had the inalienable right to treat the nurses like grunts. "And if you want to continue to have a business to run, I'd suggest you chill out. You are not the only ambulance company on the block, mister."

Fuming, I turned my back on the twins and went to the narcotics drawer to draw up the Librium. The whole time I was injecting the medication into Mr. Grennan's IV port, my switchboard ladies kept pounding at my temples, which was a bad sign; my temples were where my acute panic buttons were situated.

I ignored the feeling and continued to prepare Mr. Grennan for transport. I was putting together the transfer papers and copies of his chart when I glanced at the medication order sheet. I swallowed hard, as though I had a brick wedged in my throat. I scrutinized the order sheet again, rereading the medication order ten, fifteen times.

But no matter how many times I read it, there it was, in Dr. Cramer's miserly little scrawl, as clear as a malpractice suit is expensive: "Librium 400 mgs.—IM." I had misread the order and given the drug the more direct and effective intravenous route, not intramuscularly as indicated.

Big difference. Big mistake.

I began to hyperventilate and lost control of my knees. The feeling a nurse has when she discovers she has made a medication error could be compared to the feeling a driver experiences when he realizes he had just run over a small child and a policeman in a crosswalk.

After the initial onslaught of panic subsided enough for me to see, I looked to the patient, who was happily banging out "Big John" on his side rails, and singing along.

Thank God, he was still breathing. I ran to him, shouting, "Sing, Tom, sing! Loud as you can. Don't stop singing." A quick blood pressure revealed him to be stable, but he was beginning to slur his words and giggle, and he was having a tough time controlling his eyeballs. I interpreted this behavior as a sign of his forthcoming vascular collapse.

Sitting at the end of the nurses' desk, Les and Del were pressuring me by sulkily watching the clock. They had removed their jackets, revealing their gold rayon bowling shirts. Embroidered on the backs in red thread was the company logo: "Proctors' Ambulance Service—A Paradigm of Perfection."

Despite my hysteria, I snorted a short laugh, then promptly tripped over the wastebasket in my haste to get to the intermediate unit. At the desk, writing in his black book, sat Joe Cramer.

"Joe!" My voice was full of panic and urgency. I could feel the underarm sweat rings spread out and meet at the back of my scrub dress. "Joe, listen—I've made a terrible mistake."

Dr. Cramer's face was inflexible except for the twisted smile. "It took you this long to realize nursing isn't for you?"

"You know Mr. Grennan, the guy you wrote that Librium order for?"

Joe stared at me blankly.

"Jesus Christ, Joe, you wrote the order ten minutes ago. The big DTs guy going to St. Joseph's?"

The doctor raised his eyebrows. "Ah, yes. Mr. Big."

"I gave him the Librium IV instead of IM. He got the whole four hundred milligrams. What should I do?"

I was miserable. I wanted Joe to tell me to cancel the transfer, or tell me it wasn't such a bad mistake and not to worry.

Instead, he looked at me glumly and said, "Pray he doesn't lose his blood pressure or have a respiratory arrest before you get him to St. Joseph's."

Unable to hear over the noise of the ambulance's motor, it took a full minute before I could decipher Mr. Grennan's garbled words as, "Why, you're the little devil, aren't you?" He gave my braid a playful tug, his eyes sliding around from side to side, top to bottom.

I smiled nervously, barely able to keep the corners of my mouth steady. "What do you mean?"

"You slipped me a witty-bitty Mickey, didn't you? I can't feel my toes anymore." He giggled. I tried to giggle along with him, but the noise I made came out sounding more like a strangled cry.

Les and Del, in uptight-young-businessmen-about-town fashion, didn't turn around. I was glad about this; they might have seen how I was watching Mr. Grennan's respirations like a hawk, and become suspicious. Their unwillingness to help me transfer the patient from the bed onto the stretcher also saved me the hassle of trying to come up with an explanation as to why Mr. Grennan had zero muscle control and seemed to be three sheets to the wind.

The Proctors, as true paradigms of perfection, were the type that would have charged extra for risky transports.

The ambulance pulled into an alley in the worst section of San Rafael. The Last Chance Motel was one street over.

Les banged on the partition. "This is the place. Make it snappy. Time is money."

I was amazed the Proctors hadn't laid an egg over the unscheduled stop. It was obvious from the way Del puffed out his cheeks that he wanted to complain, to use it as a club to beat me with. I simply had to remind him that pizza dive or not, unorthodox transfer or not, it was where the money was coming from.

I took another blood pressure, which was holding steady, before shaking Mr. Grennan out of his stupor. "Who do I ask for and what do I say?"

"Vinny. Ask for Vinny. Tell him Tom zah Bomb sent youse in for zah dough."

"Okay, Tom, now do me a favor and sing some of the old songs while I'm gone."

Unable to open his eyes, Mr. Grennan slurred, "Sure, shweetheart. Tom zah Bomb'll shing youse to shleep." He opened his mouth. "Oh, when Irish lipses errr shinging . . ."

Leaving Del in charge of watching the patient's vital signs, I alighted from the back of the ambulance, rapidly canvassed the surroundings, and ran toward the door of the small establishment. Hanging from a makeshift rod of packaging string, a stained red-and-white-checked tablecloth doubled as a curtain for the glass door. In the front window, a pink neon sign read, "VINNY'S PIZZA," except the *V* and the *A* were burned out, making it "INNY'S PIZZ," if you squinted from about five feet back. Framing the sign was a burned-out string of outdoor Christmas lights.

As I stepped into the dimly lit Italian womb of Inny's Pizz, the mouth-watering aroma of cooking pizza blasted me into the front room of Scuvello's Bakery, Schenectady, 1951, any Friday night of the year. I fully expected to see the old Italian lady come out from behind the counter with a warm cannoli for me and the usual white paper bag filled with fresh pizza dough for my father.

I waited for my eyes to adjust, then sized up the room in which I stood. To my left was a small dining room, big enough for three two-person café tables. On one wall was an amateurish, hand-painted mural of a rotund gondolier decked out in his carnival best, mouth opened wide, hand to chest, eyes raised in operatic bliss. The rest of the walls were papered with old scores from Italian operas.

Dodging empty wine bottles and bunches of dusty plastic grapes that hung from the low ceiling, I took two steps to the high counter on my right. Over the top of the cash register, I saw a couple of large pizza ovens flanking the doorway of a brightly lit kitchen area.

"What's yours, lady?" The Brooklyn accent belonged to a

Danny DeVito–type guy spinning a round of pizza dough into the air. It went up once, twice, as a medium-thick crust, and came down as a large thin.

"Tom the Bomb sent me in for the dough," I said, feeling like an idiot, not so much for what I had been instructed to say, but because I had slipped into my upstate New Yorkese. ("Tahm da Bahm sint me in for da dough.")

"Dat guy's a pain in da keester," he complained, spreading the dough out on a baking board. "How much does da bum want dis time?"

"Five hundred and fifty-eight dollars even."

The man wiped his hands on the dish towel that hung from his belt and opened the cash register. He counted out the money onto the counter and handed it to me, eyeing my stethoscope.

"You his nurse?"

I nodded.

"How's he doin'?"

"You know he had a heart attack, right?"

Vinny shrugged, ladling out basil-and-oregano-spiced tomato sauce over the satiny dough. It was Italian for "Yeah, I know. So?"

"He went into DTs this morning, but as soon as he dries out he'll be okay."

"Oh sure," the man said, loading on the mushrooms and olives. "Until he starts hittin' da bottle again."

In the background, there was the short ring of a kitchen timer.

He sprinkled two generous handfuls of shredded mozzarella over the pie. I swallowed, in order not to drool when I talked. "He's got to stop drinking," I said, "or the next heart attack he has is going to kill him, you know."

I don't know exactly why I said this except that Vinny was a New Yorker: I knew about the bigger-than-life, dramatic approach.

Vinny shrugged again. "Poifect. Den my sister's gonna have a lot less heartache. She don't need no more trouble wit' dis one." He dribbled a few drops of olive oil over the top of the pie and sprinkled on an extra bit of chopped garlic.

"Yeah, well, drinkers are hard," I said loudly, hoping to cover the growling of my stomach gone wild.

Vinny walked back to the oven and pulled out a large pizza

with his oven paddle. He set it down on the counter in front of me and shoved in the one he'd just made.

He gave my face a quick, direct scan. "You Italian or what?" From the stack against the wall he took a flat piece of thin cardboard and fashioned it into a pizza box in two quick moves.

"Half." I shrugged, breaking into the staccato, sparsely worded sentence style that is New York. "My dad's family came through Ellis Island. Campobasso people. Settled upstate near Albany."

"Oh yeah?" He put the half-veggie, half-meatball pizza in the box and began to slice it with one of those round pizza cutters that always reminded me of boot spurs. "My mom come over from Naples through Ellis Island."

I nodded solemnly, as if these declarations of roots were the things that gave our lives meaning.

"You eat yet?"

"Naw, I've gotta get Big Tom up to St. Joseph's."

Vinny closed the box and slid the pizza in my direction. "For you and da drivers. You? You're too skinny. If you're gonna deal wit' Big Tom, you gotta have meat on your bones."

Normally I turn down gifts from patients or their families, but my stomach was eating itself hollow over the aroma coming from that box. I swallowed another mouthful of saliva. "Hey, thanks. It'll be gone before we hit Novato."

He made a familiar Italian salute: a subtle shrug of one shoulder, a raised hand, and a slow wag of the head from side to side. "Yeah, yeah, yeah, sure."

I checked the wad of bills in my pocket and, balancing the pizza, opened the door.

"You tell that dumb mick to call me when he gets there," Vinny said, disappearing into the kitchen. "I don't want my sister worrying herself sick no more."

"Will do." That is, if he doesn't die before we arrive.

To this day I firmly believe that pizza changed the whole course of the ride to St. Joseph's from disastrous to almost delightful.

Mr. Grennan was belligerent by the time I got back to the ambulance (just as long as he was breathing, who cared?), trying his Irish Catholic best to goad Les and Del (who were English and Episcopalian) into a fight. He had already worked one restraint off and was doggedly working on the other, promising to crush a few limey bones.

The introduction of the pizza into the scene seemed to instantly calm everybody down. Maybe it was the aroma, maybe it was the money hot in the Proctors' pockets—whatever the hell it was, we were under way before the box could even be opened.

While Les and Del devoured the better part of the pizza, I persuaded Mr. Grennan to sing his entire repertoire of Irish folk songs. As long as I could hear him singing, everything was going to be okay.

Thursday
1:41 A.M.

I sit here wondering at what point the night began to go sour. Could it have been when the Proctor twins ditched me at St. Joseph's, saying it wasn't their responsibility to give me a ride back to the hospital? Was it the hassle I had trying to find a taxi willing to go to Redwoods? Was it the supervisor's diatribe over having to fork over such a large sum to the cabbie?

It might have been the half hour I spent with Juanita in the nurses' lounge, listening to her cry and complain about Annie's three-D attitude toward pregnant nurses in CCU— distaste, disapproval, and disdain.

Juanita's obstetrician told her she couldn't continue to work night shift without putting her own and her unborn child's lives at risk. Knowing that Annie occasionally creates temporary day and evening shifts to accommodate her favorites, Juanita begged her to do the same for her until she went on maternity leave. Annie hasn't responded as yet. After Claire's last two miscarriages—supposedly caused by the stress of working nights—we can only hope Annie will let up.

So many times I find myself wondering what Jan Tobin would think of all the changes and the horseshit that goes on in this cold world that has become CCU. I wonder if she has washed her hands of us.

Anyway, if I had to bet money, I'd say that my night really went down the toilet when I retrieved my phone messages after the eleven P.M. postarrest admit was settled in.

First one was from Valerie, who chewed me out royally

for allowing the banana man to escort me to the door, call two was Simon saying that he wants to buy a motorcycle, and last but most certainly not least was David saying that he wouldn't be here when I got home because he wants to start spending more time in his own apartment.

Booooommm.

I lie here watching Mooshie try to eat the bubbles out of my club soda, and wonder why I can't laugh. My insides feel floppy, one toke over the line.

I don't know who wrote this line, but it fits: "I am left wondering and there is no one here to say yes or no."

FIFTEEN

> *"The nurse can create an atmosphere in which a reasonable and essential degree of hope can displace the panic and liberate the body's healing systems ..."*
>
> NORMAN COUSINS, *Anatomy of an Illness*

FACING THE ASSEMBLED MEMBERS of the fourth quarterly CCU staff meeting, I couldn't help but notice the difference between the expressions of the staff (excited, delighted, hopeful) and those of management (cornered—as in rats). Out of forty-five staff members, thirty-five had signed up to say they would be interested in having a ballot vote for a trial run of decentralization. Of the other ten, five wanted more information, one wrote she was too lazy to think about it, one said she enjoyed floating, one admitted she didn't like progressive change, one said it was un-American (Honey?), and one was on the fence.

Annie was having a bout of conflicting body language—smiling and gnawing her fingernails at the same time. She had made decentralization the last item on the agenda, hoping, I was sure, that we would run out of time and have to put it off until the next staff meeting in three months. She hadn't bargained on the fact that the staff would be so eager to get to it, they would gloss over everything else.

When there were no more hands for questions, I gave my spiel about how we would all have to make sacrifices until the plan was running smoothly. I was explaining where the ballot box would be, when Annie raised a nibbled hand.

"If we're going to be voting on decentralization," she said without waiting to be recognized, "I think you should all know *my* views before you vote."

The blank silence that followed made some people shift uneasily in their seats. There wasn't a person in the room who didn't fear Annie to one degree or another. Recognizing a hastily assembled stumbling block when I tripped over one, I clenched my tooth guard and waited.

Annie gave the audience her who-farted? glare and continued: "I don't think anything has been mentioned yet about what the other nurses in this hospital will think of you when you selfishly segregate yourselves from the rest of the nursing staff. This is going to look and feel like the nurses in this unit are too superior to extend a willing helping hand. How will you hold your heads up knowing that you've turned your backs on your fellow nurses in need?"

Annie's use of negative key words—"segregate," "selfishly"—was quite effective in bringing a quick rush of shame to everyone. The single Benedict Arnold reproach was pretty good also.

Skating like mad to save her deals, Annie spouted enough fancy political rhetoric to win an Olympic debate. Her shame-fingers double axel progressed into a John F. Kennedy "Ask not what your country can do for you" triple-flip back twist and ended with a you'll-be-sorry sixty-revolution superspin. The desired psychological effect was achieved; every nurse immediately reverted to the age of six and felt terribly bad and ashamed, as though she'd been caught putting the cat in the microwave. Thirty-five sets of eyes turned on me full of mistrust and accusation.

"When I did my research on decentralization," I began, "I went to each unit and floor in this hospital to explain what we were trying to do and why. As a matter of fact, several of the best points of this plan were contributed by Redwoods nurses who have worked in decentralized units in other hospitals.

"I also might add that the general consensus was, they wished us luck and are rooting for us, because if we can set the tone, ICU would like to be next, and a couple of the floors would like to try it."

Annie didn't bother to raise her hand this time, but rather forged ahead. "Before you jump off the cliff, I still think you should bear in mind that some of you will suffer for the sake of a few self-centered people." Annie stared hard at me. "Some of you may go without work. Some of you will end up working for others who don't want to carry their share of the weight."

Their eyes shifted back to me again.

"Everyone will have plenty of work," I said, managing to stay calm, "and no one is going to have to carry anyone else's share. If we all stick together and do our own fair share, this will work for everybody.

"The main thing that's changing is that we each have a choice. We'd have options as opposed to having none. We'd have some power over our own working conditions as opposed to being powerless. Please don't forget this is a trial run—nothing is set in stone. We still have plenty of room for growth and suggestions and new ideas."

People were nodding and most of the smiles had returned.

Annie held up a hand again. "I move to have the final vote announced at the next staff meeting. If you elect this plan of yours, I also move to have it put into effect at that time."

"That's three months away," objected Beth, who was sitting in the back of the room breast-feeding her son. "You've already managed to get the vote put off for six months. Waiting isn't going to change how the staff feels about this."

"Then it shouldn't matter." Annie turned and glared at her first assistant, who instantly raised her hand.

"I second the motion to wait until the next staff meeting to have a ballot vote on decentralization," she said.

"The meeting," said Annie, "is now closed."

Phoebe said we all looked tense when we came out of the staff meeting. Annie and her entourage came out behind us, their heads bent together in whispers. I started fretting about what they could possibly do to defeat the vote, then nixed the alarm; whatever was going to happen would happen. I had to trust the basic human desire for freedom of choice.

Freedom of choice was not mine at the moment, however, since I would not have freely chosen either Mrs. Fullerton or Mr. Jacobsen to be part of my assignment.

That the confused Muriel Fullerton kept trying to bite me didn't bother me nearly as much as the fully aware Jacobsen husband-and-wife team. They were into playing a sort of passive-aggressive game that, unfortunately, was an all too familiar problem to healthcare personnel. The scenario usually went something like this:

The nurse enters the patient's room with dinner tray, checks the patient, asks how he feels and if he needs anything. The patient accepts and eats his dinner, smiles, and in a chatty manner says that he feels fine and wants for nothing, thank you so much for your concern.

The nurse exits with empty dinner tray and, happy her patient is content, goes on with other duties.

Enter spouse, who immediately asks, "How do you feel, dear? You look terrible. Are you hungry? Has anyone come in to check on you?"

At this point in the game, the patient realizes the wonderful opportunities of (1) getting positive attention from the spouse, (2) creating a situation where the spouse can feel like the nurturing rescuer, and (3) being able to bond together with the spouse against a common enemy: the nurse.

The patient—in this case, Mr. Jacobsen—answers, "I feel terrible. I've got pains all over, I'm starving, and nobody is willing to do anything about it. I haven't seen a nurse for more than five minutes all day."

"Well!" says the outraged, rescuing partner. "We'll see about this!"

The rescuing partner then heads straight to the administrative offices and complains, presenting a complete list of the offending employees, along with vague threats about malpractice suits or going to Brand X hospital in the future.

Management, wearing kid gloves, gives plenty of attention to the plaintiffs. On the other hand, management knows, in its heart of hearts, there are more sides to a story. If the allegations are found to be false or greatly exaggerated, all employees coming into contact with that patient are then instructed to take care in documenting every word spoken, and every action taken, in order to protect themselves and the hospital in the event of a lawsuit.

Doing my charting, I felt like a screenwriter:

Mr. Jacobsen sitting in bed at a 45-degree angle watching Phil (program on adult men who are into infantilism).

This R.N. asks, "How are you doing?" Patient answers, smiling, "Just fine." Nurse asks, "Are you having any chest pain?" Patient answers, "None at all. Thank you for asking."

This R.N. takes blood pressure 128/76, pulse 82, respirations 18, temperature 97.6. Patient requested and received results of vital signs. Patient denied pain or discomfort of any kind several times during assessment. Lungs clear, color

*normal, skin warm and dry, no edema present, normal heart
sounds, negative Homans'. Rest of physical examination and
lab results all within normal limits (see flow sheet for details). This R.N. asked if patient needed or wanted anything.
Patient answered, "No, I'm fine," and resumed watching TV.
This nurse gave patient his four P.M. medications, explained
the actions of each medication, and asked if he had any
questions about them or anything else. Patient took medications and repeated, "No, I'm fine."*

Later that evening, Mrs. Jacobsen would write a formal
complaint stating: "My husband said that during her four P.M.
visit, Nurse Heron completely disregarded his anginal pain,
never once inquiring as to how he was feeling."

Mr. Zehger, my postcardiac-arrest patient, appeared to be as
unlike a Type A personality as you could get; his eyes and
smile fairly radiated serenity. For the forty-one-year-old CEO
of a major San Francisco advertising agency to be this tranquil
was saying something. I wasn't sure what, except perhaps that
he hid his stress well—more than likely right in his coronary
arteries.

The pale, thin man was sitting up reading *The Wall Street
Journal.* He was also chuckling—not your usual response to
The Wall Street Journal. I introduced myself and set the chart
down on the bedside table, next to a white teddy bear with a
helium balloon tied around its arm.

"How're you feeling?"

Mr. Zehger put down the paper to reveal a second teddy
bear sitting on his abdomen. "Happy to be alive," he replied in
a voice that was perfect for telling children's stories.

The bear, the reply, the eyes, and the voice led me to suspect
that Mr. Zehger was one of those people who, like Scrooge after the visitations, had been to the other side and come back
gentler, wiser souls.

I opened the chart to his history and physical and read the
first few lines. "It says that besides having a good-sized heart
attack, you had a V fib arrest at home and your wife initiated
CPR?"

Mr. Zehger nodded. "My wife and I had just taken the CPR
course at the fire station the week before. Jake and I wouldn't
be here if it weren't for that."

I quickly scanned the next few paragraphs, finding a lot

about the particulars of Mr. Zehger's MI and his prior state of health, but nothing about a Jake.

"Jake?"

"Our four-year-old. I was doing CPR on him when my heart stopped. After I conked out, my wife did CPR on the both of us until the paramedics arrived."

That my jaw unhinged in amazement set Mr. Zehger to laughing, a sound as pleasant as his voice.

"Okay," I said, sitting on the edge of the bed by his feet. "I want to hear this story. Nobody told me anything about a family CPRfest."

Mr. Zehger sighed in mock exasperation over having to tell the story *again*. Only the satisfied smile at the corners of his mouth revealed that he loved reciting every word.

"Friday before last, I had left the house to go to work, but when I got to the car, I realized I'd neglected to give Jake a kiss, so I went back.

"As soon as I walked into the living room, I saw him lying under the coffee table." Mr. Zehger stared past me at the wall, as though the scene were being played out on an invisible screen. "I knew before I even touched him that something was wrong, because he wasn't moving, and Jake hasn't been still for three seconds since he was born. I pulled him out and saw he wasn't breathing. His face was . . ."

I sat silent as dismay clouded his eyes. Lost in his private climate of fog, he'd taken on the sad, innocent quality people often wore for a time after their first intimate brush with tragedy.

"It was blue, almost purple. I did the Heimlich on him, and on the third try, a bell that had been on the dog's collar flew out of his mouth. I thought that was all I had to do, but then I saw he still wasn't breathing. That really scared the hell out of me because I realized his heart had probably stopped and I didn't know how long he'd been like that. The CPR instructor had told us that brain death occurred after six minutes without oxygen.

"I yelled at my wife to call nine-one-one and started CPR right away. About a minute or so into it, I got these chest pains like I was being crushed by an elephant. The next thing I was aware of was opening my eyes and staring up at the undersides of a bunch of sweating chins in the ER."

From his bedside cabinet Mr. Zehger took a stack of color photographs and handed them to me. The top snapshot was a close-up of a beautiful brown-haired boy wearing Mickey Mouse sunglasses and puckering up to kiss the lens of the camera. A telltale pinkish rim of sticky cherry or strawberry something encircled his mouth. The second snap was of the same child lying head to head with a buff-colored Labrador. The boy's huge almond-shaped eyes were turned toward the camera. The smile he wore was as content and full as his father's.

"That's Jake," Mr. Zehger said proudly. "Four days after this happened, he was riding his trike, talking a mile a minute."

When I came to the last photo, one of Jake wearing a set of toe separators and holding a bottle of red nail polish, I smiled and handed the pictures back to Mr. Zehger.

My curiosity turned up as strong as fifty cats sniffing at a partially opened cabinet door. "You don't have to answer this if you don't want to, but . . ." I paused. "How do you feel about this? I mean, don't you think it was all . . . remarkable the way it happened?"

Mr. Zehger nodded, running his fingers lightly over the top of the teddy bear's ears. "It's more than remarkable. If we hadn't gone to that class, neither of us would've known what to do—or if I hadn't found Jake when I did?

"I'm convinced we were spared for a purpose. Some people think we were just lucky, but I believe that Jake and I have things to do yet that will make a difference. Maybe one of us is meant to save someone else's life someday."

His eyes closed and Mr. Zehger lay back, pressing himself into the comfort of his pillows. "Who knows what fate has in store for any of us?"

I wrapped the blood pressure cuff around his arm, thinking about the unexpected twists and turns my own life had taken. I'd given up trying to predict what fate had in store for me when I was about five. The best way to handle fate, I'd figured, was to keep my eyes open and deal with the surprises as they were sprung.

Mrs. Fullerton burped. It was not the burp of a lady, albeit a 187-pound lady in congestive heart failure, but rather that of a beer-swigging, bronco-riding, barrel-chested truck driver.

"My God," she drawled indignantly, "I knew there were pigs around here, but I didn't know they were this *close*."

I looked up from my charting and laughed. For all Muriel's confused verbal meanderings, she was pretty funny. Her eclec-

tic questions and erratic discourses provided wonderful practice
for cocktail party conversation. Should I ever be invited to one,
I'd be more than prepared to engage in verbal swordplay at
will.

Careful not to get any part of me too close to her teeth, I
had released her wrist and ankle restraints to give her skin a
rest and settled in at the small writing station at the end of her
bed to do some charting. It was a nice break; not only was I
out of the chaos of the nursing station and able to keep a close
eye on Mrs. Fullerton, but I could see Mr. Jacobsen through
the window, in case he so much as looked like he needed
something.

"Novels," Muriel mused, "that have maps as frontispieces
turn me off. Why do you think that is?"

I put down my pen and considered the question. I knew exactly what she meant. "Maybe that's because they give the impression of being more like a boring textbook than some
exciting story."

Muriel began to laugh. "They should put girlie pictures in
the front of books. My husband would read them all."

"Does your husband like to read?"

Muriel got vague. I watched her mind slip out the window
and come back in wearing a whole different set of ideas. "My
husband and I are like Clark Kent and Superman," she stated
flatly. "We're never seen in the same place at the same time."

"Oh?" I said, putting aside my chart. I wanted to get some
cornstarch powder on her wrists and ankles before I reapplied
the restraints.

"He's dead."

"Oh, I'm sorry." I hurried with the powder.

"Don't be sorry. It is only the small matter that, as a woman,
I have yet to learn the secrets of earlier mortality."

My mouth twitched, wanting to smile, but wanting more to
get the restraints on. One hundred and eighty-seven pounds of
biting woman could do some major damage.

"He was buried in the lake, you know," she continued wist-
fully. "It was such a beautiful lake, except now it's all under
water, of course."

I clicked the ankle restraints into locked position and casually brought her left hand down to the side rail. She wasn't
having any of that and pulled her hand out of my grip.

"What do you think happens to all the dead bird bodies?"
Mrs. Fullerton asked this in such a way as to make me think

it was one of the more meaningful questions in life. What really got me was that I didn't know the answer. I mean, how often does one find a dead bird body lying around? Bird burial service doesn't sound right, and I doubt any self-respecting cat would eat one he hadn't killed himself.

"I don't know, Mrs. Fullerton." Again I tried to pull her hand down to the side rail.

That was when she got ahold of my little finger and gave it a squeeze. I thought she was being sweet until she twisted it back on itself and put it in her mouth.

At once her teeth crushed down and I heard the digit crack. With the first shock of pain, the switchboard ladies instantaneously projected a large-screen mental picture of my gangrenous right hand, minus the pinkie. At the knuckle joint were large, purulent Frankenstein-monster stitches. The message they sent with the visuals was that my finger remained crushed between her teeth—*do something*, for Christ's sake!

Okay, so before I passed out from the pain (my eyes were now rolled back into my head), I could twist her cheek off or bite her arm until she let go, or I could follow my gut instinct and pull my finger out, probably leaving most of it in her mouth. I didn't have anything I could use to pry open her jaw, and I didn't want to jeopardize my free fingers.

The something I needed to do came to me on a wave of nausea. "Mrs. Fullerton?" I sucked in my breath and somehow made the words happen. "Have you ever ridden the swan boats at the Boston Public Garden?"

It was the open-sesame question, for she instantly opened her mouth and answered—something about having been Leda in another life.

I had a glimpse of the reshaped, bloody digit that burned like fire before I ran to the sink and blindly doused it with antibacterial soap. I knew it had to be broken, but I didn't want to look to see if it was all there. Behind me, I could hear Muriel rolling around the bed, pulling at her leg restraints. I didn't want to look at that either.

I did look out the window, though, and saw a red-faced Mr. Jacobsen motioning for me to come to his aid. Incident report number two. The nurses' station was a zoo of doctors and nurses, most of whom were preparing for the insertion of an intraortic balloon pump. Dr. Cramer and Dr. Mahoney were conferring about the postarrest patient who had been admitted from ER, and Dr. Meyers was barking orders at Honey about getting Swan Ganz and arterial lines in on a pulmonary edema patient who was going down the tubes.

I started feeling faint, the white and blue spots blocking out my vision. As I opened my mouth to yell, I found a pair of eyes staring at me. Dr. Voorhees raised his eyebrows in question. With my uninjured hand, I motioned to him for help.

Eric rose from his chair and came toward me. It was probably a four-second walk from the desk to where I stood, but in that time, an urgent, enormous sadness broke over me and I began to weep.

The cold pack, fashioned from an exam glove filled with crushed ice, numbed my finger and part of my hand. My wrist ached from the cold. Don had taken me to the Tears and Laments Room (my new name for the Quiet Room) rather than put me up for public viewing in ER's main lobby where everyone could gawk at the whimpering nurse. The crybaby.

I was both relieved and embarrassed that it appeared I was crying because I could not handle the pain of a crushed finger. (Nurse Fallacy 46: Nurses are tough as nails; they don't even bleed when wounded.) The fact was, I wasn't weeping because of my finger—I was weeping over the general state of my life.

Insular layers of mental blindness, rationalization, and denial worked well for me when it came to facing unpleasant realities. I was doing well at ignoring my discontentment when the hot almond tea and the white plastic lawn chair incidents touched off the fuse.

But before I go into the almond tea thing, I have to explain that more than anything in the world, I hate to be cold.

Which was unfortunate, because the Bay Area seemed to be getting colder every year. It was not uncommon, on any given day between November 1 and March 31, to be scraping patches of ice crystals off the car windshield, or cutting down trees and shrubs that had been killed by frost. It was reminiscent of my early years in upstate New York.

What was even more unfortunate was that my pink cottage had one dysfunctional wall heater—purchased by my landlord at a garage sale—that had been declared a health hazard by the gas company. This left me with the fireplace for heat, which limited my living space to within five feet of the hearth.

One November morning, I awoke to the sight of my breath billowing out over my bed. From the thermos at my bedside,

I poured myself a cup of still-hot almond tea, then lay back to stare out the bedroom window (the inside of which was coated with a thin layer of ice) that faced the gravel parking lot of the psychiatrist's office next door.

For a while I lay there imagining what I looked like in three pairs of wool socks, long johns, flannel nightgown, wool mittens, angora neck scarf, and navy watch cap. I added the unappealing sight of my tooth guard and the faint white line of dried drool tracks on either side of my mouth, and understood immediately why David did not want to make love before he left for work.

From there my mind wandered to the pattern of cracks in the window and how they'd come to be. Frequently patients left the shrink's office under either emotional or financial strain (at $155 per fifty-minute hour, it had to be one of those painful payment moments). As a result of this tension, they spun their tires as they tore out of the parking lot, thus kicking up gravel which hit the window with considerable force.

Outside, a departing patient had been letting his car run for a good ten minutes (probably trying to get the windshield defrosted while chanting his inner-peace mantra). Since the exhaust pipe was less than five feet from the window, lazy clouds of blue fumes seeped steadily through the aforementioned cracks. I was concentrating on this cloud, when a sparkle drew my eye to my tea.

A blade of sunlight had sliced through the upper pane and landed in my cup. Reflected in the light were thousands of sparkles floating about in my tea.

Probably the cup was dirty, I thought, or maybe the teakettle had some rust on the inside. Braving the polar hell of that drafty, icy cottage, I shuffled to the kitchen to wash the cup and kettle and begin again with fresh water.

Still there were sparkles.

Repeating the process with a different cup, a different kettle, no tea, a different tea, didn't matter. There, in my tea, were thousands of things—some sparkling, some not; some floating, some moving under their own power.

With cup in mitten, I ran next door to the landlord, an easygoing gentleman in his seventies, who only nodded thoughtfully at the sight, handed me a recent copy of our local newspaper, and told me to read page 12.

I went back to the icebox shaped like my cottage, and upon discovering it was warmer outside than in, pulled up one of my new Price Club plastic lawn chairs and sat down to read. Page 12 told me that after a bout of nuclear testing somewhere, the government had reportedly dumped a mess of nuclear waste canisters in San Francisco Bay near the Farallon Islands. Mutated fish and other strange forms of glowing life had recently been discovered hanging around out there. It was feared by our West Coast Einsteins that maybe several of the canisters were disintegrating.

From there the article made a few journalistic hops, skips, and jumps, eventually getting around to the quality of the Bay Area's water supplies. In two and a half columns, it was reported to be in questionable shape. The article ended with the statement that the incidence of cancer in the Bay Area was on an alarming rise.

Thoroughly depressed, I put the paper down and turned my attention to the new patio chairs. With pragmatic pride, I noted they were sturdy yet lightweight, durable in case of more earthquakes, and I could leave them out, without fear of rust, in the rain that we hadn't had for six years. White may not have been the most practical color . . .

Uhn, white?

I removed my glasses and looked closer, running a finger across the arm. A well-defined finger track of white showed in the background of gray. I checked my finger—a coat of fine, black powder lay upon it like a death card.

Soot from the chimney? Perhaps. Or maybe it was more related to the highway traffic less than fifty feet from my front door. Considering that the population had tripled, and people were becoming more and more L.A.-ified—that is to say, they regarded their cars as extensions of their physical bodies—clean air in the Bay Area had nearly gone the way of Southern California air.

So, if my chairs were covered with black dust, what was happening to my lungs?

This revelation caused me to take an overview of the town wherein I had resided for twenty-three years. The once balmy, bucolic bedroom community was now overpopulated, polluted, nippy, and with single-car garages selling for $200,000, waaaay overpriced.

If environmental pollution was the tip of my iceberg, my job at Redwoods Memorial was the glacier. For the promoter of the "most incredible profession in the world," nursing was fast becoming a tedious job. I was in the land beyond burnout, and it was unbearable.

Like clockwork, migraine headaches began to plague me the day before I had to return to work, and not go away until I left the hospital for my scheduled days off. Management took every opportunity to remind me that I was inconsequential to the job and that the personal touch I, as the individual nurse, brought to my patients was replaceable.

No longer willing to be ruled by this attitude, both Pia and Nealy quit to go to other, more nurse-friendly facilities. Beth, fed up with the unequal distribution of work between Annie's pets and her peons, and frustrated by the unsafe patient assignments, gave one month's notice.

By the time I made it to work, I was usually so steeled for the daily injustice or attack, it would take hours for the coiled spring of anger to relax, only to be replaced with feelings of futility and frustration.

I cried myself to sleep after almost every shift. The nights I didn't cry myself to sleep, I spent tossing feverishly from the tortures of what the French call *l'esprit de l'escalier*, which translates literally to "the wit of the staircase"—all those clever and convincing things I *could* have said to management that did not occur to me until I was on my way down the stairwell to my car.

All in all, the most deeply felt injury was the loss of my "family." Facing work each day without the safety net of Pia's warmth and compassion, Nealy's down-to-earth attitude, or Beth's dry sense of humor and strength left me feeling isolated and unprotected. Bearing the load together had made it easier for each of us to maintain. Now there was no one with whom to share secret laughter and the ever growing frustration.

When David first mentioned that I should think about quitting nursing, I was appalled at the idea. *Me* quit nursing? It seemed as unfathomable as the Pope quitting the church to become Madonna's brassiere keeper. Still, the seed had been planted, and on numerous occasions, I found myselves arguing over the issue.

Me 1: Yeah, but nursing grounds me.

Me 2: Into the ground it grinds you. It's become abusive living, Ec. Like David says, it's killing you. The management is wearing you down. I mean, where's the joy anymore?

Me 1: But I still like taking care of people.

Me 2: There's plenty of other ways to take care of people without getting abused.

Me 1: But what else would I do? Nursing is my life.

Me 2: Nursing is becoming your death, and don't give me that crapola about what else would I do. You've got fourteen years of critical care experience—there's plenty of things you can do.

Me 1: Psssh. I'd be bored or go crazy.

Me 2: You wouldn't be bored if they locked you into a bare four-by-four box, and crazy is the norm for you. Live for the first time. Do what you really enjoy. Write, hike, do some gardening, take time to give to yourself. Try being normal.

Don brought me out of my depressing reverie by daring to take the ice pack off my finger. The two pain pills he had given me earlier hadn't really touched the pain, but made it so I didn't care much.

Before I could get up and follow him to X ray, I took a final long look at the wallpaper photo of trees and wondered why I couldn't see the forest.

In X ray, nobody gave much attention to me or my finger, which looked like a purple, tubular balloon waiting to be twisted into the shape of a miniature dog. Twenty minutes later, I was sent back to ER with the filmed verdict of a fractured phalanges.

While Dr. Kin cleansed and splinted the digit, he gave me the speech we give all patients about how a human bite is one of the dirtiest wounds, and how I needed to take antibiotics, and keep my hand iced and elevated above my head.

I nodded my way through the speech realizing that the only thing I wanted to know was how long I could be off work.

I drove home in conflicted states of pain and ecstasy. I was secretly thrilled that Muriel had chosen my right hand instead of my dumb hand to injure, although it was sad to think a throbbing, mangled finger was more than worth five days' medical leave.

Something, I realized, was very sick about that.

Wednesday
5:30 A.M.

As day breaks, I am unable to sleep for my physical and emotional pains. Wearing three sets of clothes, I sit by the fire crying and hurting out of control like a dry Christmas tree that has caught fire.

David has chosen to stay at his apartment tonight, though he did call when I got home and listened patiently to my tirade about the decentralization meeting. We soon veered off the problem of how my job was killing me, took a joyride down several conversational side streets, and eventually came to a stop at the main-artery issue of our relationship. It was the same circuitous onramp/offramp maze of *Let's keep things in this quasi-living-together-but-not-really* versus *Let's move into one place together.* The exit statement from David was, and I quote, "I love you a lot. We're great together. You're my best friend. But Ec, what is the future of this relationship?"

His question hung in the air like the last pedaled note on a piano. The man who has always been here now seems to be missing from the connection. The surrender has gone to resistance and I am feeling sad and somehow betrayed.

I stamp my foot like a child and pout. I don't want to be one of the 24,067 women in the United States who are, right at this very moment, going through one of the stages of hurt, anger, and/or depression involved with letting go of a relationship. I don't want to think about waking up without David's arms around me.

I am selfish and do not presently have the grace or good sense to walk away and go on. Strong as a rock of Jell-O, I'll let hope keep getting in the way.

On the lighter side: I received my evaluation in the mail. The last line read: "At times it is hard for Ms. Heron to back down when she believes she is right, whether it be from a physician, or nurse management."

My formal rebuttal states that I will continue to stand up for my beliefs and not be treated like anything less than a professional. I also noted they've substituted the word "customer" for "patient" on the grading sheet (it is identical to my report cards from grammar school). Couldn't they have used "healthcare consumer" at least? Waitresses and salesclerks have customers. Nurses have patients.

It is fully light outside and still sleep refuses to come for the race going on in my mind. I am so frigging tired. I think I need to take flight to somewhere else.

SIXTEEN

"To one who has been long in city pent,
'Tis very sweet to look into the fair
And open face of heaven."

JOHN KEATS, *Sonnets*

BELOW, AN ENTIRE WORLD of sparkling blue-green water stretched in every direction as far as the eye could see. A small dark shape skimmed over the waves, never falling behind. I searched the sky for the wayward bird, and finding nothing, realized the figure was the shadow of the two-seater plane in which I was currently a passenger.

For me, the original white-knuckled flyer, flying is hours of panic interspersed with one or two moments of sheer terror. That's when I'm in a big commercial jet. Here I was, in the middle of December, thirty-five hundred feet above the Caribbean Sea in a jerry-built 1956 Volkswagen Bug with wings. That it was wired together in some places, duct-taped in others, and packed nose to tail with eighteen hundred pounds of broccoli and frozen chicken parts did not cheer me, but further intensified the plane's deathtrap air.

Added to all these minuses was the fact that flying this dilapidated grocery cart was a crusty, monosyllabic bush pilot named Pinky who could have been either an extra from an Indiana Jones movie or an escaped robot from the Pirates of the Caribbean in Disneyland.

I was engaged in breaking off the broccoli spears that were rubbing against the back of my neck, when Pinky swore, worked the soggy nubbin of an unlit cigar to the other side of his mouth, and pulled loose the top of the plane's instrument panel.

A smoky electrical smell filled the cabin as wires and odd-looking mechanical parts sprang every which way over the top of the panel. Struggling out of his leather bomber jacket (the effect, with the khaki shorts, argyle knee socks, and Zoris, was definitely a "look"), Pinky reached down into the mess and began blindly twiddling around. "You mother of a whore!" He spit into the mess of wires. "Are you trying to kill me again?"

The words "kill me *again*" put my ulcer in an acid Jacuzzi and my mind into a my-life-flashed-before-me mode. How did I get myself into these Lucy Ricardo–esque situations? my switchboard ladies demanded to know.

Well, I explained, this one all began about the same time I regained function of what I had come to refer to as my Mrs. Fullerton finger. My five days' medical leave proved to be the priming of the pump. On my first day back on the job, the crippling migraine and cold sweat that immediately settled over me as I walked through the double doors of CCU made me realize how much I needed time away from the escalating strain of work. After a week of living in this state, I squared my shoulders, and asked Annie to grant me a full month of vacation time.

Thinking back on it now, I should have realized that with the decentralization issue hanging in the balance, it was to management's advantage to get me out of the way for as long as possible. Annie not only granted me the time off, but did so with a cheery "Bon voyage."

Seeing as how coincidence often plays the starring role in my life, it was not surprising that the day I was trying to decide where I should spend my time off (I had the globe out and was about to tie on my blindfold), I received a letter from a friend, "Doc" Jim, the pharmacist on St. John, who wrote to say he knew how much I detested cold weather, and by his thermometer it was 85 degrees at that very moment and only 44 degrees in San Francisco. He added that his guest cottage was going to be vacant for a month or two, and would I like to use it?

I'd never been to the Caribbean, and certainly the temperature sounded right to my numb fingers, plus the current air fare specials were about what I spent for firewood in a month. Looking out the window for further confirmation, the frosted branches of my dead rosebushes said "Yes!"

Mooshie and David both encouraged me to go in their own, subtle ways. Mooshie refused to let me pick him up, clinging to David's pant leg or shoulder each time I came near (in California, this is referred to by licensed animal therapists as dysfunctional father-pet bonding). David simply reminded me that crying myself to sleep each night and having migraines and cold sweats twenty-five days out of thirty were a pretty good indication I needed a time-out. Simon, lost in the dense fog of adolescence, wouldn't notice I was gone until he got sick of pizza or ran out of money.

Besides, I needed a tan desperately; my skin was so white, you could read by the light from my legs.

On my third glorious tropical day, James found me roasting on the white sand baking sheet of Trunk Bay Beach and told me about a pilot friend who was flying a twin-engine cargo plane to Montserrat, the Emerald Isle of the Caribbean. If I could be at the St. Thomas airport within two hours, and if I didn't mind flying with crates of broccoli and frozen chicken, I could hitch a ride down-island, spend a couple of days exploring, then hitch a flight back.

Montserrat, James assured me as I rushed to repack my freshly unpacked suitcase, was one of the most magical islands in the Caribbean. Lying in the tropics and the trade winds belt, the undeveloped thirty-nine-square-mile British colony boasted a soufrière, a mountain, an eighty-seven-foot waterfall, and ruins of old sugar plantations, all in a lush jungle setting. It was a chance of a lifetime, Doc Jim said, when I boarded the ferry to Redhook. And he was right, except it was the *last* chance of a lifetime, because I was going to die.

As he wrestled with the instrument panel, Pinky's belly, grown rotund from years of Caribbean rum, had accidentally pushed in the yoke, which caused us to nose-dive. The ocean was getting dangerously close by the time he indicated I should take over the controls before we crashed.

Dry-mouthed, I chanted to Buddha, put on my radio headset, and grabbed the yoke. From the switchboard ladies' Necessary Recollections bag, I pulled out a few dusty memories of flying instruction I'd taken as a naive seventeen-year-old (ah, those premortal days) in someone's muddy back field. Moth-eaten, with large holes between the facts, the only memories I had left of those lessons consisted of: "Pull the yoke back and you go up, push it in and you go down." The fact that I had once soloed—that is to say, I'd taken off, flown around a field, and then landed the aircraft upright and in one piece, all by myself—meant absolutely nothing to me now as the plane lost altitude.

Slowly, I pulled back on the yoke, and sure enough, up we went . . . right into a huge cloud mass, visibility zero.

Claustrophobic and imminent-death panic wires crossed in my mind and I shorted out. My switchboard ladies pulled out the reserve mental parachutes and flotation raft, then hurriedly blew the dust off the ground school memories and put them up on the screen, so that there, in my mind's eye, was the basic instrument panel of a small aircraft.

Okay, the big dial was the horizontal indicator—keep the line straight across. Synchronize the compass with the directional gyro—good. Now even out, push in, okay, keep it steady, pressure gauges in the green, fuel tanks half full, good. The vertical speed indicator told me the pitch of the nose was headed in an upward direction—this was encouraging.

It didn't take a genius to know that to get out of the cloud, I had to either climb over it or dive under it. A red sign flashed on the switchboard ladies' screen that said, "Remember, the higher you are, the more control and time you have to get out of a bad situation." I pulled back a little more and we climbed until, after what seemed like an eternity in cloud hell, we emerged in the middle of a giant blue bowl full of fluffy mashed potatoes. In front of us, a rainbow arced between two of the cloud masses.

Despite my solemn belief we were going to die that day, the sight took my breath away and gave me courage. In that moment the pure joy of living came back to me like a fond memory, and I was ecstatic in the vast heaven of sky.

While I did some fancy scud running—maneuvering over, under, around, and through the clouds—my cigar-chewing co-pilot worked on the instrument panel, sweat pouring down his face from under a shabby World War II flight cap. Once, he looked over at the instrument panel, raised his eyebrows in an expression that said, "Hey, that ain't too bad for a broad," and pointed downward. I pushed in, and slowly dropped us below the clouds.

Off the tip of the right wing was a small green island bathed in sun. The old bush pilot clapped the top of the instrument panel back into place and took over the controls. "Montserrat," he mouthed.

We made our approach, heading straight on into the side of the mountain. At the last moment (I could see the blossoms on the shrubberies growing in the crevices of the rocks), Pinky banked left and dropped to the single airstrip running alongside the beach. As soon as the propellers came to a standstill, I popped the door open and stepped out onto the wing.

Enveloped in the clean, silken air, which smelled of ocean and sun, I was immediately struck with the sense that I was finally home after a long and arduous journey. Tranquillity filled me as I headed across the field to the immigration desk.

The immigration officer, a tall and lanky Montserratian, regarded me with an air of amusement. "Why you comin' to Montserrat, sister?" His smile revealed perfect white teeth, a feature I would soon discover was common among the Montserratians.

"I'm on vacation." I smiled and handed him my passport.

"You gonna be limin', huh?"

I thought this an odd question to ask, but decided that maybe his family owned an orchard of lime trees and he was going to tell me where to buy some. "Uhn, well, sure, I suppose I might pick some limes while I'm here."

The immigration officer threw his head back and laughed at something that must have struck him funny at that moment. In rapid West Indian Pidgin English, he related his joke to two Montserratian men playing dominoes nearby. When the chuckling died down, he stamped my passport and made a lazy, half salute. "Have a good day, girl. All de best."

Pinky's mode of land transportation proved to be as questionable as his flying machine. Called a Moke, it was Britain's automotive version of what one might imagine the progeny of a golf cart and a jeep to be. Taking the main route, we headed out of the airport and began winding around the island through lush jungle terrain.

Along the road, men riding donkeys and carrying machetes smiled and raised a hand in greeting, while the women, many of whom carried large bundles on their heads, generally seemed more reticent about returning our hellos. Every child we saw was sucking a mango with its skin pulled down in strips, like a banana. From a distance, it looked as though they were eating orange sherbet out of green paper cups.

Once, when we stopped for a donkey who'd taken its rest in the middle of the road, the youngsters stormed the Moke. Untroubled by warnings about not taking rides from strangers, happy children covered every inch of the vehicle. "Ride, mon? You give us de ride?"

As we passed by a handful of concrete and wooden shacks

painted in the Caribbean colors of bright robin's-egg blue, pink, and turquoise, my attention was taken by a towering royal palm with a narrow piece of corrugated tin roof wrapped around the trunk like a paper clip. On the section trailing two or three feet beyond the tree, someone had spray-painted the word "HUGO" with an arrow pointing in the direction in which the hurricane had obviously passed.

We slowed when we entered the main town of Plymouth, a maze of narrow streets where stucco-and-stone buildings melted into each other, pushing so close together that not even the narrowest of thoughts could slip through. Green shutters, some open, some closed, held signs advertising all manner of things, from soursop coolers and goat water, to guava cheese and chicken *rôti*. But, the best sign—the one that set me laughing—read: "Montserrat Furniture—Made Fresh Daily."

Leaving Plymouth, we headed up the other side of the mountain, winding our way through the small communities of Weekes, Cork Hill, Frith, and Salem. When we came to a section of the island designated as St. Peter's Parish, we turned onto a narrow, partially paved road. Climbing upward for the better part of a mile, we passed through a stone gate that led to a circular driveway in front of a magnificent house.

While I stood in awe of the gardens surrounding the estate, Pinky produced a key with which he opened the front door. Stepping into a veritable cathedral of a living room, I took in the sight before me in stunned silence.

The entire length of the room was wide open to the 180-degree view of lavender ocean and pink sky. Sitting to one side of this panorama was a deep golden sun, changing into its evening dress behind a purple cloud.

"It's the one view in all of the Caribbean that still stops me cold," Pinky said, handing me the key to the house.

"Oh my God," I managed to whisper, "I'm home."

Pinky removed his cigar and chuckled. "I know the feeling. That's what I said when I stepped onto my first Caribbean island ten years ago."

"You *live* here?" I asked, unable to believe that someone could actually live in such a place and not die of the beauty.

"I caretake the place for the owners, who live in England," Pinky said. "But I'm never around, except when cargo is slow, and then I only get to spend one or two days a week up here. Mostly I'm flying cargo seven days a week from San Juan to the various islands. Speaking of which . . ." Pinky checked his watch. "I've got to fly over to Antigua and then to Nevis before the airport closes. I'll be back in a couple of days to pick you up—if you want to go. If not, you're welcome to stay as long as you like." He looked at me sideways. "You know anything about gardening?"

"Sure." I nodded.

A smile like daybreak crossed the man's round face, revealing a gold-capped incisor. "Great. Feel free to do as much as you like. I'll show you around the place. There's plenty of food in the cupboards, but if you need more, you can go to the Plymouth market on Saturday morning, or leave a message for me at the control tower and I'll try to pick up what you need and drop it at the airport on my way through."

The grand, though somewhat rushed, tour of the estate left me even more agog. The two master bedrooms had private baths, and two patios apiece, with magnificent views of the ocean from one and the tropical gardens from the other. The other two guest rooms, though they had only one patio each, plus panoramic views, and private baths, were larger than my entire cottage.

Encircled by tropical trees and flowers, the pool was situated in a terra-cotta courtyard that overlooked the sea. Along one edge of the pool, a lower filtering trough provided a constant waterfall. Off to the side, behind a wall of the exotic jade vine, was another courtyard, this one to a concrete-block house that served dual purposes of laundry room and hurricane shelter.

The nursery/gardening room, with its complete set of tools and potting apparatus, was to drool over. Pinky took his time there, careful to show me where everything was.

Back at the front door, the pilot pressed another set of keys into my hand. "I'll take the Moke back down to the airport. There's an old Land Rover in the garage that belongs to the house. It isn't as much fun to drive as the Moke, but it's safer."

On his way out, Pinky stopped and turned back. "Don't be afraid of the critters that creep in during the night. The only ones that are even remotely poisonous are the bufo frogs, and they're hard to miss."

Immediately I conjured up visions of man-eating frogs with fangs and tongues the length of a man's leg. "You have poisonous frogs around here?"

"Well, they have these glands on their head that make this white sticky fluid that's supposed to be poisonous, but you'd have to lick the frog to get sick."

"Gee, I'll try to hold back," I said. "It'll be hard, but I think I can restrain myself."

Pinky winked at me from the door. "And be careful of the jack-spaniards that hang out under the elephant ear leaves—they sting like the dickens."

Although I didn't have a clue, I smiled bravely and waved this away as though I knew exactly what he was talking about. Mentally, I envisioned gangs of matadors named Jack who hid in the bushes and jabbed people with their swords.

The upper and lower verandas boasted sleeping hammocks, every variety of table and chair, and mounted telescopes for looking out to sea or sky. It was a struggle to decide, but I eventually settled on the upstairs veranda, watching in awe as the sun went out in a blaze of orange, gold, and lavender. At dusk the jungle began taking on another face, of mystery and hidden dangers. Before the endless sky was completely dark, there was a rush of air near my head, and my hair was pulled. I turned in time to discover eight or ten bats soaring through a hole in the high ceiling some thirty feet up. They glided through the rafter beams and over the pool, disappeared for a few seconds, then flew in through the hole again.

Okay, so I had bats in my belfry. I liked bats; Doc Jim told me they ate three times their weight in insects each night, which was part of the reason why there were few mosquitoes and no-see-ums near the house.

Without batting an eye, I moved quickly out of their flight pattern and went to explore the rest of the house. I found the fresh linen (four closets' worth), and was making up the bed in the upstairs master bedroom when I realized the sounds coming from the jungle and the rainforest had changed from birdsong to a deafening cacophony of crickets, lizards, and . . . (gulp) frogs. In this clamor was one noise that, to my ears, sounded exactly like someone clanking a machete against the stone wall that bordered the property. I blocked out visions of savage jungle dwellers and made dinner for myself from the abundantly stocked, very British pantry (where else could one find ten boxes of tea, four jars of marmalade, twelve tins of water biscuits, and five jars of Marmite?).

I showered in the master bath under the scrutiny of a dove perched on the opened shutter. Taking this as a good luck omen, I crawled happily into bed, pulled the mosquito net down around me, and listened to the noises of the night jungle.

I pinched myself to make sure I wasn't having one of my Technicolor, full-length dreams. I, Echo, was a dweller of the jungle, miles from the nearest human being, surrounded by clean water, clean air, and the music of a tropical jungle to lull me to—

From the kitchen came the crash of pots and pans.

I held my breath, lying as still as a millstone at the bottom of a river. Then a broom fell, the handle slapping against the ceramic tiles.

Granted, it was 85 degrees, but I began to sweat profusely as I reasoned out what was making the racket. Pinky had said crime was virtually unknown on the island. The closest thing to theft might be the borrowing of a garden tool, or perhaps a set of pillowcases from your clothesline. A few months later, you would be apt to find the pillowcases washed and neatly folded on your doorstep, and the tool, honed and polished, back in its original place.

A cupboard door crashed open and something fell with a thud.

I cautiously opened the net, grabbed my flashlight, and tiptoed through the house. Before actually stepping into the kitchen, I reached around and flicked on the fluorescent overhead lights.

At the time, I was astounded that my loud and prolonged screams didn't bring hordes of people running. What I didn't know was that even if I had been heard, no one would have come near the place, since many Montserratians were convinced the trees on the estate were occupied by jumbies, or bad spirits. What did occupy the kitchen at that moment, however, I would have traded for jumbies any day, for scurrying across the walls and ceiling and sliding along the ceramic floor tiles were a platoon of cockroaches about half the size of Rhode Island. People in the southern states sometimes call them palmetto bugs, but you can't fool me, Gertrude—a cockroach is a cockroach is a cockroach.

Two seconds and one blink later, there wasn't a trace of the giant, disgusting things, and all that remained were the echoes of my screams. I don't know what I expected; I was in a tropical jungle in a house that was completely open. It was only natural that the house would have cockroaches the way California had Yuppies.

The culprit rearranging the kitchen was a large gray bush rat, who, though now cowering in a corner of the floor, did not pause for a second in pursuit of his goal of eating through the package of dried apricots I'd brought from St. John. At one wave of my arms, the rodent scampered onto the veranda and disappeared into the jungle, taking an apricot with him.

I didn't dare move my feet, afraid of what I might disturb; I didn't think I was ready yet to face any more jungle creatures. A white glob fell onto my arm. I looked up and received another wet splat on my forehead. Hanging over the rafter, perfectly aimed at my head, was the anal sphincter of a foot-long lizard known as a wood slave. I quickly dodged the third attack. At the sink, I washed myself off and noted that all the globs contained undigested portions of cockroaches. This lumped lizards in with the bats as being okay creatures. Cleaning the mess off the top of my head was preferable to cockroaches any day.

First lesson of the jungle: Never leave garbage or food exposed to the insect or rodent public. I put a tight cover on the garbage pail and refrigerated whatever food had been opened, all the while keeping a close watch on the whereabouts of the wood slave above. It was okay; he was busy stalking a moth whose wings spanned ten inches and were like silk canvases painted with the intricate designs of a Persian rug.

The activity going on around the kitchen light drew my attention. Along those three long fluorescent tubes, hundreds of moths had gathered—some tiny, some as big as the one being stalked by the wood slave. The cloud of fluttering bodies and wings in colors of neon orange, white, lime green, pinks, and reds changed constantly, like a kaleidoscope. It reminded me of the parking lot of Jumpin' Jack's, a summertime hangout for teens in my hometown.

I got right up next to the light to study some of the strangest-looking flying things I'd ever seen; one moth was shaped like a coffin, another like a prehistoric monster. The one I named the Zoot Suit Rasta moth had a head covered with shiny black dreadlocks and wore fuzzy checkered pantaloons on its legs. I was concentrating on the prehistoric monster moth exploring under my fingernail with its antennae, when I glimpsed a flick of red out of the corner of my eye.

I whipped around in time to see a hairy red tarantula drop ten feet down from the rafter onto the counter I was leaning against. The body, which was the size of an oatmeal cookie, hit with a plop two inches from my elbow.

It is a certainty that I had never moved so fast, nor screamed so loud in all my years on this planet. I was cowering against the broom closet when I saw the King Kong of arachnids hop—yes, I said hop—toward me.

Mobilizing at the speed of light, I ran into the living room—backward.

The damned thing hopped after me.

Terrified, I could only think to go down to the lower master bedroom and seal off the room. Halfway down the stairs, I glanced over my shoulder, only to see The Thing hopping, stair by stair, right on my heels.

I made it to the master bedroom and slammed the door, still screaming. Ten minutes later, I opened the door cautiously.

The red tarantula sat waiting patiently. In one hop, it was inside the room and sitting on my bare foot.

For the frozen four or five minutes that followed, I watched The Thing—and I'll swear to this on anybody's Bible—stare back at me while it checked me out with its antennae—or antlers (they were big enough). When it was satisfied, it hopped off my foot and onto the wall in search of whatever it was it ate—a cow or a sheep maybe.

I beat feet upstairs, turned on the beside lamp, got into my bed, and pulled the mosquito net around me. As I lay hyperventilating, my heart pounding, I realized I was no longer in paradise; I was in Jungle Terror Scream Hell.

With this thought still going through the old synapses, a furry black thing, caught in the mosquito netting above my head, struggled to get free.

It was during the scream that I realized it was only a bat.

I pulled the layers of netting apart and freed it, but being blind as a bat, instead of flying out the patio doors, it kept crashing into the wall and knocking itself to the ground.

After the flying mammal repeated this stunt ten or fifteen times, I finally pulled the sheet off the bed, threw it over the thing, and shook out the sheet off the deck. Of course, it took off like a bat out of hell.

Back to bed. Turn off the light. But wait . . . .

A bump in the surface of the nightstand moved. Focusing, I saw a small lizard scurry from the oak stand to the light blue wall. Within a minute, it changed from a light oak color to light blue. Up close, small round gold eyes stared into mine. I cocked my head; the chameleon cocked his. I moved my head to the left, and his eyes followed. I began making a variety of insect noises in hopes of getting some kind of communication going, until the tiny lizard began to take on an expression of pity.

Back to bed.

I had actually gone as far as to doze off, when I awoke to a rustling of cellophane—similar to the noise you hear behind you at the movies as someone delves into a package of red licorice. Except I recognized this as the sound of someone opening my package of rice crackers, followed by the rhythmic chewing of someone eating my rice crackers.

"Look, whoever you are," I said in a clear, strong voice, "go ahead and take the whole package. There's two more boxes in the breadbox in the kitchen, but watch out for the roaches."

The rustling and crunching stopped for a minute, then resumed. Getting up steam, I reached through the mosquito net and turned on the light.

I wonder, even now, if anyone was listening to the bouts of intermittent screams that night or on the nights that followed. I would love to have heard just a few of the stories that must have gone around.

There, on the pillow next to mine, sat a huge black land crab. In one claw was my package of rice crackers, in the other a half-eaten cracker. The ugly thing eyed me with a sour expression and took another nibble.

I made a grab for the package, and the crab scurried sideways off the bed and onto the ceramic floor tiles. Making a noise like a tap dancer on a glass table top, it clacked its way across the floor to the bathroom.

By the toilet, we commenced to have a tug-of-war with the crackers. During the tussle, it became clear the land crab was stubborn as hell and quite strong. It wasn't until he lunged at my leg with his free claw, though, that I really got angry. I wouldn't argue about the crackers, but one of us had to leave. Using the toilet brush, I slid the crab (was he ever!) onto the deck and closed the jalousie doors.

Back to bed.

This time I slept for maybe an hour, until someone turned off the sounds of the night and replaced them with birds. Thus I had passed my first night in the jungle.

After a quick breakfast of yogurt and fresh mangoes, I dressed and headed toward the garage to negotiate the Land Rover, a British-built mechanical wonder that looked, handled, and ran very much like a military tank or a cargo truck.

I am here to tell you that driving with the wheel on the right-hand side of the cabin, having to shift with one's left hand, while driving on the left, is an experience any dyslexic masochist might like to give a whirl. Town was only seven miles away, but the drive took thirty minutes. This was partially due to the fact that the Land Rover was hard to steer for a 108-pound weakling, partially because the roads were narrow and curvy, and partially because of the pointers.

Within the first mile after I had found and turned onto the main road, I came upon a group of five adolescent boys all shouting and pointing excitedly to the trees down the way. Slowing down to a crawl, I craned my neck to see what must surely be some true wonder of nature just in front of me.

The teens ran to the Rover and piled in. When they realized I was totally at a loss to understand their Pidgin English, the young man sitting in front pointed in the direction of town.

" 'S all right, sister. We ridin' to town."

Wanting to show goodwill, I smiled and after a few grinding attempts managed to find first gear, and off we went with a lurch.

Another half mile down the road, at Salem, three women carrying what looked like bags of laundry on their heads, heard the Rover (besides driving like a tank, it sounded like one too) and began pointing into the trees.

Once again, I slowed to see if I could glimpse what they were pointing at, and the same scene was repeated: The three women piled into the rear and took seats. There were rounds of " 'S all right, sister, 's all right, brother," and we lurched forward yet again.

I finally got up the nerve and turned to the boy next to me, whose name, as far as I could tell, was Denver. "What is everyone pointing at?"

Everyone in the Rover howled with laughter. When the sounds of glee subsided, Denver explained. "When de people want to ride, dey point to where dey are goin'. We all pointin' to town."

The light dawned. Instead of the American hitchhiker's thumb, the Montserratians pointed to where they wanted to go. I laughed until I wheezed, which got my hitchhikers all to laughing again.

In Cork Hill I picked up six more pointers—four men, a secondary school student, and a very old woman. The boys in the front moved around to the back to stand on the bumper, two of the Cork Hill men squeezed into the back, and two climbed over the hood to sit on the top of the car. The women sat in front with me. More " 'S all rights" all around and lurch again.

By the time we reached Plymouth, I was pouring sweat (94 degrees and climbing at ten A.M.). Each time I made a passenger drop-off, there was a shout of "Thanks, sister. All de best." Now pointerless, I found my way to the waterfront, parked, and ventured into the town on foot.

The first thing that struck me was the absence of Christmas flash and trash. Thank little baby Jesus for that! Instead of strings of gaudy lights hanging from outdoor trees, children dressed in bright colors swung from the branches of mango trees, looking like so much overripe fruit. Instead of Salvation Army Santa Clauses and bassinets strewn with hay and halos, there were colorful, ten-feet-tall mocko jumbie figures who raced through the narrow winding streets scaring children and superstitious adults.

Making my way into a small variety store that put me in mind of a five-and-dime from the 1940s (certainly the stock was at least that old), I was told by an unsmiling cashier that they did not accept U.S. currency; only East Caribbean money would pay for my bottle of coconut oil. The six other people in line behind me didn't grumble the way Americans might have done, but they did take on very serious expressions. I searched through my fanny pack, hoping against hope that some E.C. might magically appear. When it did not, I slapped my forehead in exasperation. "Gosh, I'm really sorry, but I think I left my mind at home hanging in the closet."

The clerk covered her mouth and giggled. Pretty soon everyone in line was at least smiling. Without another word, the clerk took my U.S. bill and exchanged it for E.C. The woman in line behind me took my hand and walked me next door to the bank. She pointed to the window that said "Currency Exchange" and gave a rather lengthy, animated speech, not a word of which I caught. From that day forward, whenever dealing with Montserratians, I tried to play a role that was a combination of Bozo the Clown and Woody Allen. This more often than not earned me the respect of the Montserratians, though wary glances from the British.

I wandered through the streets waving lazily and " 'S all right"-ing everyone I saw. On one corner, an old woman sitting under an awning reached out and gently wrapped her hand around my ankle as I passed. Taking two oblong packages wrapped in white parchment paper from the covered basket in front of her, she handed them to me. "You skinny girl, eat my *rôti*. Dey fatten you up. Only two dollar."

I gave the woman two dollars E.C., which was about seventy-four cents, and headed down George Street toward the waterfront where several groups of men sat playing dominoes under the clock tower next to the post office. From a green-shuttered window, I purchased a soursop cooler and sat on a stone fence nearby.

Throwing caution and my vegetarianism to the winds, I bit into a delicate homemade pastry dough filled with potatoes, onions, carrots, and shreds of (I think—I hope) chicken, all swimming in a thick, curry gravy. The foamy, ice-cold soursop was orgasmic.

I inhaled the meal, not caring that several of the men had stopped playing dominoes and were having a good laugh over my gluttonous passion. When I'd licked the paper and the inside of my cup dry, I started back up the mountain.

I picked up eight pointers and dropped them all at Cork Hill where, from what I could gather from the slower-spoken of my passengers, a "jump-up" was in progress. The event itself seemed to get its lifeblood from a wall of some twenty-five speakers. A sort of West Indian reggae/rap/steel drum music blared from tweeters and woofers, vibrating loud enough to shake bananas from the trees. Literally.

A cluster of twenty or so Montserratian men swayed and danced to the beat, while the women stood in a wide circle around them, talking to each other with downcast eyes.

Thirty minutes later, I pulled into the circular drive and almost hit one of the six goats that came bounding off the front veranda. Telltale shreds of bird-of-paradise stalks hung from the mouth of the leader. One baby, too small to make the jump, backed into a corner and bleated its newborn heart out.

Taking the trembling puppy-sized kid into my arms, I followed the bleat of its mother into the dense part of the jungle. When we were close enough, I released my squirmy bundle, watching it trot unsteadily toward Mom. I walked on for perhaps another half mile, until I began seeing long rope vines—like those used by Johnny Weissmuller as his main transportation in the old Tarzan movies—hanging willy-nilly from the trees. Seizing this as the perfect opportunity to live out my childhood fantasy of swinging from tree to tree, I took one end of a good-sized root and headed toward a sunny rock covered with what, in my myopic haze, I thought were exotic turquoise plants.

At once the "plants" turned into full-grown iguanas, some as long as two feet, and disappeared into the underbrush as fast as the cockroaches had the night before. This fostered only a small scream. I was improving.

When I tired of my Tarzan swing, I lay down on the lower part of the rock and stared at the sky. Halfway to achieving a 1960s kind of contact nirvana, I was brought back to the living dream of the rainforest by a presence. As if in a slow-motion movie, I turned my head to my immediate right.

Standing over me was an old West Indian man with his machete raised, ready to bring it down.

I gasped and opened wide for the scream, but stopped when he put his fingers to his lips. A second later, the machete blade sliced the air an inch from my ear and struck the crevice where the rock and the ground met. In a crouched, hyperventilating position, I jumped up and backed away from the man, who was now hacking wildly at the underbrush. Who knew what his problem was? Maybe he was pissed off because I was lying on his private rock, or maybe he was having one of those bad voodoo jungle days.

Seeing my fear, the old man reached into the underbrush and pulled up two halves of a three-foot black snake. The scream, waiting impatiently, came out of me like the operatic wailing of Turandot in act two.

He dropped the dead reptile halves and waved his arms. "Rest yourself, sister, rest yourself. De snake gone. He not hurt you, but de Bible say de snake is evil."

I stopped screaming abruptly. Not knowing what else to say, I said, " 'S all right?" and sat down.

The black man grinned and held out a weathered hand for shaking. "I'm Salem. You de pilot's new woman, huh?"

I shook the man's hand, noting that around his neck he wore a silver chain with a crucifix, a stick, and a black stone hanging from it. "My name is Echo. I'm just visiting at the house while Pinky is gone."

The man nodded, and sat down in the underbrush, careful to make sure all snake parts were thrown far and wide. "Woppin'?" he asked.

And I thought we'd been doing so well communicating.

"Woppin'?"

"Oh, dis goat over in de ghaut, he givin' me trouble. Woppin' you?"

Woppin'? Woppin'? Think abbreviated with an accent. Ah! What's happening. "Ah, I'm hanging out enjoying the jungle."

"Limin', huh?"

There was that strange question about the limes again. "Well, no, I haven't found the lime trees yet."

The old man looked at me curiously for a few seconds and shrugged. "You know where de avocado tree be?"

"No."

"You know where is de soursop?"

"I have a soursop tree in that yard?" I asked, my taste buds suddenly interested.

"Sister, you got three acre of all de fruit and flower. I de mon who plant dem twenty year ago." He got up, hacked a few times at some of the taller underbrush, and began to make his departure. "I come another day, show you where de fruit grow." He looked back over his shoulder. "I got to get me goat home before de old woman lock de door."

"I'd really like to know about the plants," I said to the retreating figure. "I hope to see you soon, and all de best."

"All de best, sister. Go home before de dark come an' bring dem snakes lookin' for dey brother."

Day 5, Montserrat, West Indies
3:00 A.M.

I am writing this by candlelight in the closet of the downstairs master bedroom. Outside, the wind is howling like a wounded beast and shoving the metal patio chairs around as if they were feathers. Earlier, one was blown into the pool and now rests at the bottom. The rain is so heavy that I cannot see much beyond two or three feet when I dare to open the Dutch door jalousies.

At one A.M. the wind was so strong that there were whitecaps two feet high in the pool, so I ran around the house securing all the hurricane shutters. There was no electricity, of course (third time this week). Salem says the "lectric" is trying to escape from Montserrat because it doesn't like to be trapped in the cables. I found three kerosene lanterns and a half dozen candles from the hurricane emergency supplies. Thank God Pinky thought to show me where they were kept.

Salem stopped by around four P.M. to say his "inside"

mind (I think he means his intuition) was telling him a storm was coming. I got so caught up in the gardening, I completely forgot about his warning. When I went to bed I was aware that something was "off," but didn't pay any attention to my own intuition. Had my mind been present, I would have realized how unnaturally still it was. Even the creatures were silent. It was hotter than usual and there wasn't so much as a sigh of breeze. The noise woke me at midnight. The second I opened my eyes, I saw that the royal palm in the front garden was bending at an alarming angle, and a flowered bedsheet flew across the yard like a decked-out jumbie. A pair of men's pants caught in the breadfruit tree, and the legs were dancing like a stoned-out Rastafarian at a jump-up. Talk about jumbies—I won't be able to get Salem to come near the place.

The violence of this force is frightening, but there is a wild force of my own that wants desperately to run out into the middle of it.

I doubt the new hibiscus or the lamb's-tongue ferns will be anywhere near where I planted them—probably find them on the roof (if there is a roof).

Besides my nerves, my ears are getting the worst of this. The noise is deafening, plus my ears hurt from the pressure changes . . . similar to those I experience when flying.

In abstract, the island reminds me of a woman who has just washed her long hair and is vigorously shaking out all the water. I cannot even imagine what a full-blown hurricane must be like. Salem said Hugo was the worst thing he had ever experienced in his life (he has not been off the island since the day he was born sixty-seven years ago), but when I told him about the earthquakes in San Francisco, he said he'd rather be blown up to heaven than fall down a crack into hell.

I know where Betty Crocker lives. Everything I bake or cook comes out just as good as anything Aunt Martha ever made. My corn bread is as fluffy and light as a picture, and I made the creamiest, most wonderful yogurt from dry milk. It must be a combination of the water, the heat, and the humidity.

Jack-spaniards, by the way, seem like your everyday wasp. I've also seen a few bufos—almost stepped on one the other evening when I went out for a walk. They look like our frogs back home in Scotia.

Oh, and limin'? It means lying back and relaxing.

I am passionately in love with this place—critters, wild weather, and all! How good it feels to breathe clean air and drink fresh clean water. I have not had a migraine since I landed. All in all, I feel the same way about finding Montserrat as I did that time, during the pyromania phase of my childhood, when I found a full pack of matches under a pile of dry leaves.

When Pinky checked in, I asked if I might stay on in the house until the end of the month, provided I did a few hours of gardening or housework each day. He was delighted by the deal. I thought it was an even shake, considering the condition of the house and the garden. During the cleaning process, I found several types of nests in the kitchen cupboards, and at the bottom of one of the bedroom closets I came upon two green velvet mounds. The mounds turned out to be a pair of red and yellow Tony Lama boots under three inches of mold. Leather and dark fabrics don't do well in Montserrat's tropical climate; my leather belts both turned fuzzy within the first week, and my black tank top resembled a camouflage shirt.

Every few days, Salem suddenly appeared from out of the jungle, announcing himself by clanking his machete against the stone wall that surrounded the estate. For the price of a malt beer and a basket of limes, I received a crash course in both tropical gardening and bush medicine.

On the two and a half acres of mature, tropical garden, Salem had planted a living produce market of breadfruit, avocado, lime, tamarind, guava, lemon, orange, banana, papaya, mango, soursop, passion fruit, and cashew trees. The basil, oregano, and lemon-grass, he told me, had been planted by the wind.

My second day in the garden, I learned that gardening without proper gloves, shoes, and long pants is a perfect setup for trauma. First my arm turned numb and swelled from the sting of an unknown black wasplike thing with neon-orange antennae; then I stepped, barefoot, too close to a centipede.

Salem appeared as I was soaking my very swollen and painful ankle in iced salt water. He immediately went off to gather "bush" and came back ten minutes later with an assortment of plants and roots which he boiled down and made into a poultice. The leftover oily black "tea" he gave me to drink.

As soon as my cup was drained of the vile, bitter liquid, Salem smiled as proudly as a child with a gold star. "You never gonna be bit by de centipede no more."

"Why do you say that?" I burped up the unpleasant after-taste of bush tea, concerned about the alarming noises my stomach was making. It sounded like it was moving, trying to claw its way out.

"In de bush, I crush up de old grandfather centipede. Now you got him inside, de other ones smell him and run away."

Day 10, Montserrat
10:00 P.M.

I find it distressing that I still cannot understand a word of the Montserratians' version of English. After asking them to repeat themselves for the fourth or fifth time, I finally just nod and smile. God only knows what I'm agreeing to. Sometimes, though, the odd way they look at me when I answer really gets me worried.

I went down to the Emerald Café yesterday afternoon and gave up being a vegetarian again for the sake of adventure: I ordered mountain chicken, which turned out to be frogs' legs the size of turkey drumsticks. Someday I'd like to see one of those suckers in the living skin. Then again, maybe I wouldn't.

True to their name, they tasted like a light chicken with a slightly slippery texture. The goat water stew doesn't even remotely tempt me, though the salad made almost entirely from flower petals was exquisite. The hot pepper dressing would have blown my socks off had I worn any, and I got a major sugar rush off the coconut pie with homemade mango ice cream.

On the way home, I was so involved in watching the sun-set that I drove the first mile on the wrong side of the road. Dyett, the mechanic down at Happy Hill, waved and laughed from the side of the road. As I passed, he shouted out, " 'S all right, sister, but you gotta do better den dat if you gonna wake up in de morning."

Pinky temporarily traded the Moke for the Rover, since he had some big loads of produce to deliver to private buyers. This toy jeep is definitely more fun to drive, but I found major drawbacks: it seems the British, in all their automotive wisdom, built the distributor directly in front of the engine, next to the open grille. So every time it rains (on an aver-

*age of three times a day), the thing gets wet and stops dead
in its tracks. After I was almost run over, I found an old
margarine tub and covered the stupid distributor.*

*The best for last: I was pruning the poinsettias and cut-
ting back the elephant-ear plants yesterday, when I uncovered a mossy footpath, set with pieces of bright ceramic tile.
The afternoon shower had begun, but I used one of the cut
elephant-ear leaves as an umbrella and made my way down
the narrow trail along the side of the mountain, until I came
to a rock alcove.*

*Someone—I suspect someone close to the God within
himself—had cut a chair into the rock. At the foot of this
chair was carved a perfectly square kneeling platform that
was covered with a cushion of velvety moss.*

*In the chair, which was overhung with orange and purple
bougainvillea, I turned my mind toward the boundless panorama of green sea and pearl-gray sky. I stayed there on
heaven's doorstep until a spray of shooting stars reminded
me I was earthbound and it was time to come to bed.*

The day was glorious. Taking up the walking stick Salem
had fashioned for me, I left my garden behind and set out
early, walking the trails of St. Peter's. In a section of road
flanked only by tall trees and bushes, a muscular young man
wearing nothing more than a pair of tattered cotton pants came
out of the jungle and walked steadily toward me. Swinging
from his hand was a fair-sized machete.

As we passed each other, we smiled and bid each other a
good morning. A gardener perhaps, or a farmer going to or
from his vegetable (or perhaps, ganja) fields in the mountain.

It occurred to me that there were very few places in the
world where I could have experienced this same encounter
without feeling fear.

By the time I reached the district clinic, I was exhausted. I
found the shade of a mango tree and sat down to rest and sip
some Gatorade. An old woman came out of the one-room
schoolhouse used for the preschoolers and motioned that I
should come to her.

"Come, come, girl," she said. " 'S okay. Come to me."

Like an obedient child, I went, and as I approached, she
stepped very close. "Good morning," she said, barely smiling.
"I love your face. Me love you."

The warmth of surprise and pleasure and love moved me to

tears. My first impulse was to hug her, but I stopped myself, knowing that the Montserratians conveyed their feelings with words and actions rather than touch. I thanked her and, sensing the beauty and wisdom of her spirit, returned the compliment.

For want of a better place to take the conversation after that intimate lead-in, I asked about the small group of preschoolers who were busy playing with the chickens in the yard.

The woman half smiled, shrugged, then stooped to pick a piece of tall grass. I was getting used to the slow, careful Montserratian method of answering questions, which seemed more satisfying than the quick blurting of the first half-formed thought that came to mind.

"Oh, dey play now, but after, dey study de lessons," she said, and as if to demonstrate, turned and sternly called the children back to their places on the wooden porch of her schoolroom.

I moved on, hearing her call out the alphabet as their little voices repeated in unison, "A, B, C . . ."

Day 25, Montserrat
11:00 P.M.

Pinky will be here tomorrow to fly me up to St. Thomas. If ever a place has gotten ahold of me, Montserrat has woven its magic into every fiber of my being.

It has been the perfect last day. I drove the Rover (my biceps are back to what they were when I drove the '57 Chevy wagon) down toward Galway's, and once I found the trail, went as far into the ghaut as I dared. When the trail got too hilly and rough, I set the brake and hiked into the gorge. I was beginning to think I was going to be one of those people who wander into the jungle and are never seen again, when I heard Great Alps Waterfall.

What a sight. What a feeling—I let the water beat down on my back until I felt like a piece of tenderized meat.

When I returned to the jeep, I decided I could not leave the island without mastering the claustrophobia that has kept me from going all the way to the center of Galway's Soufrière.

I drove to the head of the soufrière trail, not dwelling on the fact that the volcano is still active. I decided that if the tons of soft clay that made up the narrow crater walls of the soufrière were, by that long, long chance, to fall in on me, then so be it.

I took off my shoes and followed the warm, milky stream toward the steam clouds in the distance. Intimidated and exhilarated at the same time, I stopped at the first sulfur steam vents, removed all but my shoes, then steamed myself until my skin felt like velvet. Still, by the time I got to the pockets of bubbling mud and sulfur deposits, I was having to concentrate to keep from hyperventilating. About thirty yards farther, the iron oxides streaked the mud deposits with red, blue, yellow, white, orange, and black stains. To take my mind off my panic, I painted myself from head to toe in designs I remembered from pictures of American Indians. Fully decked out in my mud masque paint, I kept going until the walls narrowed down to an opening that barely permitted me to squeeze through.

My fear took me to every confined place I have ever fled. I stopped, closed my eyes, and breathed—if I was going to dance, it had to be right then. So, like the commercial says, I just did it, squeezing through that high, narrow passageway like the devil's army was on my tail.

When I opened my eyes, I was standing within the heart of the volcano, steam billowing into the air from a caldron of bubbling earth. I sat down near the edge and cooked in a silence that was almost as deafening as the waterfall. The clouds of steam created an atmosphere of tranquillity that was otherworldly. Had Buddha or Jesus or Isadora Duncan floated by, it would have seemed perfectly natural.

The rest of the day was no less dreamlike. By the time I made it to Plymouth, the sun was setting. Not wanting to miss my last sunset, I got out and walked along the waterfront. I had just asked for a sign that I would return to this magic island, when I looked toward the horizon. The sinking sun exploded in a neon-green burst. I'd thought people were pulling my leg when they told me about the "green flash." Still don't know exactly what causes the phenomenon, but I know it doesn't happen often.

For old times' sake, I had a scream relapse tonight. After dinner I was washing the dishes, when I heard the oven racks rattling. Not knowing what to think, I turned on the oven light and looked through the viewing glass.

On the top rack were two good-sized bush rats mating away like mad. Had I pulled up a chair and made some *popcorn, it would have been like watching rodent porn. The humor of the situation was wasted on me at the time, however, for I lost my head and hunkered down to scream my guts out.*

I have come a long way, though. At first I couldn't stand to even look at cockroaches; now I smash them between my bare fingers or toes, glad for the popping noises they make.

As I write this, Stanley, the red tarantula, has come out to say goodbye. Above, the wood slave's aim is getting better. I think I must have a bull's-eye painted on the top of my head.

Salem doesn't believe I'm actually leaving. The closest he could come to a farewell was to say he'd look in on the garden while I was away.

I dread going back to live in that crowded, polluted place. I dread going back to go through the long and painful process of letting David go. I dread going back to a job where I don't make a difference, and where everything I try to do is questioned and criticized.

In this living dream, a warm breeze wraps me in silk while the full moon has turned the ocean into one large moonglade. I hear a dog bark over in Providence and smell the ylang-ylang tree from the side yard. The sky is alive with stars.

Christ. What a dream I have had.

"Let's count those hands again."

"We've already counted them twice, Annie," I said, my nostrils flaring so wide, I'll bet I could have fitted a shot glass up one side. "It isn't going to change."

Annie stared at the room, looking pale. Her several attempts at turning over the final decentralization decision had failed. I thought the way she'd changed the date of the meeting to the day before I was scheduled to come back from the West Indies was a cheap shot. That I had come back two days early must have greatly disappointed her, but the fact that most of the decentralization supporters were working or in school still gave her an edge. Out of forty-five staff members, only twenty-three had shown up for the meeting, and a good portion of those were Annie's brownnosers.

Annie visibly blanched when I made my appearance, and quickly went into a huddle with her three management assistants. I don't remember exactly what I thought at the time, but I do recall that the slippery smell of trickery was in the air.

We counted out the ballots in front of everyone—thirty-seven voting in favor of decentralization, eight voting against. It was there before all our eyes in black and white: thirty-seven signatures right next to the checked boxes under "Yes, I want a six-month trial run of decentralization in CCU."

Then, like a bad accident, everything happened so fast, it took me days afterward to sort out how things went so wrong.

Annie stood and cleared her throat. "I think that since most of these ballots are more than a month old, and in light of the new information that's come up, we should take a revote now. A couple of the people who turned in ballots don't work here anymore, and I don't think it's fair that the rest of us should be saddled with the decisions of others who won't have to pay the penalties if this system is instituted."

"Wait a minute!" The force of my voice startled several people in the front row. "*What* new information has come up?"

Annie turned on me, fighting to stay in front. "While you were off on vacation"—she said the word "vacation" with an accusatory tone, as though I'd been away killing puppies—"some of us have been talking about instituting self-scheduling. It's a much less drastic measure than decentralization, and we thought it should be at least discussed before we get ourselves into this other mess."

I swallowed hard, trying to get the bile down. Annie was going to throw in the self-scheduling issue as a way to confuse matters and take focus away from decentralization. "Before I took this vacation, which, for everyone's information, was the first I've had in three years, it was decided by the unit that we would vote on decentralization, not self-scheduling. Exactly *who* thinks that self-scheduling should be discussed, and has everyone been told about it?"

Leslie, one of the new staff nurses, raised a hand. "I saw Annie's notice about it, but it was confusing. I don't think I really understand how it works and what it has to do with decentralization."

Chris, a decentralization supporter, stood. "They had self-staffing in the last hospital I worked, and it was a disaster. It's why I quit. Only a few favorites got the schedules they wanted."

Dennis, a marginal yes vote, raised a hand. "I'm going to school," he said defensively. "I can't take a chance on not getting my regular schedule. Decentralization sounds okay on paper, but what happens if people don't carry their own weight, or if there isn't enough work to go around? This self-scheduling thing doesn't sound so great either. I don't want to take the chan—"

J.B., one of Annie's team, interrupted. "Well, I think decentralization benefits only a privileged few." Here, she narrowed her eyes and turned to stare directly at me.

People began to look confused. Some were shaking their heads and talking to each other. I saw what was happening and my heart sank.

Annie came on strong again, capitalizing on people's fear, and suddenly the whole meeting began to stink of tactics used in Orwell's *Animal Farm*. "You know, with the economy the way it's going, you may want to think twice about the fact that with decentralization, you *aren't* going to be assured of getting work. If you're a single parent with a mortgage or rent, you'll end up having to take a second job to cover your basic expenses."

"That's *not* what is going to happen, people!" I pleaded. "You will have as much work as you want. The only thing that's changing is that you'll have a choice of where and when you want to—"

"Not true," said Gail, another management hopeful. "The people who need full-time work will be forced to float."

More heads began nodding in agreement. Without backup from the stronger staff members, defending the issue was like swimming up Niagara Falls. I sorely felt Beth and Pia's absence; they would have easily kept the meeting in our lane.

"First of all," I said as levelly as I could, "let's drop the you're-all-going-to-starve kick. Secondly, when the census drops, everyone will have their choice of what they want to do. There will always be people who want the time off, and those who want to float. Decentralization benefits all of us. According to these ballots"—I waved the stack of papers in the air—"the majority of us have already agreed on this."

Heather, an eloquent speaker and a longtime management supporter, raised her hand, and I kissed hope goodbye. "Personally, I think decentralization is a solid idea, and I agree it does give nurses more of a choice . . ."

Both Annie's and my jaws dropped.

". . . but I'm still confused as to how it will actually work for CCU. It seems so complicated."

"Like any new system, it's going to seem complicated at first," I said. "The basic idea of it is to bring the scheduling decisions to unit level rather than having all the decisions made at upper-management levels. If you read the—"

Annie held up her hands. "It sounds to me like you folks aren't at all sure of what you want. There are too many questions about this issue. I move that we have a revote."

For one brief moment Annie glanced at me. In those eyes I thought that I saw a fleeting glimpse of shame, that the old Annie, the nurses' champion who had once personally taught each new staff member the ropes of cardiac nursing because she *cared*, was saying she was sorry.

"All in favor of decentralization, raise your hand."

Thirteen hands went up.

"All voting against decentralization?"

Ten hands showed.

The gavel was about to come down, when Annie and her three management nurses raised their hands faster than bullets could fly.

"Fourteen against," said Annie quickly, "thirteen for. The decentralization issue has lost. Meeting adjourned."

"We agreed management would not vote on this issue!" I yelled over the noise of scraping chairs and end-of-meeting confusion.

A few people stopped talking and turned around, but the point went unheeded. I thought about jumping up on the table to make them see the injustice that had just taken place, when I realized nothing would change the end result. I suddenly knew that even if we had unanimously voted decentralization in, management would have said they had to have administration's approval, and it would have died there. The whole voting issue had been a sham. The choice had never been ours.

When I think about it now, I realize Annie actually did us a favor by saving our time and energies in a no-win situation.

Friday
10:00 P.M.

Simon called today to say he'd stop by to say hello when he could. I have to reason with myself not to feel hurt when I don't see him for weeks. He has his own life.

Then again, I have to laugh at myself; I remember when he was younger, there were moments when I wished for the

*day he would grow up and be out of the house. It's true—
you must be careful about what you wish for.*

*I am staying at David's until the cottage's water pipes are
repaired. The day I got home from Montserrat, they all froze
and burst. I've been here for only three days, and already
David is showing those ancient signs of bachelor irritability
over having a woman in his space. Rather than pulling
closer ("Absence makes the heart grow fonder" doesn't
seem to apply here), he has grown more resolved about not
living together. Last night he briefly mentioned something
about needing to be single.*

*A wiser woman would say pay heed to the death bell toll-
ing in the distance. But it seems to be all words, for in daily
practice, we're still loving and laughing as always.*

*Okay, David—so if we need to "move on" from each
other, why are we still slow-dancing in the living room?*

*What took place today at the staff meeting kicked the guts
right out of me. It was so unfair, it hurt. What really has me
puzzled, though, is how people like Annie sleep at night.*

*I'm starting to feel like the blind person who finds the
fruit salad just a bit too confusing. Man oh man, when did
life get so weird?*

SEVENTEEN

> *"I heard a nurse say that just getting through
> an eight-hour shift was a heroic deed. It's
> true; nurses who take part in that life-and-
> death dance each day subject themselves to
> visual, emotional, mental, spiritual, and some-
> times physical assaults. Even though we de-
> rive deep satisfaction from what we do, I don't
> know one nurse who doesn't suffer daily from
> a battered soul."*
>
> LAURA GRAY, R.N.

WINTER WAS LIKE A RETIRED ACTOR making a comeback in an
old play; it kept drawing out lines and milking scenes long after the curtain should have been brought down.

Northern California had now entered a new ice age which
had yet to be announced. Each morning, I faced the challenge
of changing from my one set of long johns and three layers of
sleepwear into running long johns, earmuffs, gloves, and two
layers of sweats before any part of me was frostbitten. Running with my mouth and nose covered by a heavy woolen
scarf was a new kind of experience in anaerobic training.

To keep my mind off the cold while I ran (I kept having this
unpleasant vision of my lungs freezing into a block of ice and
cracking), I started listening to cassette tapes. Within a short
time, however, it was apparent that there were drawbacks to
musical tapes. I could not listen and run at the same time; either I'd try to sing along and end up inhaling wool flaps, or I'd
unconsciously start to dance and run to the beat at the same
time, which whacked the hell out of my pace.

Enter the books-on-tape addict. Whenever I ran, I listened to
everything from blood-tingling thrillers to children's stories.

Not only did it take my mind off the weather and my now constant headaches, I'd get so involved in the readings that I'd run
an extra mile or three before I realized how far I had gone.

It was the beginning of March, and the small patches of thin
ice cracked under my shoes as I made my way along one of
the southeastern ridges of Mount Tam. In the earphones,
Bernie Siegel read sections from his book *Love, Medicine and
Miracles*. This tape was not a random choice, as my selections
usually were. Three of my friends had recently been diagnosed
with cancer, so I figured if this guy had a new angle on getting
them and myself through the process, it was worth an auditory
read.

I was coming around the last curve of the fire trail, when Dr.
Siegel explained how he asked patients what they would
change about their lives if they knew they were going to die in
a day, a week, or a year. This, he said, was a way to give people an immediate awareness of how they felt.

I turned off the tape and asked myself what I would do if I
had six months to live. The answer came without a second's
hesitation—quit nursing and get out of the rat race.

I ran to the edge of the hill and took in the panoramic view
of Mill Valley, Sausalito, and San Francisco. Through the
pinkish-brown haze of smog, I could barely make out the
Golden Gate Bridge. A mile away, bumper-to-bumper freeway
traffic snaked along the coast with a constant, dull roar.

After a moment, a desperate desire to be free from my life
as I knew it worked its way into my throat and stuck there as
a kind of permanent sadness.

"Whoa, wait a minute," I said, looking at the assignment
board. "April Fools' Day was *last* week. Who's the joker?"

Kate, one of the new orientees to day charge duties, gave
me a woeful glance. "No joke," she whispered. "Annie made
them out herself. She said if there were any complaints, to address them to her personally."

At that moment, one of the four nurses assigned to float
walked in, saw the board, and swore as she stormed off in the
direction of the stairs. I felt no sympathy; she was one of the
nurses who had voted against decentralization.

The patient assignments for each of the three nurses left in
CCU were heavy and unsafe. Yet again, we had shortchanged
ourselves to keep the budget safe for the big guns.

The old fury started to rise, then died. I silently renewed my promise that I wouldn't get involved; I wasn't going to do that to myself anymore. I walked into report mentally repeating my usual "I only have two arms and legs" battle cry. I would not play supernurse. I would not kill myself for a management that did not care about its nurses.

Grim and silent, Jeffrey and Yolanda—the two other nurses on the battlefield—took report, not daring to complain for fear Annie would hear about it and come down on them. Listening to the patient descriptions, I thought how absurd it was to expect that the three of us could handle that many acutely ill people and still do our jobs well. Not even a narrow margin had been left for new admissions, and it was a full moon; there'd be more than one.

I began my initial assessment rounds imagining I was in a field hospital in Vietnam and we'd lost most of the staff in a bombing raid. All around me, soldiers were bleeding and dying, crying out for help.

It wouldn't be so bad, I thought. I could stretch myself—at least until the next bomb dropped.

Phoebe approached carefully. I'm sure my tight expression was enough to intimidate anyone. As a nurse with a purpose and eight patients depending on her, I didn't find it easy to smile. In the background, no fewer than six call bells were ringing—and had been ringing for some time. Having to tend to the more pressing priorities, Jeff, Yolanda, and I ran, grim-faced, in and out of patients' rooms. For me, the moment's priority was making up a lidocaine drip for Mr. Hartquest, who'd just had a run of ventricular tachycardia along with his chest pain.

"Ec?"

I pulled the plastic valve cover off the IV bag with my teeth and grunted to let her know I'd heard her and wouldn't bite.

"A nurse from three south brought this up for you." Phoebe waved an envelope in front of my eyes. "She said it's important that you read it tonight."

" 'Ead it," I said, the plastic tube clenched between my teeth.

"Hey, eat it yourself," Phoebe said indignantly, and started to walk away.

I took the plastic cover out of my mouth. "Read it. I said read it, not eat it. I can't read it—my hands are full." I held up the two IV bags and the tangled mass of tubing.

Phoebe smiled slyly. "Oh Ec, why don't you just admit that you never learned to read or write? Don't you think we know the real reason why your handwriting is completely illegible?"

"Ha ha. 'Ead it, 'Ebe."

Phoebe opened the envelope and shook out the single piece of notepaper. "Okay. It says, 'Dear Miss Heron, my name is Rachel and I'm a patient on the Big C Ward. I was reading your book when my nurse informed me that you worked here. I am having surgery tomorrow morning, and would like to talk to you before I go. If you get a break, could you please stop in? Don't worry about waking me if it's late.' It's signed Rachel Goldsmith."

I thanked Phoebe for the message (" 'Ank 'ou"), grabbed an IV insertion tray, and ran back toward Mr. Hartquest's room. On the way, I glanced into Mrs. Rubinstein's room. Her call bell had been on a long time, and any length of time for an eighty-four-year-old on diuretics was too long. My fear was confirmed when I caught a glimpse of her struggling to get out of bed.

I wanted to stop and help her to the commode, but Mr. Hartquest's chest pain and arrhythmias were priority in the order of medical attention. The worry that the old lady would fall and end up with a broken hip—or worse—settled into my temples.

"Stay in bed, Mrs. Rubinstein," I shouted to her. "I'll be there in a second to help. Don't try to get up."

Two doors down, Mr. Ruez, my seventy-eight-year-old congestive heart failure patient saw me fly by and held up a hand. "Miss? Please, miss, I need . . ." The look of distress on his face as I yelled, "Hold on, Mr. Ruez!" made my stomach squeeze.

Running into Mr. Hartquest's room, I simultaneously saw the ventricular tachycardia on his bedside monitor and his body arched back in seizure.

Down the hall, Phoebe yelled, "Hey, somebody! Mrs. Rubinstein fell and there's V tach in room thirty-two."

I lowered the head of the bed and was delivering a precordial thump to the center of Mr. Hartquest's chest, when I saw Jeffrey and Yolanda easing the patient in the room across the hall to the floor. The man was turning blue as horrified family members looked on. Yolanda hit the code button one second before I hit mine.

And all around us, the call bells went on ringing without being answered.

"The float team has been cut from the budget," Nan repeated, slipping in a second IV on the semiconscious Mr. Hartquest. I hung a dopamine drip and hooked it up to the fresh IV port while Yolanda ventilated his lungs with the oxygen bag. Phoebe, bless her little monitor tech's heart, was comforting the family, trying to explain what had happened.

We jockeyed the gurney and two IV pumps out the door on our way to the acute side of the unit, where a ventilator, but no nurse, waited for Mr. Hartquest. Nan was trying to get back some of the CCU staff floated out, but what she was going to do in the meantime was beyond us.

"Why did they cut the float team?" Yolanda asked in new-hire innocence. "I've never worked at a hospital that didn't have a float or an IV team."

"It was determined they weren't needed," said Nan.

"Not needed?" Yolanda's eyes went wide. "Why? Are we supposed to wait until somebody dies to prove we need extra house staff?"

Dr. Cramer came out of Mrs. Rubinstein's room and joined in behind our entourage. "We need to get Mrs. Rubinstein down to the scanner. X ray said if we could get her down right away, they could fit her in."

"Well then, you're going to take her, Joe, because none of us can leave the floor. In case you haven't noticed, we're short-staffed again." I glanced over at Nan, who looked away.

Joe checked the wall clock. "I'm signing off to Meyers in four minutes. If I'm not home on time, my wife's going to leave me."

"Then Mrs. Rubinstein isn't going to get her scan tonight," I said, steering Mr. Hartquest's gurney into the acute room. "It's really simple. We can't spare the nurse."

Joe turned red and his neck grew stiff. "I am so tired of this crap!"

We each grabbed a part of the pull sheet and transferred Mr. Hartquest to the bed.

"Then admit your patients to another hospital, or complain to administration," I said. "You keep saying how sick and tired you are of it, Joe, and yet you never do anything about it. I've told you before—don't wait for the nurses to do something.

We've been bound and gagged when it comes to getting things changed. We don't have a—"

"Please. I need help." A pale and trembling Mr. Morales, my resolving pulmonary edema patient, stood in the doorway, holding on to the wall. His robe fell open and our attention was drawn to the blood dripping from around his urinary catheter. "I'm bleeding. Nobody has answered my call bell, and I . . . I . . ."

The man started to cry.

I gave Joe a see-what-I-mean? look and helped Mr. Morales to a wheelchair. Rushing him back to his room, I passed Mrs. Rubinstein's niece, who was screaming at Phoebe that she wanted to speak to the person in charge. From the distension of her neck veins and the timbre of her voice, it was obvious she wouldn't deal well with the news that there wasn't anyone in control, let alone in charge.

Five more call lights were on, and I could hear Mr. Shackman, my sixty-two-year-old angina patient, yelling for help from down the hall. The dinner trays, delivered some forty minutes before, were sitting in the carts, congealing. Yolanda and Jeffrey were zipping from one room to the other as fast as they could go.

Hurriedly, I threw a fresh bath towel over Mr. Morales's blood-soaked bed and removed the old catheter. I handed him a fresh gown and washcloth with the promise that I'd be back as soon as I could to insert a new catheter and clean him up.

On my way to Mr. Shackman, Jeffrey ran past me with a syringe of morphine. "Mrs. Vernon is heading down the tubes," he said. "Keep your ears open for the code bell."

Yolanda, on the run with three trays stacked on top of each other, was making an effort at getting people fed. "Mrs. Raimer pulled out her IV," she said. "Her hemoglobin is in the panic value of low and she needs two units of blood ASAP. Can you restart her IV?"

"I can't, Yolanda. Have Phoebe call—" I stopped, realizing there wasn't anyone to call. "Sorry."

Mr. Shackman was having chest pain, and his rhythm was tachycardic. "Where the hell were you?" he yelled, clutching at his chest. "I've had that goddamned bell on for ten minutes. Get me a nitroglycerine. What the hell's wrong with the nurses up here anyway?"

I opened my mouth to placate, then stopped. Mr. Shackman was the CEO of a large company; placating wasn't the way to go. I gave him oxygen and took his blood pressure before giving him a nitro. While the nitro dissolved under his tongue, I sat down on the bed. "Sorry about this. We're having a problem with staffing tonight. How's the pain?"

"Still there, but not as bad as before." His anger obviously subsided, he sank back into his pillow as though his spine had collapsed. "Sorry I yelled, but this is no goddamned way to run a hospital, I'll tell ya. You can't screw the customer and not screw yourself out of business at the same time."

I popped a second nitro under his tongue. "Well, I hope you write a long letter to the administrator when you get out of here and introduce them to that idea. I'm sure they'll find it quite novel. I've got to do something right now, but I'll be back in five minutes. Can you hold on?"

Mr. Shackman closed his eyes. "Okay, but just don't forget about me this time."

Heading back to Mr. Morales, I saw Joe wheeling Mrs. Rubinstein out of the unit and pinched his arm. "Don't worry, your wife won't leave you. If you want, I'll write you an excuse. 'Dear Mrs. Cramer, Joe couldn't come home on time because the suffering and the understaffed needed him. Enclosed please find his Eagle Scout badge for completing his nurses' aide service.' "

Joe didn't acknowledge my presence, let alone my attempts at humor. He just kept on walking, mumbling in a way that put me in mind of Lurch on *The Addams Family*.

At the monitor banks, Phoebe answered the constantly ringing phones. She looked exhausted. "There's an admit in ER," she said as I passed the desk. "What'll I do?"

"Call Nan. That's all you can do. Don't let it get to you yet. It's only seven o'clock."

Mr. Morales was silently weeping. He had not changed into the fresh gown I'd given him, nor had he attempted to wash himself. As quickly and gently as I could, I sponged him off and changed the bloody sheet on his bed. As I helped the frail man into a clean gown, he took my hand. "I'm sorry," he said.

"Why?" I asked, surprised.

"Because I have taken so much of your time."

I put my arm around his shoulders. "Don't be sorry. You deserve better care. You shouldn't have to come and find a nurse because you're in pain. It's just that—" I shot up as though I'd sat on a hot coal, remembering Mr. Shackman's pain. "I'll be back to reinsert that catheter in a minute, Mr. Morales. Hold on."

Sprinting back to Mr. Shackman's room, I saw Sarah, hands on hips, arguing with Nan in the hallway. They stood on either side of an ER gurney that held an obviously ill woman. The patient, pale and glistening with perspiration, was vomiting into a much too small emesis basin.

I was mentally trying to reprioritize so the new patient could at least be taken out of the hall, when I came upon Mr. Shackman on his hands and knees on the floor at the end of his bed.

"What'd you lose?" I pulled him to his feet.

"Nothing. I'm trying to make myself pass some of this damned gas."

Instantly my sixth sense of impending disaster set my switchboard ladies to pulling alarms. Mr. Shackman was that particular shade of grayish white, and his nose was the color of putty. I broke out in a sweat, experienced some chest pain of my own, and pushed him toward the bed.

"Get into bed please, Mr. Shackman," I said, managing to get the blood pressure cuff around his arm. His skin was cool and clammy.

"I don't feel well."

"Please, Mr. Shackman, get into bed."

Mr. Shackman got into bed all right—he fell over onto it.

Without needing to look at the monitor, I hit the code button and began CPR.

We got Mr. Shackman back, then lost him, then got him back, then lost him for good. It was during the final resuscitation attempt that I remembered Mr. Morales and felt like crying.

Prioritizing had become painful. Should I catheterize Mr. Morales first or should I give out my six P.M. medications, which were almost two hours late? The new admit was still in the hall waiting for a nurse to admit her. Twice, the woman's husband had threatened to take her home.

Mr. Shackman's wife and son were still in the waiting room. The chaplain was busy with the evening service, and there was no one available to tell them what the procedures were for releasing the body. I wasn't even sure if they knew Mr. Shackman was dead. Should I comfort them first, or wait until I dealt with Mr. Morales and passed out the medications?

Mrs. Rubinstein had put her bell on for the bedpan twenty minutes ago, and I figured she'd probably wet the bed long before I could get to her. That would mean a linen change and a bath, and that meant turning her, and that meant causing her more pain. I wouldn't have time to do eight o'clock rounds and assessments, but I had to go through all the patients' eight P.M. meds to figure out which ones should be given stat. Mr. Ruez's infiltrated IV needed to be changed, and then there were the incident reports to be written about the codes and the missed doses of six P.M. medications.

The moment Dr. Meyers called off the resuscitation efforts on Mr. Shackman, I stopped doing chest compressions, washed my hands, and raced back to Mr. Morales's room. In the hall, Mrs. Silvers, an angina patient of Jeffrey's, was tending to the basic needs of the woman on the gurney, who was yet to be admitted. Trying to help, Phoebe had put a telemetry monitor on the woman and given her a warm washcloth.

Phoebe looked up as I passed the desk. She seemed less upset, almost lost to the excitement of the war zone.

"I put Mrs. Rubinstein on the bedpan," she whispered. (Cardinal Rule 12: Monitor techs do not have physical contact with the patients.) "She peed to the line that said two hundred cc."

I made a sign of the cross over her and sailed into Mr. Morales's room, where I found his telemetry monitor carefully wrapped in tissue paper on the bedside table. Pinned to the tissue was a note:

Dear Nurse,

Gone home for a few hours to get some dinner, take my pills, and relax. Don't worry about the heparin lock, my wife will take very good care of me and your equipment. I have urinated since the catheter came out and it's okay—no blood. Left urinal in bathroom for you to measure.

I'll be back in a couple of hours when you aren't so busy, so don't you worry about me either.

Bert Morales

My first impulse was to run for the chart and call him at home to demand that he return immediately. I would have to impress upon him all the procedural and legal problems that would now have to be dealt with. Then I realized that things

wouldn't be any different for him if he did come back. Mr.
Morales would get better care and more healing rest at home.

I sat down on the bed, anger, guilt, and sorrow rising like a
tidal wave. Urges to call Annie, the chief of medicine, Nan . . .
anybody who could listen and change things so that the patients didn't have to keep going without, and the nurses didn't
have to keep feeling helpless.

Reading Mr. Morales's note again, I realized that the bottom
line for me as a nurse—as a human being—was caring for
people in need. Constantly having to prioritize patient needs by
what was the most urgent duty to be performed in order to
keep that person alive was not being a healing caregiver. I had
become a triage officer, leaving no room for even a loving
touch. I felt like an automaton, programmed with a medical da-
tabase and designed to administer basic services to the greatest
number of paying customers I could physically accommodate.

I could vow all I wanted that I would not play supernurse or
stretch myself, but I knew that when faced with the patients'
need, I, like most nurses, would stretch until I broke.

Phoebe came to the door. "Mr. Morales is off monitor," she
said, looking around for him. "And the new patient's husband
just picked her up and carried her off the unit saying he was
bringing her to Brand X hospital. Dr. Meyers is screaming his
head off, and we have another admit downstairs in ER ready
to come up for a temporary-pacemaker insertion."

The clerk came over and gave me a brief pat on the shoulder. "I wish there was something more I could do to help out."

The code bell sounded, then stopped. Someone had hit the
panic button by mistake. Phoebe and I, having run out into the
hallway, were adrenaline-charged and wild-eyed.

All around us, call bells were lit and ringing. An isolated cry
of "Help, someone please help!" came from somewhere down
the hall.

Without thinking, I ran in the direction of that thin plea,
dodging the bombs that kept falling.

I hesitated in the doorway, listening to the rhythmic breathing of the sleeping patient. It was after two A.M. and I was arguing with myself as to whether I should wake the woman.
My pragmatic nurse side was appalled at the idea of waking a
woman who was set for surgery in less than five hours. My
healing side knew that complying with her wish would be

more beneficial to her peace of mind and body than eight hours of unbroken sleep.

I lowered the side rail and sat down. Beneath me, the mattress was still warm from the heat of her body. Her jaw was clenched as she slept the fitful sleep of a warrior on the night before the first day of battle.

Studying her face, I tried to imagine what she was like. Her black hair was of the thick curly type I found so attractive, although the person that kind of hair belonged to rarely ever thought so. Despite her furrowed brow, the corners of her mouth were etched with laugh lines, giving the overall impression that she frequently resided on the lighter side of life.

From a cursory check of the chart, I knew that she was a thirty-two-year-old veterinarian's assistant, was unmarried, had no children, and was recently diagnosed with uterine cancer. Of course, everything on the chart pertained to her body and her disease; nowhere was there so much as a word about her emotional or mental state of health.

"Rachel?"

The jaws unclenched and the dark lashes opened quickly, as though she hadn't really been asleep, but waiting with her eyes closed. "Echo?"

"Hi."

Automatically, the woman pulled her arm out from under the covers and took my hand, grinning like a maniac. We sat like that for a while, until we both started to giggle. After a couple of seconds, the corners of her mouth pulled down and the laughter turned to silent weeping. Lightly stroking her head, I waited.

"Sorry," she said, sitting up. "I don't know what comes over me lately."

"That's okay. Your life has been turned upside down—you get to cry any time you want. Let me know when the anger phase hits, though, so I can get out of the way."

She smiled. "Oh, the rage has already hit—big-time. I'm really pissed about this." Rachel tried to pour a glass of water and found the pitcher empty.

"You're NPO for surgery," I reminded her. "That means you can't have anything to eat or drink."

Rachel tapped her forehead. It made a surprisingly hollow sound. "Forgot to put the contents back in after Halloween," she said dryly. There was a short silence. At last she said, "Thanks for coming down. I know this is awkward. I mean, you don't know me, but I wanted to ask if you could . . . well, like in your book, your friend Jan? She depended on you so much to keep her going. You gave her hope." Rachel paused and checked my eyes to see if I understood what she was trying to say.

"I'm scared. Ever since I found out I've got cancer, I've felt as though I'm down in this hole alone and no one can get inside and be with me, no matter how much they love me. I'm . . ." She turned her dark eyes on mine again, looking earnest. "Do you know what I'm talking about?" The question was not whether I understood what she was saying, but more, could I please explain to her what she was saying.

I nodded. "I think so. But first I have to tell you that I can't take the credit for knowing what Jan needed—it's more like Jan knew what she wanted from us and asked for it. Her cancer was long and tough. She went in and out of remission so many times over so many years that she considered herself a professional dying person. She could have given seminars on the finer details of dying well."

Rachel played with the corner of her pillowcase, nodding slightly. Waiting.

"And you're right, Rachel." I sighed. "When it comes down to it, we're all ultimately alone. Nobody can be in there with you no matter how much they love you. This is your lump of clay, handed to you by fate. It's up to you how you want to go about molding it."

"But I don't want to die," she said. "I'm not ready for that."

"Then make sure you don't. Hell, don't stop living to make room for your fears. It's exactly the other way around." I crossed my legs, and one knee made a popping sound that made us both smile briefly.

"Educate yourself to all the possibilities and take the battle a day at a time, a lab test at a time. In between rounds, do everything you can to enjoy your life. Treat yourself the same way you'd treat a new love—pamper, spoil, be frivolous, go the extra length. . . . Each of us should do that whether we're sick or not. We should look forward to each day, instead of—" I shut up.

What a hypocrite. Wasn't I that woman in the mirror who was being eaten up from the inside out?

Rachel read my mind. "Do you live like that?"

I shook my head. "No." I sighed again. "My life's not feeling well right now." Uncomfortable under the woman's scrutiny, I got off the bed and put up her side rail. "Tell me what you thought I could do or say that would change things for you."

Rachel thought for a minute. "I wanted you to tell me everything is going to be fine and I'm not going to die."

"Can't do that." I secured the rail lock. "I can only tell you not to stop living, and to make the most of everything you have right at the moment."

"Yeah." She yawned. "I've been pretty stingy with myself—the majority of my life is a collection of lost opportunities."

"Well, it's time for some reprogramming."

"I know, I know," she said. "I promise, when I get out of this hospital, no matter what the verdict, the first thing I'm going to do is get an hour-long foot massage and straighten my hair."

At once a hard lump formed in my throat and I had to fight back tears. I'm tired, I thought. I'm tired and low and I can't do this for much longer.

Rachel, who had been staring at my profile, squeezed my arm. "What about you? What are you going to do when you get out of the hospital?"

All the light conversational answers made a rush for my mouth, but were stopped by a set of clamped jaws. Like the Montserratians, I thought about Rachel's question, waiting for the right answer.

"Live," I said after a while. "I'm going to try to learn how to live for me."

At three A.M. I awoke screaming from a dream. It was one of those dreams in which I was trapped in the equipment utility room, unable to move or fully wake up. I kept crying out for help, but my voice was lost in all the other cries of my patients who had been left unattended for the whole shift. All I could think was that someone was going to die and I was the only one who could prevent that from happening.

With a herculean effort, I summoned up the scream and awoke.

Wednesday
3:30 A.M.

Tired of making tossed salad out of my sheets, I lie here watching David sleep, and I realize I must come to grips with my life. In my own words, I have to take the clay and do some molding. Here I am giving out all this advice and taking none of it myself.

On those who did not quit living before they were dead— the show of Risen's deathbed sketches has drawn much attention and critical acclaim. The papers are saying the show will go on tour. I hope he knows what is happening. He so loved to have people enjoy the fruits of his talents.

Hmmm, I wonder if he and Jan have started a cardiac clinic for departed souls?

From his perch on David's face, Mooshie just gave me a look that clearly said, "You worry too much. Turn off the light and join us in sleep." The tip of his pink tongue is hanging out of his mouth, which tells me he is in a high state of feline bliss. And why not? He is safe and overfed, kept warm and vibrated by the muffled snores coming from David's mouth.

The sight makes me laugh and at once I cannot fathom my life without David and his laughter. Why must there be this conflict? Is it really true that what is best for his life means I cannot have him in mine? It seems too brief a time that we have shared our lives. Am I awfully selfish to want more?

Oh, God, why have you played this little trick?

Can I let go of everything at once? Do I have the courage to change my life? Scary, sister. Very scary.

EIGHTEEN

"A nurse's career is typically a roller coaster ride between enthusiasm and burnout, fulfillment and frustration. Eventually, she will reach an end point. Once she is finally there, either she can flounder in the sea of bitterness and trepidation or she can free herself and go on. It is a gross misperception that the test of a true nurse is the test of time."

LINDA STONE, R.N.

THROUGH THE RED HAZE of my nylon car cover, I watched the three Jehovah's Witnesses who had invaded my front porch ring the doorbell a fourth time. With propaganda booklets ready to be sprung on the hapless victim who answered the door, they were persistent—as only God peddlers can be—showing every sign that they would wait forever if necessary to launch their verbal crusade.

Chuckling to my un-Christian self, I went back to my stack of mail, satisfied in the knowledge that another interruption had been diverted.

I suppose spending the majority of the day inside a car that was shrouded by a car cover may have seemed strange to others, but I couldn't have been more thrilled; it was the closest I'd come to being invisible. (I am one of those people who constantly ask themselves: Would you rather be invisible or be able to fly? Since I do so much flying in my dreams, I usually go for invisibility.)

Necessity is the mother of invention. This had been proved the afternoon my hands were rendered useless from the cold. The fireplace wasn't doing the job, and warm water was only a temporary remedy. When the tips of my fingers turned deathly white, I made an unconscious migration to the car and, without removing the red nylon car cover, opened the door a crack and slipped inside to instant silence and heat.

A natural solar heater, the cabin was an even 80 degrees from late morning until late afternoon. True, the nylon cover gave everything a reddish glow that left my color perception tinted with green and purple hues for hours after I left the car, but it was a small trade-off for the warmth and invisibility I so desperately needed in a think tank and writing space.

As the Witnesses went for a fifth press of the bell, I flipped through the envelopes, until I came to a letter from Janey and one from the same elderly man in Maryland who had advised me how to go about asking for a love for my life some years before.

I opened Janey's first and found a greeting card that bore a Rubenesque painting of a genital-less Adam and Eve in the Garden of Eden. Standing before them was God in His flowing robes, hands outstretched. In one of His hands lay a human brain, in the other a set of male genitalia. The caption under this illustration read: "Okay, people, I've only got one of each. You choose who gets what."

Inside, Janey had written, "Ain't it the truth?"

I opened the second letter with apprehension, not sure whether I wanted to know what the future held.

> ... Had to write, dear child, because my time is getting short and I want to encourage you a last time to use your writing gift to crusade your cause instead of continuing active nursing. It is time to let go; you have served your time in purgatory. Let the younger ones do it and learn the hard and wonderful way you did.
>
> This is frightening to you, I know, but you will find that you will continue to make a positive difference through your written words. Most forms of love, such as romantic love, have no guarantees, but healing love lasts forever. Shake the tree that is your life. To move forward, you must bear the pain of change.
>
> If I may be so bold as to offer advice: Accept opportunity, for it will lead you to a positive end.
>
> I doubt I will be in this phase to read any more of your work, but I will see it from a different plane. Do not give up the good fight, lady.

While I doodled idly on the windshield with my big toe, the man's words ricocheted around my head—"purgatory," "let go," "move forward." I took in their true meaning and after a while they began to stir the long-dormant elation called possibility.

San Francisco was having one of its surprise warm days wherein the north winds had died down just enough to allow us humans to unthaw for a day.

It was, I thought, a good day for going to the empty well.

My appointment with Annie was for one P.M. As I entered the stairwell, the noon whistle went off, letting me know I was way too early, but then again, I had a bad habit of being early for appointments that were vitally important to my life.

On the first flight of stairs, I passed Dr. Cramer, who was so absorbed with writing in his black book, I was surprised he was negotiating the stairs as well as he was. To see how he would handle the opening of the basement landing door, I glanced back over my shoulder. His stethoscope, I noticed, hung by an earpiece from the back pocket of his scrub pants, lazily swinging back and forth—like a tail. The image came to mind of a page from the *New England Journal of Medicine* with a photo of Joe as I saw him at that moment and a caption reading, "The civilized medical animal." I laughed quietly, and continued climbing upward.

At the second flight of stairs, the sound of weeping disturbed the silence of the stairwell. On the top step of the third-floor landing, I found Sarah.

I sat down and put an arm around her shoulder. "Hey, what's wrong?"

Sarah quickly disengaged my arm. Bitter sadness left no room for coddling. "Insensitive assholes!"

"Okay," I said. "So other than George Bush, Rush Limbaugh, and Nancy and Ronald Reagan, who are we talking about here?"

"It doesn't matter," she said, wiping her reddened nose with the shredded remains of a Kleenex.

I picked a piece of Kleenex lint from her upper lip, felt in my jacket pocket for the folded sheets of toilet paper I usually carry with me, and handed over the few measly squares.

Sarah wiped her eyes and studied the two wet smears of mascara while the shuddering, involuntary gasps that follow a hard cry rhythmically shook her.

"If it's enough to make you feel this bad, Sarah, it matters. Talk to me."

We waited until she could speak.

"About three years ago," she began, her lips moving clumsily, "a woman came in with her husband who was dying from cancer. He was so far gone, we put him in the end bed and just did comfort measures until he died a couple of hours later.

"Nell refused to leave him right up until the mortuary came." Sarah glanced at me sideways. "Not many people know how to love like that, you know.

"I asked if we could call someone to be with her, but she didn't have anybody, so I asked if she wanted to come home with me." Sarah shrugged. She was now rolling the toilet paper into tiny balls between her forefinger and thumb. "That was the beginning of a relationship where she became as much a part of my family as my own mother.

"But"—she sighed—"you know how it goes with the good people—she was diagnosed shortly afterward with sarcoma in her lungs. We've been dealing with that okay, up until a couple of days ago when she called and said she couldn't breathe.

"She looked like death when I brought her into ER—her hemoglobin was down to six. Anyway, I go to register her, and when I come back, I find this stupid administrative nurse in charge of services standing over Nell, who's fighting to breathe, verbally battering her, telling her she needs to have a psychiatric consult to determine if she's competent enough to make her own decisions about her treatment.

"It was such a cruel thing to do to somebody, I lost it—I ordered her out of the ER and told her if she came near Nell again, I'd charge the hospital with harassment."

"Jesus, Sarah, I'm—"

Sarah held up a hand, her voice coming stronger. "Then her doctor orders an abdominal scan for yesterday, which was my day to work twelve hours, right? I begged the people over in X ray for an early appointment so I could have enough time to bring her in and then home again before I had to be on duty.

"The way it turned out, the scan ran overtime and I was going to be about thirty minutes late for work, so I called the ER supervisor and told her what had happened and that I was going to be a half hour late, and could they cover me for those thirty minutes?"

As she gathered herself up, the flat look in Sarah's eyes turned to piercing anger. "This . . ." Sarah's mouth worked furiously, the negative adjectives bunching together but not coming forth. "This person that *I* trained when she was a know-nothing rookie tells me that Nell is *not* my mother and if I come in late, she'll write me up.

"She knows what Nell means to me. She knows I have never once in twenty years called in late and that I give more of myself to that department than anyone. But of course, none of that makes one goddamned bit of difference.

"I ended up screaming that compassion was mightier than the pen, and hung up. Meanwhile, Nell's crying because the doctor has dumped the information on her that he suspects she has lymphoma in her liver and spleen but he doesn't have time right then to explain to her what that means. She's begging me not to leave, and I'm going crazy because I can't stay, because some unfeeling jerk is going to make my life miserable if I'm so much as a minute late."

Someone opened the second-story door, and Sarah quickly hid her face in her hands. When the footsteps went in the direction of the first floor, she sighed, but did not uncover her face.

"I've been in ER for twenty years," Sarah said slowly, as though she were feeling every year. "In all that time, when someone was needed to stay overtime until things got smooth, I never complained—I just did it. I'm the only one who remembers people's birthdays, or brings in holiday treats, or arranges parties for special occasions. I'm the only person who cares enough to . . ."

Sarah began to cry again. In the filtered light, I could see the small carotid pulse in her neck beating rapidly, like that of a wounded rabbit.

Abruptly, she sat up. "But you know what? That's all going to stop. It doesn't get you anything except hurt. I won't ever again . . . I'll never . . ."

I pulled her head onto my shoulder and let her cry her hurt out.

"Sarah, there are people in our profession who stop feeling and go on autopilot. You're one of the ones who can't let that happen, because every time you see someone in need, you'll forget that it's time to go home, or that your back is killing you, or that you haven't eaten in ten hours. You'll go until you drop."

"Oh great," Sarah said finally, wiping away the rest of her

eye makeup. "Someday they'll find me in the dirty utility room with the bedpans, dead of the nurse's curse."

The rhyme potential of her last words was too much to be ignored. "What could be worse?" I recited, tapping out the rhythm on her knee, "than to be in a hearse, bloated to burst, with a nasty case of the nurse's curse?"

Disgusted, Sarah sighed. "Jesus," she said, "what *could* be worse than to die a nurse?"

"Well," I said slowly, "I suppose we could die like Normal People."

Idleness led me to my locker and my mailbox, but it was intuition that told me to purge the two boxes of the entirety of their contents. Three pounds of mail and four pounds of odds and ends (one clean scrub uniform, six forks, two antique butter knives, four toothbrushes and two tubes of paste, deodorant, three odd running shoes, and a red Dairy Queen apron) were removed from my locker and stuffed into my carryall bag. Placing the lock and key inside, I left the locker door open. Ever since a forgotten tofu carton had exploded, the inside had turned ranker than the insoles of Simon's Air Jordans.

The Robert Redford (sigh) photo stayed pasted to the door for posterity.

Walking past the nurses' station on my way to Annie's office, the day charge nurse, a woman I'd never seen before, hailed me over to the desk and in an officious manner asked if I needed assistance.

True, I was out of uniform, but the fact that we did not recognize each other, and I knew only one nurse on the unit at that moment, made me sad and a little resentful. Management had at last succeeded in creating a "corporation" ambience among the caregivers.

I swallowed the feelings and smiled into that cold face, saying simply that I had an appointment with the head nurse and I could find my way.

The paper clock tacked to Annie's office door indicated she would return in ten minutes. Taking a seat, I commenced watching the CCU Cavalcade of Chaos from a totally detached position. The staffing was slightly better than on evening shift, but there were still too many call lights going unanswered despite the flurry of nurses running in and out of the rooms.

Somewhere down the hall, a thin voice crying for help did not cease.

Through the double doors, Annie hurried into the unit. With a short apology for being late, she invited me into the inner sanctum of her office, a cluttered ten-by-eight closet that housed two large file cabinets, two desks, and three chairs. The place was a claustrophobic's nightmare.

Under Annie's desk was a pair of running shoes. "Those yours?" I asked before she could get all the way out of her coat.

Annie nodded.

"Put them on," I said. "Let's get the hell out of here and go for a walk over by the creek."

Making our way down the walking path that ran along the water, we spoke briefly of the everyday things that, in the old days, we had once spent time discussing at length: gardening, Jan Tobin, dogs, Simon, her house, my writing, nursing. When we were exactly one mile away from the entrance of the hospital, we momentarily paused to watch Buchanan College's rowing crew glide by.

Annie stood poised, expectant. "Okay Ec, so what's this all about?"

I took a deep breath and relaxed my shoulders. "I've got to get out of nursing for a while, Annie. I'm tired. I'm at the end of my rope. I want . . . I need a six-month leave."

Expressionless, Annie stared straight ahead. "No can do. The administration doesn't give out personal leaves anymore."

"Oh come on, Annie, I've been here fifteen years—doesn't that count for something?" I swallowed the lump that had formed in my throat. "I need a break. Every time I come to work, I get sick worrying about what bullshit is going to be pulled on the staff, or if one of the patients will die because we couldn't get to him fast enough. Then I go home so wound up, I don't sleep."

Obeying some invisible signal, we started walking again.

"It's not the nursing itself," I continued. "I love taking care of people. But the politics are killing me. It's criminal not to be able to take care of—"

"Then you're in trouble, Ec," Annie said dryly. "Because it's going to get worse. There's going to be more budget cuts, and the tighter our belt gets pulled . . ." She stopped, then resumed in a firm, this-is-the-way-it-is tone.

"Redwoods Memorial is a business."

(Didn't I know that.*)*

"We're here to serve *and* make money."

(But at whose expense?)

"Take me, for instance . . ."

(Seventy thousand a year? More?)

"I love my job . . ."

(At that salary in these times, who wouldn't?)

"I trust management's changes . . ."

(I would hope so, since you're the one who makes a lot of them.)

"You're so negative about the management . . ."

(Sometimes the truth hurts.)

"But [sigh] if you really don't like what you see . . ."

(Now for the bottom line, folks.)

". . . then why don't you quit?"

(Was the unspoken end to that statement ". . . and give everybody a break"?)

"Regardless of what you may think of my politics, Annie, I *am* a practical person for the most part. I don't want to quit and then find out that I've done the wrong thing. I want some time out to get myself together. If I still feel this way by the time I have to come back, then I'll quit."

Silent, we resumed walking while bits of California's incongruous nature played themselves out around us: Yuppie joggers zoomed by with their golden retrievers while the homeless people of Killer's Cove slept on the creekbank alongside picturesque herons and ducks.

"What about a medical leave?" Annie asked suddenly.

"I'm not sick."

"But you're under stress caused by your job. There are medical leaves available for that sort of thing." Annie picked up a slimy, chewed-up tennis ball that had rolled in our path and threw it toward a wagging retriever. "I'll see what I can do. When do you work next?"

"I'm on duty this weekend."

Annie thought for a minute. "Okay, I'll run it by personnel and leave a note on your timecard."

It may have been Annie's sudden smile or the new spring in her step, but as we walked into the hospital, my switchboard ladies were sending peculiar signals that I was about to be diddled.

Back in Annie's office, I picked up my carryall and said I'd talk to her later. That she gave me a hug and said a very deliberate "Goodbye, Echo," instilled such an uneasy feeling in and around my throat that at the double doors, I turned and

looked at the unit with the distinct feeling I was seeing it for
the last time.

Nothing had changed. The nurses still ran, the call bells still
buzzed, and at the end of the hall, that pitiful wail for help still
sounded, but all at once I wanted to run to Annie's office
shouting, "I didn't mean it. It was all a joke."

What had I been thinking about? I didn't want to leave nursing. Who would I have to take care of? What would I do without all those adrenaline rushes? I would feel like I was out on
the end of a kite string, with nothing to fulfill me.

"Move, please!"

The command came from one of the new grads, who was,
at that moment, at the other end of a gurney that was bearing
down on me at great speed. The gurney was filled to capacity
with a mountain of a man who appeared to be having a hard
time breathing. As the front wheel slid into my Achilles tendon, I reached out and grabbed the woman's arm with enough
force to stop her *and* the gurney. "Slow down!" I began to
shake as the pain traveled up the back of my leg.

"I told you to move!"

I gritted my teeth and straightened to my full height (although I am over five feet six inches tall, I usually slouch
down to around five feet four). "The nurses who work in this
unit try not to go out of control even in the worst of circumstances." I glanced at the patient, who was speedily turning
dusky about the jowls. "Get some oxygen on this man and on
your way past the clerk's station, tell them to call for blood
gases stat and get someone to follow you to his room with the
crash cart."

As I shoved the gurney through the double doors, I heard
the girl grumble, "Who are *you*, anyway?"

"I'm a senior nurse here," I called after her, "and I would
strongly advise that if you—"

The double doors closed on me and my advice with a soft,
hydraulic hiss.

The call from the newly re-formed, smoke-free health office
(Miss Milks had been given a gold-plated cigarette case/
cigarette lighter set and an honorable discharge) came less than
twenty-four hours after my walk with Annie.

"Hello, this is Judith from Redwoods's health office. Is this
Ms. Heron?"

Four hundred fear-laden thoughts crossed my mind in the

split second before I answered. Had Miss Milks given me the wrong HIV test results? Had I come into contact with the plague or tuberculosis? Had Annie smelled my locker and thought it might be contagious?

"Uhn, that depends." I was clearly reluctant.

"We've just spoken with Annie, your head nurse from CCU?"

"Yeah?"

"And I'm calling to tell you not to bother coming back to work. Redwoods can't risk the chance that you'll further injure yourself and bring a lawsuit against us."

"Excuse me?"

"Your six-month medical leave is effective immediately. You'll need to contact personnel for details on the proper paperwork and releases."

"You're actually going to call temporary burnout a medical problem?"

"Oh yes."

"Well, Jeez, what exactly did Annie tell you?"

Judith hesitated. "I'm sorry, but I'm not at liberty to discuss that with you, but I will tell you that she's very concerned that you get this leave."

"Well, can you at least tell me if the words 'rabble-rouser' or 'troublemaker' came up?"

There was silence in which I could almost hear the woman grin. Then, "I think, Miss Heron," said Judith from the health office, "you shouldn't look a gift horse in the mouth. Good day."

In regard to my life, I know better than to question anything that has to do with fate or coincidence. So, a week after my leave was granted, when the call came from London asking if I would consider being the full-time caretaker of the house in Montserrat, I said yes.

I didn't think about it; it was an answer that had been waiting for the question.

After all, why start following the rules now?

When I look back on it, I think the happiest aspect of leaving, besides the idea of escaping from the pollution and the overcrowding, was getting out of that refrigerator of a cottage and selling twenty-five years' worth of junk I'd collected and convinced myself I couldn't live without.

The shocking parts were things like sending in change-of-address forms, and turning my old blue Honda (with car cover and its secret of invisibility) over to Simon. Giving up the phone number I'd had for twenty-two years was like selling the Statue of Liberty to the Japanese.

The majority of my friends were skeptical about the move. Just because I liked to douse my morning oatmeal with ketchup and horseradish, most of them felt I was other-directed, but now they were convinced I'd lost my mind because I wanted to leave the land of sun (ha!), surf, and sophistication. Among themselves, they made bets about what would get to me first: Loneliness? Strange insects? Lack of conveniences? Voodoo?

I thought my therapist explained it perfectly, however, when she stated that going off to a remote island was the eccentric's way of dealing with midlife crisis.

I spent a good deal of time packing up what was left of my household—putting half in storage and shipping the other half to Montserrat. When I wasn't packing, I was running around the Bay Area taking photos of certain places. To be sure, this was a strange group of pictures, but each had special meaning to me—like the one of the chemistry work station at Buchanan College laboratory where Janey and I first met; the sidewalk square with Simon's hand print in the corner from when he was three; Sadie the spider and her two hundred new babies in the corner of the living room windowsill; the front seats of the Honda, where I edited a major portion of my books and where Simon and I had our most serious heart-to-hearts; the chair by the fireplace where David and I first kissed.

The sledgehammer to the heart, of course, was Simon and David. Simon and I discussed Montserrat almost every time we were together. He was encouraging, taking the stance that I should do what I wanted with my life, and if this adventure was what I wanted, great . . . just as long as he could come and visit.

David and I were another story. Living in denial, neither of us ever even mentioned my leaving until the day David walked into the living room, bare except for ten or fifteen packed boxes, looked around, and asked in genuine surprise, "What's going on here? Where's all the furniture?"

Had we been only parting lovers, it would have been hard enough, but losing a best friend was unbearable. Every time we tried to talk about it, we choked up before even a few words were out, making it impossible to take the conversation anywhere.

I returned to the hospital only once, to sign some papers. Although it had been just a few days since my interview with Annie, I found that my mailbox had a new name on it, and my locker was occupied by some stranger's neatly folded uniform and an air freshener. The photo of Robert Redford was gone, and in its place hung a photo of Fabio.

Thinking I would take a last look around, I had gotten as far as the double doors to CCU when my stomach balled into a knot. The pneumatic doors I had passed through so many times were now an impenetrable barrier that I couldn't bring myself to cross. I no longer belonged to the world on the other side.

January 16
11:00 P.M.

It is my last night in this house after twenty years, and the memories are rolling through my mind one after the other: the nights I enjoyed a cozy fire while imagining I was in Paris at the turn of the century, the months Daniel and Kathleen lived in the haunted front bedroom, all my Christmas Eve open houses, the night Simon almost died from his asthma, the times we laughed ourselves sick, the day we brought Mooshie home, the day David came to my door, the thousands of hours in that small sunny room where I wrote my heart out.

Yesterday I said a final goodbye to Mary Dale, Pia, Tom, Kaye, Beth, and Phoebe—all very concerned and excited for me. Phoebe said to remember that this is what people's fantasies are made of.

Fantasies? I'm terrified. This morning (I have a different "feature" fear each A.M.), I actually broke into a sweat at the thought of Mooshie encountering one of the bufos. I cannot get used to the idea that I will not be working in the hospital. Although I am sometimes ecstatic, phantoms of guilt haunt me daily that I am betraying my purpose for living by leaving nursing.

Relocated Sadie and her babies to the toolshed. I hope she makes it. She's been in that sill for as long as I've lived here.

After dinner I went to David's, where the TV never sleeps (I told him he was going to turn into a vidiot). Desperate to keep myself from thinking about the reality at hand, I watched the news. The stories came in this order: There are only fifty-two California condors left, because the rest have been killed off by hunters, lead poisoning, and pesticides.

Next came the discovery of NAMBLA (I can't bring myself even to write what the initials stand for) meetings in the San Francisco library building. This is an organization of men devoted to molesting and having sex with young children. The former leader of NAMBLA had boasted of molesting or raping countless young boys. He was tested as HIV-positive.

This was followed by the story of a S.F. woman who was arrested for killing her infant twins a week ago. She had been arrested and convicted for child abuse before, but at the time of the killings was a county-appointed foster mother for a large number of children. The spokesperson for the foster home agency stated that they couldn't always check out their foster parents due to lack of funds.

The news ended with a story about a child who was accidentally shot to death during a gang war in south San Francisco.

Simon came to say goodbye. We discussed his courses at Buchanan, and while he played David's guitar, I was struck by what a handsome, gentle man he has become. He left with the words that I should relax and enjoy myself and that he sure was going to miss my pasta e fagioli.

Then Jack called to tell me Janice died yesterday. It has been a year and a half since the first time she told me her symptoms and her frustration over not being taken seriously by the doctors in her HMO. I remember crying afterward, knowing that the private doctor I referred her to would find colon cancer and that she would not survive. Her life slipped through our fingers despite all our ferocious tenacity to hold on. My poor Janice—you had such a hard road all your life, though Jack said he thought at the end you finally believed you were loved.

Janice? You were and are loved. Keep the corn bread and clabber warm for us.

Weirdest things are going through my head at the oddest times—like an ongoing show of This is Your Life. And the dreams? The one I keep having over and over is David driving out onto an ice-covered lake and sinking through the ice.

I am on the beach, powerless to help him, and the grief is overwhelming.

It feels as though I have made a wide, gaping cut down the length of my soul, and yet I had no other choice. I feel like a homeless person, but at the same time, free. I am excited and tortured, depressed, frightened and ecstatic, wanting to run back and wanting to run forward—a neurotic's waltz complete.

I'm going to turn out the light now and fold into David's arms for the night.

David, heart of my life, what will happen when I awaken from one of those four A.M. nightmares and you are not there to hold me and tell me it's only a dream?

Thursday
?? P.M.

I am somewhere over the Bermuda Triangle, and having fears upon fears over what I have done. Under the seat, Mooshie has stopped yowling and the carrier box has finally stopped rocking. God only knows what I'll find when I open that box.

The drive to the airport was avoidance at its best. I thought about movies I'd seen, flowers, shopping for cat food. David cried, though I know better than to think the tears are for my departure—parting a man and his cat is a crime for which I shall never be forgiven.

Reality, stay away from my door until I have more strength to stand on.

Tomorrow I meet Pinky in San Juan. From there he will take Mooshie and me to our new home. He was kind to give the owners my name and phone number, but, as he said, it was a crime for that house and grounds to go unattended for so long.

I calm my fears with the thought that this is an adventure and planes do fly both ways. These are my escape route messages. I suppose this is related to my need to know where the fire escape routes are in hotels and theaters.

During my layover in Atlanta, I had my worst attack of doubt. I began looking around for a ticket counter for San Francisco, but called David instead. At the sound of his "Hi sweetie," I broke down.

Turbulence has set in, and I need to put this away so I can give my fear of flying some proper attention.

I will hold on. I will—if just to see what is around the next cloud.

EPILOGUE

June 5

Dearest Janey,

I don't know how it happens, but there don't seem to be enough hours in the day to get everything done. One day slips into the next, and before I know it, I'm lost in the simple routine of living day to day. When I awoke this morning, I had to count on my fingers to figure what the date was, only to realize it's my birthday. However, I don't remember which one it is and I don't care enough to get into more complicated mathematics. Paradise and age have a way of making those once important numbers inconsequential.

Except for Mooshie, you are the first to know that this morning, exactly fifteen years to the day after I was hired at Redwoods Memorial, I finally freed myself from the Chair of Forgetfulness—I called Annie and told her I will not be returning to work.

She needed a reason for the official records, so I explained that one day about four months into my leave, I woke up feeling like a human being again. The old joy I had for living had been renewed, and I knew then and there I would not be going back.

Do you think she'll actually put that down as my reason for terminating?

As the recession deepens, I am sure this would be considered a foolish—actually, a really stupid—move, but I can't go back to that nightmare yet. I'd rather starve here in peace. From here it's easy to see how management, with all the policies and rules, wears down a person's morale.

The world of high-tech medicine—and my part in it— seems very far away, although I honestly don't know how long I can stay out of bedside nursing. In the meantime, I'll keep my fingers in the pie with my literary efforts and the lecture circuit.

Within a day of my arrival, a thirty-two-year-old Montserratian woman who clerks in one of the town liquor stores stopped me on the road to say she'd heard I was a nurse (news and gossip take about five hours to be known to every man, woman, and child on the island, giving some truth to the jungle drums stories). She was taking a blood thinner but didn't have a clue as to why she was taking it or even what kind of drug it was. After I explained it to her, I spent an hour answering her questions about basic preventative healthcare for her and her six children.

A week later, another Montserratian girl showed up at the door with her child asking if I would check him over. The two women were so trusting and appreciative, it made me feel I'd really done something worthwhile. In "payment" for my services, one woman gave me two jars of hot pepper jelly, and the other left three ripe soursop on my doorstep.

The main medical problems among the Montserratians are the same as our African-American population's in the States—high blood pressure, diabetes, asthma, heart disease and the resultant pulmonary problems. Every once in a while, there are runs of some tropical plague or other; at present, there are two reported cases of dengue fever on the island, and a cholera alert has been posted.

I miss hands-on patient care and have been pursuing the idea of volunteering for one of the district day clinics. So far I've not had a lot of luck, as there seems to be a good deal of red tape involved for a non-Montserratian trying to work there. This is such a disappointment. Like most nurses, I am addicted to that need to touch people.

Gardening has become a time trap. I could work on it for twelve hours a day and not scratch the surface, for no sooner have I cleared away a vine from some wondrous flowering tree than it is grown back four days later. And the goats here are worse than the deer back home. However, gardening is the best healing therapy in the world, plus the rewards of frangipani, ylang-ylang, shell orchids, sky flow-ers, pride of Barbados, hibiscus, ixora, red ginger, chenille, poinsettia, bird-of-paradise, and jasmine keep the ten or so vases I have around the house constantly filled.

I, the grower of fifteen-pound zucchini and one-pound to-matoes, cannot get one measly vegetable to sprout to save my life. The seeds rot in the ground from all the rain, or if the shoots do make it out, they succumb at once from a wide variety of hostile forces such as heat, insects, goats, or agouti—a weird rabbitlike rat thing the sight of which would absolutely freak you out.

You asked what I do for entertainment. Call me the Jane Goodall of insects. Each night I sit on my ladder under the fluorescent light in the kitchen, making sketches of the var-ious flying critters. It's like watching a National Geographic special. So far I've come up with thirty-four varieties of moths.

It is much hotter here than I imagined. This morning, for instance, I awoke at six A.M. to 90-degree heat. Dehydration is a problem for us white women with blood pressures of 90 over 40, so to remind myself to drink fluids, I keep a plastic irrigation bottle of Gatorade tied to my belt at all times. Pinky said the Montserratians at the airport wanted to know what evil jumbies I was warding off by wearing a jug of urine.

Speaking of hot air and urine, Mooshie loves it here. He sleeps all day, then comes alive around ten P.M. to chase the cockroaches and the slower lizards. He is terrified of the pool monster, however—won't go within ten feet of the edge. Unfortunately, the goats don't affect him one way or the other. I was hoping he might scare them off with his cater-wauling.

The lingo is coming slowly. I still don't know most of what is being said to me, but there are certain phrases I love. For instance, Beware of Dog signs become Bad Dog signs. A friendly dog is referred to as a "play dog." To neuter or spay an animal is to "change the nature," and if you are thinking of someone, you say your mind is "resting on" or "running after" them.

Other than what is produced on the island, food can be pretty expensive, since much of it has to be imported. Imag-ine paying $1.50 for a fist-sized head of lettuce, or $6.00 for a small block of cheese. Fresh vegetables, when not in sea-

son here, are scarce. I must admit, though, that the conspicuous absence of junk food and sweets—overabundant in American food stores—is refreshing.

While I find that many items—fabric, hardware, household gadgets, skin creams, shampoos, soap, over-the-counter medicines—are quite reasonably priced, the cost of a basic washing machine is beyond prohibitive. However, I am trying hard to adopt the foreigner's commandment, "Thou shalt not compare or complain," so this afternoon I am going to teach myself how to make a passable cheese from my home-made yogurt, and will put my mechanical aptitude to the test by taking apart the dinosaur of a washer I found in storage to see if I can make it work. If I fail, I shall buy a washboard and experience laundry the way my grandmother did. As for a dryer, there's a natural one on the upper deck.

The locals are geniuses at making use of everything so that nothing goes to waste. Watching these people work is a lesson in recycling at its finest. Plus, there is no litter—the Montserratian saying is: "Stow it, don't throw it."

Accepting an occasional pan of my yogurt corn bread and a roasted chicken dinner as bribes, Pinky supplies me with lettuce, Gatorade powder, tofu, and broccoli. He doesn't understand why I don't want newspapers, but although the isolation is something to be dealt with, I still have no desire to connect with the outside world. It would be sacrilegious to be reading endless accounts of violence while in this peaceful place.

By the way, Pinky has agreed to let me use his PO box in Puerto Rico, since mail sometimes takes a coon's age to get to and from Montserrat. He flies the mail down about once a week, so I can at least be assured of hearing from you guys back there in the civilized (this adjective is used tongue in cheek) world.

At $1.20 per minute, calling the States is a rare treat. I can't tell you how much pain a silent phone can cause.

Besides lettuce and big baking potatoes, I sometimes miss good old American efficiency. Making a simple transaction—either banking, or purchasing something, or paying a bill—takes three times the amount of time and hassle here. It is sometimes very difficult to get things done. For instance, last week I needed some Scotch tape and went into town. No one had tape. They were totally at a loss to under-

*stand the concept of Scotch tape, clear tape—it was all a
mystery to them.*

*Oh well, it is exactly as Dr. Cramer said—it's all in the
game of trade-offs: no pollution, but mediocre roads and a
scarcity of cars; no earthquakes, but hurricanes; no pesticides or food additives, but no big heads of escarole either;
no migraine headaches, but dealing with the do-it-next-
week, make-do mentality.*

*There is some racial conflict here, although not like in the
States, and certainly not as bad as on the islands where
there is a large tourist trade. The Rodney King verdict has
left a sore spot and is causing some antiwhite sentiments to
surface.*

*I must tell you that being part of the minority has caused
me to look at racism in an entirely new way—like from the
other side of the fence. This old bleeding-heart liberal is
getting a real education. At my first tiny taste of racial discrimination, I fell apart, full of resentment and feelings of
injustice. It sent yours truly scurrying through her tape collection for the Martin Luther King speeches in a hurry!*

*It is now clear to me on a very small scale what keeps the
struggle for equality fueled, when in my outraged question
"Why is this bag of potatoes only two dollars for him, and
five dollars for me?" I hear echoed, "Why is this college
only for whites, and not for me?"*

*And while we're on related subjects—to be a single white
woman in the West Indies is a difficult undertaking. Gloria
Steinem would have a stroke. I have spoken to women here
who believe that their greatest goal in life is to be "given"
a baby by a man. If someone can't remember a woman's
name, she is referred to as "So-and-So's woman."*

*Yes, there are a few Montserratian women in government
office, and several who run businesses, but there is also a lot
of machismo going on. Consider: When I tried to open a
checking account at the local bank, cash in hand, I was told
I had to have a letter from a Montserratian man stating that
I was "worthy" to give the bank my money.*

Needless to say, I am presently paying in cash.

*I get lonely. Being miles from the nearest human being
suits me in some ways, but there are moments when I have
a longing to make that human connection. I miss the simple
pleasures of sitting around laughing and talking with a comfortable old friend. As a longtime recluse, I thought being*

this isolated would be a blessing rather than a problem. I was wrong about that.

It wasn't until the day I unpacked my clothes that I got a sense of the move being long term. That was when the thought of not seeing the people closest to my heart for so long a time took root and blossomed into a deadly sorrow that is the epitome of my unrest here.

Like dust bunnies under a bed, these sad feelings breed so that sometimes I get to worrying about things like, What is going to happen? Then I realize the grieving and worrying is as dumb as lying on your deathbed worrying about what it's going to be like to die. Still, some days, instead of exercising, I find myself spending fifteen minutes crying in place.

All in all, Janey, I have begun to take a long look at myself. Sometimes I wonder how far I can go with this. One day I think I have made the worst mistake of my life, on another I think I am brave, and on yet another I revel in the tranquillity and the turmoil simultaneously. In a quiet struggle for survival in my isolation, I have had to reach deep down. And God, the manner of things I have pulled up! Secrets, strengths, pain, fears, and wits that I did not know I harbored. Facing my demons has been, to put it mildly, a complex and bizarre experience.

In the end I cannot deny that there is a peace that surrounds me such as I have never known before. The voice coming from this newly built inner room is urging me to take advantage of this feeling while I am here.

Ha! A bush rat just walked over Mooshie's tail. The retarded feline fool raised his head long enough to yawn and then went back to sleep. Inches from his dormant body, two small lizards play a hide-and-seek game. Well, it is 100 degrees and humid, without any breeze. But look out, creatures, when ten P.M. rolls around with a cooling rain and breeze—the panther awakes.

Last night the jump-up drumming rocked the jungle until three-thirty A.M., when it came to an end with some interesting outright screaming. This morning the hymns from St. Peter's could be heard all the way up here.

I look over the jungle that stretches out before me, all sultry and tropical mystery. If I raise my sight an inch, I can see that the rest of the world is nothing more than an expanse of ocean and sky framed by the bright red flowers of *the royal poinciana trees. It is hard to tell where one stops and the other begins.*

In this dark orange sky, a silver sun has come out from behind a purple cloud. For one moment, I was confused as to whether it was the moon or the sun.

I must turn off the tape player now; Baez is beginning to sound nasal, and I want to hear the birds' sunset songs instead. Give hugs all around and write when you can. I love you dearly and wish that joy and peace surround you.

Until next epistle, I remain,

> *Your jungle-trampling friend,*
> *Echo*

*Now, at a time when the spotlight is turned on
health care and what goes on in hospitals,*

Echo Heron

has written

TENDING LIVES
Nurses
on the Medical Front

a compelling collection of real-life medical
dramas experienced by nurses throughout
the country.

Each nurse has a chapter, every chapter written
in his or her own voice. Their experiences range
from inspiring to tragic to downright funny. And
the stories are charged with the issues that affect
nursing care today.

TENDING LIVES

is a moving, inspiring book about a noble profession.

Published by Ivy Books.
Available in bookstores everywhere.

The Adèle Monsarrat, R.N., medical thrillers . . .

by Echo Heron

PULSE
When sweet young Chloe, everyone's favorite nurse, dies in the recovery room after a routine appendectomy, it's the third sudden death among the hospital staff in a year, and Adele Monsarrat's suspicions are aroused.

PANIC
Only hours ago teenager Iris Hersh was in perfect health. Now she hovers near death, pulse racing, temperature soaring, ravaged by a virus that medical science has never before encountered—and doesn't know how to stop.

PARADOX
A beautiful young woman with amnesia lies in Ellis Hospital, remembering nothing about where she was driving when her car plunged over a cliff—or the identity of the dead child in the backseat.

Published by Ivy Books.
Available in bookstores everywhere.